Disabled Clerics in the Late Middle Ages

Disabled Clerics in the Late Middle Ages

Un/suitable for Divine Service?

Ninon Dubourg

Routledge
Taylor & Francis Group
LONDON AND NEW YORK

The publication of this book is made possible by a grant from the University Paris Diderot (Ecole Doctorale 382 and Laboratoire ICT) and the FRS-FNRS.

First published in 2023 by Amsterdam University Press Ltd.

Published 2025 by Routledge
4 Park Square, Milton Park, Abingdon, Oxon OX14 4RN
605 Third Avenue, New York, NY 10158

Routledge is an imprint of the Taylor & Francis Group, an informa business

ISBN: 9789463721561 (hbk)
ISBN: 9781041178200 (pbk)
ISBN: 9781003694045 (ebk)
NUR 684

Cover illustration: Ill in bed bishop writing a letter, illustration of the Decretum Gratiani, Bologna, fourteenth century (Bibliothèque Nationale de France, NAL 2508, fol. 144v)

Cover design: Coördesign, Leiden

DOI 10.5117/9789463721561

Table of Contents

List of Figures

Preface

This research began in Montpellier, in the south of France. I wanted to work on medieval disability, following a long family history that made me very curious about this issue in pre-modern times. A meeting with Mr. Julien Théry, who introduced me to supplications and papal letters, in which I found a formidable cache of material for the cultural history of the medieval period, marked the beginning of the long path that is the writing of a book. I 'go up' to Paris to meet Mr. Henri-Jacques Stiker, whose book, *Corps infirmes et société*, was always at my bedside. He introduced me to Mr. Didier Lett, in whom I found a thesis director, in the noblest sense of the word. His help and advices allowed me to give substance to my ideas. I would also like to thank Mrs. Maaike van der Lugt, Mrs. Irina Metzler, Mr. Charles de Miramon, and Mrs. Myriam Winance, who did me the honor of reading and discussing this work.

This book would never have seen the light of day without the financial, but also human and logistical support of the University of Paris Diderot, and more particularly of the ICT laboratory and its successive directors, Mrs. Liliane Hilaire-Pérez, Mrs. Anna Caiozzo, and Mrs. Charlotte de Castelnau-l'Estoile as well as Mrs. Laurence Griffoul. I particularly thank the ED 382, its former director, Mr. Jean-Pierre Guilhembet, and its former co-director, Mrs. Florence Binard, for the training I received during the thesis. I would also like to thank the students of the University of Paris Diderot for the pleasure I took in teaching them medieval history, historiography, and historical methodology. I feel honoured to have seen them grow and flourish in contact with the teaching staff and their nascent or already affirmed passion.

My research benefited from three grants from the École française de Rome, during which I was able to build up my corpus of documents. I would like to thank Mrs. Catherine Virlouvet, Mr. Pierre Savy, and Mr. Stéphane Gioanni for having welcomed me, as well as those in charge of the library of the French School, Mrs. Annie Coisy and Mr. Clément Pieyre, for their letters, which allowed me to enter the Vatican Apostolic Archives. I took great advantage of the ideal setting offered by the French School, which gave rhythm to my research during my stays. The staff of Vatican Apostolic Archives and Library have always been of great help in consulting the primary material of this research. I thank them here for their precious advice, as well as the archivists of the National Archives of Paris and the Bibliothèque Nationale de France.

I must mention the names of all those who answered my questions as I worked on this book: Mr. Olivier Canteaut, Mr. Arnaud Fossier, Mr. Armand Jamme, Mrs. Élisabeth Lusset, Mr. Olivier Richard, and Mr. Laurent Vallière. I would also like to thank Mr. Jean-François Ravaud and Mrs. Isabelle Ville who welcomed me to their workshop *Handicap et Sociétés* and to the network of the same name. I am also grateful to the members of the *Homo Debilis* network for the fruitful meetings they have organized periodically: Mrs. Bianca Frohne, Mrs. Jenni Kuuliala, Mrs. Irina Metzler, Mrs. Cordula Nolte, Mrs. Wendy Turner, and so many others, have contributed greatly to the theoretical and practical framework of my research. My warmest thanks also go to my editor at Amsterdam University press, Mrs. Shannon Cunningham, and to the editors who kindly proofread my text, namely Mrs. Alicia Spencer-Hall and Mrs. Vicki Blud.

The writing of this book allowed me to meet wonderful people, of whom it is impossible to make a complete list. Each of them, in his or her own way, has helped me to carry out this research and has served as a reference point in both happy and difficult moments. The unfailing support of my friends and my family and in-laws, far from the world of research, must be underlined. May they all find in these anonymous thanks my most sincere gratitude and affection. Finally, the immeasurable support of Kevin (and Windy) could only be sketched. I will therefore remain silent about him, as I am at a loss for words.

General Remarks

I wished to respect the language of the Latin sources used, but I have sometimes simplified the spelling and restored the capital letters where possible, as well as adjusting punctuation to facilitate the reading. The translation of this type of Latin document being very complex, it was mostly not done word for word but rather with the aim of reproducing the idea contained in the document.

Introduction: A Formal Dialogue

Abstract
The introduction presents the main historical context to the study at hand, with an in-depth focus on the corpus: the petitions sent to the popes and the letters written in answer by the Papal Chancery. It investigates the identity of the petitioners, alongside procedures and regulations relating to the written documents themselves. Most writers were members of the Italian and French high clergy, though individuals from all levels of the Church are represented in the petitions. The correspondence between such clerics and the Papal Chancery depended upon established writing and regulatory processes, both in terms of the rules put in place by the Chancery to guarantee its intervention and the mechanisms available to supplicants for reporting their impairments and making an effective case for dispensations.

Keywords: Petition; Papal Letters; Experiences; Methodology; Discourses

> And if thy right hand offend thee, cut it off, and
> cast it from thee: for it is profitable for thee
> that one of thy members should perish, and not
> that thy whole body should be cast into hell.
> – Matt. 5:30 KJV

Using this sentence, Pope Leo found much-needed biblical justification for an act that appeared senseless to all those around him. Shortly after his election to the papacy, Leo had encountered a beautiful woman who, with due reverence, kissed his hand chastely. This unleashed within Leo, as legend has it, a fleshly temptation so powerful that he had only one option to staunch its fire: to cut off his hand, as prescribed in Matthew 5.30. Whilst this may have resolved the new Pope's internal spiritual struggles, it generated another set of problems entirely, even threatening his position as leader of the

Dubourg, N., *Disabled Clerics in the Late Middle Ages. Un/suitable for Divine Service?*
Taylor & Francis Group, 2023
DOI: 10.5117/9789463721561_INTRO

Church. Following canonical regulations on clerical impairment, his distal forearm amputation rendered him ineligible to perform Mass. The clergy openly voiced their dissatisfaction with a pontiff who could not fulfil one of the most basic, one of the most important, clerical tasks. Their disparaging sentiments were shared by the Roman laity, who threatened a revolt against Leo's religious authority. And so, Leo turned to another beautiful woman to resolve his situation: he entrusted his misfortunes to the Virgin Mary and prayed to her for a miraculous remedy. She dutifully appeared to him in a vision, restored his hand and explicitly authorized him to celebrate Mass. The story of Leo's amputation circulated widely in the Middle Ages, and experienced particular popularity in the mid-thirteenth century, featuring in numerous collections of miracles and *exempla*, in poems, and even songs.[1] Gruesomely entertaining and spiritually educative, it is little wonder that it gained such currency. Its utility as an *exemplum* is not limited to medieval audiences, however. It serves as an excellent primer on the main themes at play in a study of clerical disability in the Middle Ages.

Despite clear evidence of interest in clerical disability in the medieval period, the clergy has been all but forgotten in the discipline of disability history, an area of research that has recently undergone tectonic shifts in scholarly approach.[2] For many years, the topic had been studied almost exclusively from the perspective of social history. This approach privileged the construction of disability as physical anomaly, and analysed such difference in terms of marginality, poverty, and deviance.[3] In this, scholarship followed the contours of public policy that conceived of disabled people as indigents, patients, and/or objects of charity, a stance predicated on the medical model of disability.[4] In the 1980s, however, the issue of accessibility became crucial. Scholars and activists alike emphasized the distinction between impairment and disability, developing the social model of disability.[5] Whilst impairment is a biomedical fact, disability is a condition created and imposed upon non-normate bodies by an ableist society which does not offer equal access to all. The social model enacted a radical shift in conceptualizing disability,

1 This narrative can be found in the miracles collection of Bartholomeo of Trent (see MS 1794, University of Bologna, and Dondaine, "Barthélemy de Trente O.P,"); in the *exemplum* collections of the *Tractatus* 37, the *Tabula exemplorum* 5, the *Alphabetum narrationum* 20 and the *Scala Coeli* 31 (see Delaune, Le handicap dans les *exempla* médiévaux); but also in the poems and songs from the *Cantigas de Santa Maria* (see the Oxford database).

2 For a more complete historiography, see Dubourg, "European Medieval Disability History".

3 Stiker, Ravaud, and Albrecht, "L'émergence des disability studies", p. 48.

4 Masala and Petretto, "From Disablement to Enablement", p. 1236.

5 Barnes (eds.), *Implementing the Social Model of Disability.*

yet it still had, and has, its limitations, especially in terms of definition(s) of disability itself.

Academics in the 2000s recognized more clearly than ever that the meanings, and thus the experiences, of disability changed over time, and within and between cultures; hence, the need for a cultural model of disability.[6] The documents used in developing this model, however, typically relate to the substance of laws, rather than their application. In other words, these sources fail to shed light on the real-life experiences of disabled people.[7] Notwithstanding such weaknesses in the literature, close attention to cultural and temporal context remains paramount in understanding disability history. From 2005 onwards, disability has been conceived of as a socio-cultural phenomenon, that which diverges from culturally constituted 'norms' at a given moment in time.[8] More recently, in the past decade or so, researchers have called for further refinement of this model, foregrounding the significance of intersectionality. In an intersectional framework, disability is understood as only one of the elements of identity that collectively governed an individual's lived experiences in medieval society, alongside gender, race, sexuality, and so on.[9] Researchers using an intersectional, cultural model of disability examine the ways in which a given society produces its own norms, including those from which the disabled body notionally deviates. Of prime importance are the ways in which an individual's experience of disability depends on their multiple subject positions, not just their physical ability or lack thereof. Such work is fundamentally interdisciplinary, thereby offering a comprehensive approach to disability and impairment as historically contingent cultural phenomena.[10] With this methodology, it becomes possible to analyse disability as a specific phenomenon, all the while considering the many social mechanisms which produce the non-normate, and the multiple contexts in which disability, as a category, is embedded.[11] Scholars have been all but unanimous in urging for this kind of methodological innovation in disability studies, yet its adoption has

6 Turner and Pearman (eds.), *The Treatment of Disabled Persons in Medieval Europe*; Metzler, *Fools and Idiots?*

7 Metzler, *Disability in Medieval Europe*; Eyler (ed.), *Disability in the Middle Ages*; Turner and Butler (eds.), *Medicine and the Law in the Middle Ages.*

8 Nolte (ed.), *Homo debilis*; Collard and Samama (eds.), *Handicaps et sociétés dans l'histoire*; Metzler, *A Social History of Disability in the Middle Ages.*

9 Goodley, *Disability Studies.*

10 Burghardt, "The Human Bottom of Non-human Things", p. 5; Shildrick, "Critical Disability Studies", p. 30.

11 Waldschmidt, "Warum und wozu brauchen die Disability Studies die Disability History?", p. 26.

been slow, particularly in historical research. Only a few historical studies have thus far taken into account this interdisciplinary, intersectional way of thinking.[12] Nevertheless, several publications have recently aimed to contextualize historical experiences of disability. They have contributed to a deeper understanding of disability in the premodern era and of the body in medieval Christian thought, by adopting a rigorously focused analytical gaze.[13] Eschewing generalized surveys, such enquiries concentrate on a delimited geographical region, and/or a specific primary-source corpus, including using material from papal registers. This is illustrated by the work of Friederike Stöhr on disabled German and Scandinavian clerics, which leveraged papal petitions dating to the fifteenth century, preserved in the Apostolic Penitentiary.[14] Stöhr built on the earlier work of Jussi Hanska and Kirsi Salonen, who consulted the same set of primary sources in their book-length analysis of clerical careers from 1458 to 1471.[15] Such scholarship demonstrates the productivity of studying papal documents and religious experience in terms of disability history.

Following a post-structuralist approach, this book proposes that disability is constituted by social and cultural processes, mechanisms which likewise integrally shape representations of the impaired body.[16] Disability is polysemic; as a concept, it is both diachronic (mobilizing concepts or structures that evolve over time) and synchronic (revealing structures, ideas, or cultures from a specific point in time). From a synchronic perspective, the language of disability is common to all contemporaneous narrators at a deep and unconscious level.[17] The cultural model, as sketched above, makes it possible to reconceptualize disability in this mode, by taking into account the specific cultural contexts which produce the disabled body and the lived experiences of disabled people.[18] Impairment, understood by its direct link to the body and physical difference, is culturally constructed in a similar fashion. It has its own symbolic dimension in which illness, old

12 Krötzl, Mustakallio, and Kuuliala (eds.), *Infirmity in Antiquity and the Middle Ages*; Turner and Lee (eds.), *Trauma in Medieval Society.*

13 Kuuliala, *Childhood Disability and Social Integration in the Middle Ages*; Scarborough, *Viewing Disability in Medieval Spanish Texts*; Künzel and Connelly (eds.), *New Approaches to Disease, Disability, and Medicine in Medieval Europe*; Baker, Nijdam and Land (eds.), *Medicine and Space.*

14 Stöhr, *Körpermakel – Arbeits(un)fähigkeit – Kirchenrecht.*

15 Hanska and Salonen, *Entering a Clerical Career.*

16 Hughes and Paterson, "The Social Model of Disability and the Disappearing Body", p. 326.

17 Metzler, *A Social History of Disability in the Middle Ages*, p. 4.

18 Shakespeare, "Cultural Representation of Disabled People".

age, accidents, and so on contribute to its social construction.[19] Within this framework, the body becomes a social and historical object: it must be re-centred as the primary object of analysis.[20] The cultural model demonstrates that society, as a capitalist and materialist system, is not the only 'disabling' agent. What becomes clear is that biological factors and the socio-cultural perception of the impaired body are inseparable, and intertwined, in the understanding and lived experience of disability. Impairment is not only a medical condition, but an experience, and a discursive construction. Consequently, it is as much social as it is biological.[21] Consideration of impairment and disability in concert allows us to discern the various aspects of physical and/or mental handicap in a given society. In that respect, they function in the same way as other analytical metrics, such as age, gender, or social status.[22] In short, impairment and disability exist first and foremost as shifting cultural constructs that change across time and between places. The signification ascribed to these constructs also varies according to more immediate, or narrow, social and/or environmental context(s), and may therefore change depending on the documents studied.[23]

In petitions written by disabled clerics and pontifical letters, studied as the primary corpus for this book, the 'impairment' turns into a 'disability' in relation to the pontifical institution because of its consequences. Indeed, within the supplication process, 'disability' appears because 'impairment' prevents clerics from fulfilling their social role, which requires a particular kind of 'fixing' from the pontifical institution. In this material, clerics with a range of impairments – including physical conditions (e.g., limb loss, bodily weakness, disease), sensory impairments (e.g., blindness, deafness), and mental infirmities (e.g., senile dementia, epilepsy) – encounter similar or comparable difficulties in fulfilling some of their ecclesiastical duties and benefiting from their associated rights. These individuals, then, experienced disability as a social, religious, and cultural phenomenon, in terms of the way in which their impairment(s) were framed as barriers to their full participation in the Church.

Normality is defined at a cultural rather than an individual level. As such, any study of the representation of a specific group of disabled people, such as clerics, must be grounded in a more generalized understanding

19 Siebers, "Disability in Theory", p. 739.

20 Gleeson, *Geographies of Disability*, p. 67.

21 Thomas, "Disability Theory: Key Ideas, Issues and Thinkers", p. 52.

22 Krötzl, Mustakallio, and Kuuliala, "Introduction", p. 5.

23 For examples, see Hsy, Pearman, and Eyler (eds.), *A Cultural History of Disability in the Middle Ages*.

of the bigger picture of disability, including its complexity, in medieval society as a whole.[24] To this end, it is necessary to determine the way in which physical and mental conditions were perceived on the basis of the knowledge and practices of the period.[25] When referring to 'the body' in medieval society, we refer more accurately to the *Christian* body, for religion was the primordial signifying framework in which the body was embedded and was its principle regulatory agent.[26] The prescriptions set out in dogma were not just spiritual, but physical. For example, Christians were instructed on an array of appropriate practices, including those regarding food (e.g., Lenten fasting, ingestion of certain foods on certain days), sexual intercourse (e.g., approved positions, prohibition during menstruation), sleep (e.g., structured according to canonical hours), and work (e.g., the timing of rest).[27] Moreover, ecclesiastical authorities explicitly legislated the idealized form of embodiment, the 'perfect body' required of all clergy. The impaired bodies of clerics exhibiting 'defects' of body or mind (*defectus corporis* and *mentis*) fell short of this normative standard, and thus were judged to be 'irregular'. Clerical impairment as a category of experience is, thus, integrally contingent: inseparable from the power that legislates its form(s), and the culture in which it is produced. For this reason, this book establishes a critical dialogue between norms and practices. As the sources demonstrate, norms can and do shift, thereby changing an individual's (experience of) impairment, even as their physical condition(s) may remain the same. The norms decreed by pontifical authority, such as statutes in canon law, could be endorsed, modified, even overruled, on a case-by-case basis, as the Papal Chancery responded to individual cleric's petitions, in letters written and sent in the name of the current Pope.

This book approaches medieval disability on the basis of correspondence received and issued by one of the most powerful medieval authorities in the Western world: the papacy. Concentrating on sources from the eleventh to the fourteenth century, this study tracks the papal monarchy's formation, its glorious heyday, and its eventual decline.[28] This tumultuous period saw the emergence of a papal theocracy (a political system whose nature is based on power from God), founded on legal concepts but also on administrative

24 See Linton, "What Is Disability Studies?", p. 518; Meade and Serlin, "Editors' Introduction", p. 4.

25 Van Trigt, Gross, and Söderfeldt, "Historicizing the Social Model", p. 95.

26 Hutchinson, "Disabling Beliefs?", p. 11.

27 See Bynum, *Christian Materiality*.

28 Whalen, *Dominion of God*, p. 3.

organization. The book starts on the theoretical foundations laid by the Gregorian reforms that advocated the assertion of papal power and stated a stronger separation between the laity and the clergy. One of its manifestations was the Investiture Controversy, which tried to define whether the king (temporal power) or the Pope (spiritual power) had the legitimacy to appoint the prelates of the Church. Elected in this context, Paschal II (1099–1118) is the first Pope we encounter in the corpus. He was the first pontiff to attempt to resolve the thorny issue of antipopes, 'competing' Church leaders that had long been an issue, with the present interlopers installed by Henry IV.[29] During the late Middle Ages, the papacy was in conflict with various secular forces around these issues of delimiting its temporal power, to the point of having to flee Rome and take refuge in Avignon from 1309 to 1378. The study ends with the pontificate of Gregory XI (1371–1378), which marked the return of the papacy to the Eternal City. Yet Gregory's reign also saw the beginning of the Great Western Schism that divided Christians into two factions for some forty years. This *terminus ad quem* corresponds to the end of the period in which the papacy, in Rome as in Avignon, had strenuously attempted to solidify and centralize its authority.

The popes developed the administrative centrality of the Church around their person in the Curia (the popes' court and central administrative government) in order to strengthen their power. They created a colossal volume of diplomatics in pursuit of this goal, forming the rich corpus of material that furnishes the present study.[30] From the twelfth to the fourteenth century, the ecclesiastical institution exercised temporal, as well as spiritual, supremacy over the whole of Christendom. Its role in defining impairment and disability cannot be overstated. The real-world power of papal letters to settle clerical or religious problems across Europe lay in the pontiff's own ability to grant graces – the prerogative of the greatest monarchs of the medieval period – and the letters' function as a vehicle by which to transmit that grace. Grace, in this context, typically refers to grants of permission to ratify, edit, and/or exceed rules and established norms, issued in response to an individual's petition. Taken as a corpus, then, the papal letters bear witness to a 'dialogue' between the lived experiences of disability (specific clerics; petitions), and the structures which constructed disability as a category (the

29 Ullmann, *The Growth of Papal Government.*

30 This moment in ecclesiastical history, difficult to study given the great diplomatic output of the multiple Chanceries (Avignon, Rome, Pisa), reveals the problems of power around which the question of pontifical grace crystallizes.

papacy, as Church authority; papal letters), allowing historians to grasp the complexity of such interchanges.[31]

Disability and impairment are socio-culturally structured as deviance, that is, the inability to conform to the bodily and/or mental norms produced by one or more authorities.[32] Indeed, the very materiality of the body is challenged by knowledge power.[33] Dominant discourses, for example medicine and law, orient the body and render it 'intelligible', at least partially. In Foucauldian terms, these authorities determine a baseline of 'normality', thereby producing impairment and disability.[34] Accordingly, categorizations of normality and abnormality ultimately serve to establish who has the right to be part of society and who does not.[35] The necessity of first defining normality in a given context, in order to discern and define otherness, has become ever more clear, as more and more researchers have begun to examine disability across cultures and time periods.[36] We must seek out the 'perfect', 'normal' body in a given culture to bring into focus the 'imperfect', 'abnormal' body, following the discursive logic of ableism.[37] From this point of view, studies of disability highlight the fact that disability and normality are, to some degree at least, fluid concepts and states.[38] The medieval Church had the prerogative of transmitting, revising, and applying canon law. With pontifical letters, the institution issued pronouncements on all, and any, issues relating to the ministry, religious obligations, and Christian life. The Church's epistolary policy had a notable impact on the lives of the clergy and laity alike as its authority grew stronger during the thirteenth and fourteenth centuries, particularly in the papacy's official acts.

This study operates according to two fundamental principles. Firstly, the impaired body is understood as both the product and target of social anxieties. In medieval society, as arguably in our own, physical and mental impairments are linked to abnormality. This gives rise to legislation and regulations which exclude disabled people from social roles, services, and more. This is equally true of the situation within the ecclesiastical institution,

31 Millet, *Suppliques et requêtes*. It was rather about presenting a petition in a right form so that the popes could accept it than a real and developed 'dialogue' but it could also lead to a series of epistolary exchanges.

32 Thomson, *Extraordinary Bodies*, p. 6.

33 Foucault, *Surveiller et punir*.

34 Shildrick and Price, "Uncertain Thoughts on the Dis/abled Body", p. 234.

35 Meekosha and Shuttleworth, "What's so "Critical" about Critical Disability Studies?", p. 65.

36 Kudlick, "Disability History", p. 560.

37 Titchkosky, "Disability Studies", p. 219. On ableism, see Campbell, *Contours of Ableism*.

38 Frohne and Horn, "On the Fluidity of "Disability"", p. 28.

since impaired supplicants were obliged to seek dispensations from the Pope himself on account of their 'abnormality'. Petitions and papal letters therefore illustrate the typical anxieties of medieval society about impairment. Secondly, this corpus elucidates ecclesiastical attitudes towards 'abnormality', attitudes which are fundamental to a medieval understanding of disability more generally. This point is essential to grasp. The Church, as an institution, imposes (or attempts to impose) its authority on the whole of Christian thought. What's more, it proposes a normative definition of impairment – that which diverges from the 'perfect body' – upon which our analysis depends. These primary sources do not merely offer us information, fleshing out what we already knew, but rather inspiration: this study is guided by what these rich documents have to say on the matter of disability, using such findings to expand our conceptualization of the categories at hand. The Papal Chancery is charged with measuring impairment and deciding whether or not a person is capable of fulfilling the duties associated with his ecclesiastical office based on the severity of his 'infirmity'. As such, impairment becomes a disability.

This book hypothesizes that clerical disability emerges in the moment that an individual's impairment was recognized as such by the Church, that is, in terms of the relationship of a given body with an institutional authority. In this context, physical or mental impairments considered to be disabilities justify the receipt of pontifical grace. Indeed, the use of the Latin word *defectus* to describe the irregularity of the impaired clerical body allows us to characterize bodily difference as a crucial identity marker within the supplication process. Impairment could be a potent conduit, even remedy, for social anxieties, insofar as individuals could leverage their impairment as a pretext to justify modifying their identity, achieved through the supplication process. If recognized as disabled, individuals acceded to an established role in the community, one that could have certain advantages.[39] This papally approved transition was achieved chiefly through adapting petitioners' ecclesiastical duties, and thereby updating their social identities, according to their current level of in/ability.

Responding positively to petitions, the Papal Chancery recognized the condition of disability and – without erasing the impairment itself – erased its *institutional* effects, by enacting, modifying, or softening the application of relevant laws. In fact, granting of papal grace allowed supplicants to be

39 Calvez, "Le handicap comme situation de seuil", p. 84; or Willett and Deegan, "Liminality and Disability". See the foundational works of anthropologists on rites of passages and ritual processes, who include Arnold Van Gennep and Victor Turner.

included in an environment from which they would usually have been excluded. The Church, as the authority which defined bodily 'abnormality', could and did act as an agent both of exclusion *and* inclusion, flexing its power to produce both disability and ability on a case-by-case basis. It appears that defining disability constituted a fundamental act of governance – tinged with political value – for the papacy.

Petitions and Papal Letters

Petitions and papal letters are a uniquely rich source, offering almost unparalleled documentation of clerical impairment in the Middle Ages, from both individual and institutional perspectives. This material was the output of the Papal Chancery, an institution that underwent a dazzling evolution from the eleventh to the fourteenth century, with the epistolary apparatus playing a central role in attempts to legitimize papal authority, when granting of pontifical grace through letters became resolutely political. The archives demonstrate a noticeable uptick in the number of letters received, sent, and kept by the Curia from the reign of Paschal II (1099–1118) onwards, alongside more stringent regulation of the diplomatic format itself. The so-called Gregorian Reforms, the reign of Innocent III (1198–1216), and the promotion of *plenitudo potestatis* all explain, and justify, this new zeal to preserve correspondence.[40] Faced with the administrative chaos of an ever-growing mass of documents, the popes and the Holy See were obliged to revolutionize the organization of the Chancery, and the tools at its disposal, from the beginning of the thirteenth century.[41] From the eleventh century onwards, the influence of pontifical power expanded significantly, coinciding with the institutionalization of papal grace. The Chancery's remit broadened, and the authority with which its letters were invested was strengthened. Exchanges between petitioners and Chancery continue to be recorded to this day, and can be found alongside the medieval examples in the Vatican Apostolic Archives' registers.[42]

40 Kiedi Kionga, *Dispenses en droit canonique*.

41 Montaubin, "L'administration pontificale de la grâce", p. 321.

42 To find out more about the places where the Vatican Archives are kept, from the Lateran in 649 to the Palatine Hill in the eleventh century, to the archives we know today, set up by Pius IV (1605–1621) during the Napoleonic parenthesis of 1810 and opened to researchers in 1881 by Leo XIII (1878–1903), see Coombs, Yakel, Carlen and Gill, *Vatican Archives*, or Gachard, "Les archives du Vatican".

A Hybrid Corpus: Regulation, in Theory and in Practice

Some petitions were lodged by the laity in order to absolve a sin, commute a vow, or allow prohibited acts, such as marrying a cousin. The majority of the corpus, however, deals with issues specific to the clergy which fell under the exclusive remit of the ecclesiastical hierarchy, in professional as well as spiritual terms. This includes, for example, requests to become a priest despite the canonical impediment of *defectus*. Such a 'defect' could relate to age (*defectus aetatis*, if an individual were underage), to legitimacy (*defectus natalium*, in cases of illegitimate birth), and, crucially for the present analysis, to physical or mental conditions (*defectus corporis* or *mentis*). The presence of any defect could disqualify a man from joining the Church's ranks entirely.[43] But defects of body or mind also concern those already in the ecclesiastical community, clerics whose condition(s) now prevented them from fulfilling their responsibilities in performing religious rites (such as Mass, Eucharist) and duties (Lent, pilgrimages, and so on).[44]

Petitions and papal letters form a productively hybridized corpus, situated at the intersection of authorized, institutional policy and (auto-)biographical testimony, chronicling the lived experiences of disabled people in the Middle Ages. As such, they constitute an excellent analytical laboratory in which to study medieval impairment in its relation to the papacy as an institution, alongside the impact of official ecclesiastical judgments on disabled lives. The corpus of petitions and papal letters on physical and mental impairments under discussion in this study consists of 142 petitions, preserved for the reign of Clement VI (1342–1352), Innocent VI (1352–1362) and the first four years of the pontificate of Urban V (1362–1370), as well as 743 letters (for at least 753 petitioners) from the twelfth, thirteenth, and fourteenth centuries.

The petitions followed a complex and costly path before reaching the Pope, to whom all of the Church's *causae majores* (matters of major importance) were sent. They were addressed to the Pontifical Curia by clerics or lay people from all over Europe, reflecting the growing push to centralize ecclesiastical power. This was emphasized, for example, in Gregory VII's influential (though unofficial) treatise *Dictatus Papae*, which affirmed that the Pope alone held jurisdiction over all Christendom.[45] With few exceptions, the

43 Metzler, "Then and Now", p. 465.

44 See Parlopiano, "*Propter Deformitatem*".

45 Schuster, *Der Dictatus Papae*.

original petitions have been lost.[46] Their contents, however, were copied by the Chancery for archival purposes.[47] Petitions in this study's corpus have been preserved in the first 46 registers of the Vatican Apostolic Archives (VAA), known collectively as *Registra Supplicationum* (RS). Whilst papal bulls have been the object of fairly comprehensive research, the petitions have long been neglected, a fact that is reflected in, and explains, the dearth of published editions.[48] Things appear to be changing, however. Since the beginning of the twentieth century, the petition registers, as a collection, have been amongst the most frequently consulted medieval sources in the entire VAA.

Papal letters were written by the Chancery on behalf of the Pope in response to supplications.[49] These acts are known variously as rescripts of privilege, indulgence, dispensation, exemption, grace, or benefice, according to their content and function.[50] Dispensations relating to impairment were case-specific, authorizing a modification in the application of canonical law for a specific petitioner, without changing the legislation itself.[51] Such grants of grace remained strictly exceptional and constituted 'a temporary softening of the rigour of the law because of the necessity of time or the usefulness to the Church', to quote Bernold of Constance, a Benedictine chronicler and supporter of the Gregorian reform paraphrasing Gratian's *Decree* (*Decretum*).[52] The pontifical letters are therefore neither constitutions (which are matters of law and discipline), nor encyclicals (letters addressed to the episcopate), nor decrees (regulations valid for the whole Church), nor decretals (documents which deal with particular cases before becoming jurisprudence). Papal missives in this study's corpus are preserved in the 290 Vatican Registers (VR) spanning the years 1198–1378.[53] Some were kept in 172 Avignon Registers (AR) recording activities in the period 1309–1378.[54]

46 See Van Moé, "Suppliques originales", and Gasnault, "Une supplique originale".

47 Completed in 1899, the fund amounts to 7,365 volumes since 1342.

48 Zutshi, "The Origins of the Registration of Petitions".

49 Zutshi, "The Personal Role of the Pope", Herold (eds.), *Vom Nutzen des Schreibens*.

50 Durand de Maillane, *Dictionnaire de droit canonique*, IV, p. 360.

51 Vallerani, *Medieval Public Justice*, p. 312.

52 My translation of Bernold of Constance, *Epistola* 57, *in* Migne (ed.), *Patrologia Latina*, vol. 161, p. 326, quoted in Hoareau-Dodinau, *Le pardon*, p. 346.

53 This number rises to 2,042 for the whole series of RV (up to 1605). See Boyle, *A Survey of the Vatican*, p. 106.

54 RA run to 349 volumes and were used to record the missives of the Popes of Avignon from 1316 to 1378, then the antipopes from 1378 to 1416. See op. cit., p. 107. Under the pontificate of Clement VI, a double recording system was introduced: the first rapid and discursive, much abbreviated, on paper (AR), and the second with the hand laid down on parchment registers

Selections of this material have been published relatively frequently, edited by various European teams through history.[55]

Above all, papal letters highlight the Pope's *plenitudo potestatis*: they manifest, and act as a conduit for, the pontiff's access to grace. This was central to the papacy's legitimacy as an institutional authority, and its effective administration of the Church's affairs. Grace served as a mechanism by which the Pope could adjust, even contravene, established ecclesiastical standards, norms, and functions, by softening the application of law.[56] These documents allow petitioners to disobey notionally universal rules that, in theory, should apply, due to their physical and/or mental impairment(s), without fear of punishment. In this way, they demonstrate Weberian 'material rationality': the law is neither fixed nor entirely objective, in terms of an equal, fixed application. Broader social contexts and extra-legal concerns directly influence legal outcomes.[57] The law was ill-equipped to deal with the material effects of clerics' physical and/or mental impairments, a weakness which did not similarly affect the efficacy of pontifical grace. The latter provided the means to surpass legal authority, ensuring necessary social adjustments were put in place for disabled clergy. In concrete terms, the petitions and letters illustrate how divergences from the norm compelled institutional responses and affected, perhaps even transformed, institutional practices. This compelled, in turn, a shift in the standards by which the norm was constructed, responding to the social needs of medieval people. This is entirely in line with medieval thought, which held that neither a general rule of law nor absolute predictability of legal solutions were possible: the law lies in the particular.[58] Between the twelfth and fourteenth centuries, the Papal Chancery became something like a factory churning out case-by-case exemptions to norms, issuing countless grants of grace to disabled petitioners. Yet these 'exceptional' accommodations would, ultimately, reshape the norms to which they originally responded, gradually modifying what would be taken as normal, and permissible, for future clergy.[59]

when the document was ready to be sent (VR). However, ten years later, during the reign of Innocent VI, the Chancery made it a practice to copy only part of the letters in the VR: the two series therefore remain complementary even today.

55 This book contains unpublished papal letters. For a list of published documentation, see Bibliography.

56 Claustre, "La grâce et la norme", p. 175.

57 See Miramon, "L'invention de la Réforme grégorienne", p. 288, quoting Weber, *Rechtssoziologie*.

58 Leveleux-Teixeira, "Fabrique et réception de la norme".

59 Indeed, over time, the missives became integrated within the canon law. On this process, see Cerutti, "Normes et pratiques".

A Grounded Approach to Medieval Clerical Disability

This study employs a blended methodology, using a combination of quantitative and qualitative approaches to interrogate the corpus. Relevant information has been extracted from the textual sources, producing a database which facilitates statistical processing.[60] Quantitative analysis offers an expansive overview of the totality of cases found in the corpus, and reveals patterns in the dataset, thereby providing macro-level findings about clerical disability. Examination of a corpus of homogeneous documents can testify, for example, to continuities or differences in terms of the representation of the same phenomenon in different individual contexts. This approach illustrates the constructed-ness of impairment, as it makes visible the norms most frequently mobilized by the ecclesiastical institution in determining clerical disability, or lack thereof. Likewise, through the comparative study of the contents of the letters, we gain ever more detail regarding the lived experiences of medieval disability, especially in terms of the diversity of conditions represented. In a complementary fashion, this study offers qualitative case studies that focus more narrowly on individual petitions, and the traces of the lives of the disabled clerics they transmit. Case studies, if an appropriate case has been selected and analysed with sufficient rigour, allow historians to explore in depth aspects relevant to the research project more generally, bringing to light an individual example of a discourse or an experience that can then be generalized.[61] This approach is akin to micro-history, and is one of the most effective methods for excavating the authentic reality of situations in which rhetorical stereotyping has been used against groups of people. The generic features of a singular object are thus revealed, permitting an empirical approach.[62] In this way, serial analysis and the usage of case studies are mutually reinforcing methodological tools.

The interweaving of these two approaches is a hallmark of grounded theory, a framework first developed by anthropologists and sociologists.[63] This theory is based on the systematic analysis of all available data on a given subject. Following an inductive and grounded methodology, this book draws on several types of supplementary sources which, in various ways, all speak to the specific nature of 'normality' in the period, in order to understand the law justifying the writing of papal letters and to highlight the cultural

60 Brown, "Methodological Paradigms", p. 146.

61 Morley, *Theories, Models, and Concepts*, p. 8.

62 Passeron and Revel (eds.), *Penser par cas*.

63 Glaser and Strauss, *The Discovery of Grounded Theory*.

norms in which disabled supplicants were oriented more generally. This documentary base comprises dogmatic texts which upon which key Christian concepts depend and in which they are contemporaneously anchored. It includes biblical writings (Old and New Testaments) and foundational theological works (e.g., patristic writings and the works of theologians).[64] It also embraces legislative writings (including ecumenical and provincial or diocesan conciliar decisions) and monastic texts (e.g., constitutions, rules of orders, or customs specific to certain monasteries).[65]

This book also engages with the legal compilations that were produced as part of the drive to officially codify canonical legislation from the eleventh century onwards. Between the twelfth and fourteenth centuries, the way in which law was enacted evolved. Thanks in particular to the compilation of letters sent by the Pope, the general law became gradually incorporated into particular legislative collections. The spread of collections of decrees such as the *Decretum* (*Collectarium canonum*) by Burchard of Worms (965–1025), the *Decretum* and *Panormia* by Yvo of Chartres (1040–1116), and the *Four Books of Sentences* by Pierre Lombard (1100–1160) during this period bears witness to this change in the construction of canon law.[66] These volumes anticipate, and contribute to the formation of, the Corpus of Canon Law (*Corpus Iuris canonici*).[67] This collection of texts, compiled around 1500, contains various canonical writings and pontifical decrees. Of particular interest to the present study are: Gratian's *Decree* (*Decretum* or *Concordia discordantium canonum*), compiled between 1140 and 1150; and Gregory IX's (1329–1378) *Decretals* (or *Liber Extra*), compiled by the Dominican Raymond of Penyafort (c. 1175–1275) in 1234. Similarly, the works of various decretists, decretalists, and glossators offer invaluable context to the investigation at hand, most notably Raymond of Penyafort's own writings.[68] The oeuvre of Thomas Aquinas (1225–1274), will also be used, particularly but not exclusively the *Summa*.[69] These texts, to a greater or lesser extent, draw from real cases

64 The Church Fathers are Hilary of Poitiers (c.310–367), Ambrose (c. 340–397), Jerome (c. 345–420), and Augustine of Hippo (354–430). According to Le Goff, *L'Europe est-elle née au Moyen Âge?*, p. 13, the theologians are Boethius (c. 477–524), Cassiodorus (c. 485–585), Pope Gregory I (c. 540–604), Isidore of Seville (c. 560–636) and Bede (c. 673–735).

65 The rules of St. Benedict and St. Augustine are mainly invoked, as well as the additions of the Cistercians, the Franciscans, and the Dominicans.

66 *Decretum* of Burchard of Worms, edited in Migne (ed.), *Patrologia Latina*, vol. 140, col. 537–1058; *Decree* of Yvo of Chartres, edited in Migne (ed.), *Patrologia Latina*, vol. 161, and *Panormia* of Yvo of Chartres, edited in Migne (ed.), *Patrologia Latina*, vol. 141; Silano (ed.), *The Sentences*.

67 Friedberg (ed.), *Corpus iuris canonici*.

68 Rius Serra (ed.), *Summa iuris*.

69 Thomas D'Aquin, *Summa theologiae*, and *Somme contra gentiles*.

dealt with by the popes,[70] and served as the basis for numerous publications during the late thirteenth and fourteenth century.

With the aim of accounting for the diverse, overlapping ways in which social norms were established in the medieval era, the epistolary primary corpus is also brought into dialogue with a range of secular texts. This includes, for example, scientific writings (medical and surgical treatises, medical recipes, and health regimens) and linguistic writings (etymological lexicons, dictionaries, and encyclopaedias). Such texts are particularly productive for reference, in order to identify typical terminology used in descriptions of a given impairment or known symptomology, within the relevant discourse. This makes it possible to highlight linguistic norms and descriptive conventions that are operative, or not, within the papal corpus, and thereby to identify the harmonization of discourse. Finally, literary portrayals of physical and mental impairment – such as those found in hagiography and fictional narratives (e.g., courtly novels, allegories, and tales), demonstrate the range of attitudes towards disability in the Middle Ages from another perspective, rendering in finer detail the complex web of signification in which the papal letters and petitions are embedded and to which they implicitly respond.[71]

Writing Processes in Action

A grounded methodology supports the excavation and appropriate contextualization of heretofore overlooked information about physical and mental impairment in the primary corpus. By considering both petitions and their corresponding institutional responses, we find ourselves eavesdropping on authentic, albeit highly structured, 'dialogues' that took place between petitioners and the Papal Chancery. On the one hand, petitioners fashioned a narrative of their disability, choosing their words carefully in order to meet institutional expectations and thereby increase the chances of their request being approved. They called upon powerful intercessors and strategized

70 Hartmann and Pennington, *The History of Medieval Canon Law*, p. 9.

71 The hagiographical documents produce models to be followed and disseminate the norms, especially those produced by the pontifical institution. See Isaïa and Granier (eds.), *Normes et hagiographie*; and, for some examples, Kuuliala, *Childhood Disability and Social Integration* and Kuuliala, Peake, and Räisänen-Schröder (eds.), *Lived Religion and Everyday Life*. On the courtly novels, see for example Godden, "Prosthetic Ecologies". On allegories, consult Gianfalla, "Discours of Disability". On tales, see for instance Delony, "Alisoun's Aging" or Hsy, *The Open Access Companion*.

the best time to submit their supplication. In turn, the Papal Chancery verified supplicants' testimony with tests carried out by trusted proxies, and appointed notaries and scribes to rework and standardize their speeches. Though strongly codified in terms of its rigid epistolary style, the interaction between petitions and the Chancery nevertheless allowed the Curia to be flexible, by modifying established norms to better suit individuals' specific circumstances. This was not, however, an entirely magnanimous undertaking. The process of supplication proved to be a formidable instrument, wielded by the popes to increase their control over Christian society in the late medieval period. As I explain below, each step in the construction of the petitioner–papal dialogue served the pontifical authority. No matter what they personally gained from the interaction, everybody involved, from the petitioners to the scribes, ultimately contributed to strengthening the Pope's power.

From Real-life Experiences to Formalized Discourse

Can we ever access the real-life experiences of disabled people in documents produced by an institution, especially one that is largely responsible for constructing disability as a category in the first place? This is the question that animates the present study. Authorship is a central issue, due to the complex workflow involved in the drafting of petitions and papal letters. Bonaventure, commenting on the prologue to Pierre Lombard's *Book of Sentences*, distinguished four collaborators in the *modus faciendi librum* (composition of a document).[72] The *auctor* (author) was the most important participant, since they provided the raw subject matter, their personal observations. The *scriptor* (writer) transcribed the *auctor*'s musings. The compiler (*compilator*) then stepped in, to enrich the text with relevant references, citations, and so forth. Alternatively, or additionally, the *commentator* added their own responses and critique. In this way, the raw material supplied by the *auctor* was refined, translated into the appropriate discourse for a given context. Within the framework of the Papal Chancery, the clerics wrote the petition and sent it to the popes. The Curia's staff read the petition and wrote back a papal letter that recapped the text from the petition. We sometimes have access both to the petition and the papal letter. Because the latter notionally contains extracts from the petition, we can compare the petitioners' initial input and the official output. By comparing

72 Lett, "Des compilateurs au travail", quoting Ad claras aquas (ed.), *Opera omnia*, t. 1, 1882, pp. 14–15.

the two documents side-by-side, we may find fragments of individuals' own words and experiences.[73]

Careful framing, and rewriting, of a cleric's request began in the earliest stages of formulating the *petitio* (Fig. 0.1: § 1).

Figure 0.1 Life cycle of a petition, from supplicants' initial testimony to administrative registration

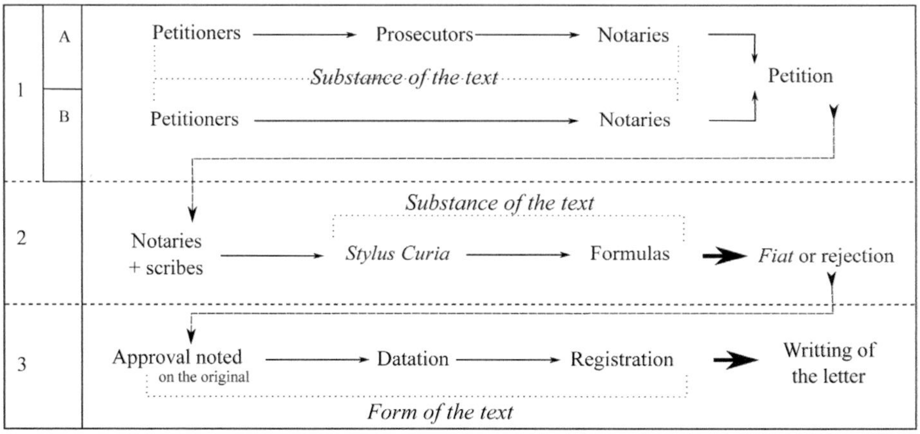

In the first instance, the *Vorurkunde* (preparatory document) was drafted by the applicant himself (Fig. 0.1: § 1A) or by a public prosecutor (Fig. 0.1: § 1B). Prosecutors were usually clerics or monks, mandated with an office or an individual in order to manage their affairs at the Curia.[74] The prosecutorial ranks steadily increased, with 40 in post during Clement VI's tenure, 68 in Innocent VI's reign, and 72 in Urban V's pontificate. Although they were not employed by the Curia directly, they were dependent on pontifical power and deeply embedded in the institution.[75] They pursued legal training similar to that of the officers of the Curia and were in daily contact with the pontifical entourage.[76] Prosecutors thus acquired the necessary expertise to ensure that no essential information was omitted from petitions, with their curial know-how offering clear benefits to the petitioners that sought out their services. The stringent submission process, to which all supplicants had to adhere, was controlled by the Chancery. This obliged the intervention of another

73 Tock, "Auteur ou impétrant", p. 216.

74 Zutshi, "Proctors Acting", p. 16.

75 Brundage, *The Medieval Origins*, p. 210. See also Makowski, *English Nuns*, p. 36.

76 Berthe, *Les procureurs*, p. 482.

layer of administrators when the petition entered the Curia: scribes and notaries. Unlike public prosecutors, notaries and scribes were not recruited by the supplicants.[77] They were agents of the Curia in charge of standardizing petitioners' testimony for administrative purposes.[78] During Boniface VIII's reign, 113 copyists served six or seven notaries.[79] Whilst scribes knew how to copy legal acts, the notaries' role, as defined by the apostolic authority, was to redraft petitions sent to the Pope into the appropriate style and format. Only once this work had taken place would petitions be presented to the popes and registered.[80] Notaries and scribes can thus be termed *petitionarii* (petitioners) in a technical sense: they rewrote submitted petitions, implementing the requisite *stylus curia* for all requests addressed to the Pope.[81]

Petitioners' own words were thus mediated by external parties, be that a prosecutor and/or notaries and scribes. Since the thirteenth century, the format of petitions had been formalized. They opened by identifying the petitioner, and someone who could possibly intercede on their behalf. There followed a statement outlining the request, supported by any details that the supplicant wished to provide. Though recounting personal, even intimate, details in order to justify their request, the petitioners' disclosures were phrased with due formality. All such material was presented in the style of the Curia, according to fixed rules and formulas (Fig. 0.1: § 2). These rules, in essence, signified the document's origins in the Chancery, and established the nature of a given act. The regulations and formulas were set out in so-called 'Chancery books', such as the *Liber Cancellariae apostolicae*, written in the 1380s by Thierry of Nieheim (1340–1418), and gained in importance between the twelfth and fourteenth centuries.[82] Collections of form letters composed by those close to the Curia on various subjects – including petitions – circulated, operating as stylistic aide-memoires.[83] Made available to supplicants, intercessors, public prosecutors, and notaries, these anthologies quickly became essential to the functioning of the administration, as they made it possible to standardize requests, and thereby optimize the task of processing them.[84] It was thus essential that the 'original' text of a petition

77 Heckel, "Das Aufkommen". For practical examples, see Cheney, *Notaries Public*, p. 89.
78 Garcìa y Garcìa (ed.), *Constitutiones Concilii*, constitution 38.
79 Digard, Fawtier, Faucon, and Thomas (eds.), *Les registres de Boniface VIII*, p. xvi.
80 Zutshi, "The Office of Notary", p. 667.
81 Barraclough, "Formulare für Suppliken".
82 Tangl, *Die päpstlichen Kanzleiordnungen*, pp. 53–316.
83 Erler, *Der Liber cancellariae*.
84 Schwarz, "The Roman Curia", p. 209.

respected formal constraints, to the extent that scribes used those documents as models for the pontifical letters.

Petitions concluded with a pontifical sentence (Fig. 0.1: § 3). If the popes approved the request and signed it, they were subsequently annotated with the word *fiat* ('done'), and, on occasion, further relevant details. This information was subsequently recorded in the registers in a prominent place, although only *accepted* petitions were recorded. Finally, petitions were not dated according to the date the request had been written or submitted, but instead when it received papal approval by the Pontifical Administration. Such dates are, in this sense, fictitious, since they reflect only when the petition was bureaucratically processed.

Once a petition had been authorized by the Pope, staff in the Papal Chancery proceeded to write a formal response (Fig. 0.2: § 1).

Figure 0.2 Life cycle of a papal letter granting grace, from composition in the Papal Chancery to receipt by petitioners

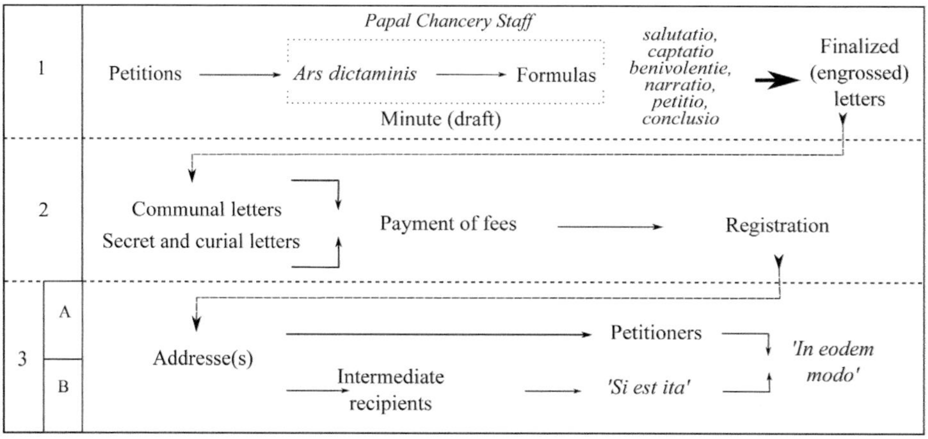

The most common process for drafting such letters, the *expeditio per cancellariam* (expedition by the Chancery), comprised four distinct stages carried out by different offices, under the direction of the Chancellor.[85] In the first office, the 'minute' (draft) was drawn up by scribes according to the basic information contained in the petition: addressee's location, status, ecclesiastical benefice held, subject of the request, and so on, as well as the date the request had been approved by the Pope.[86] At this stage, scribes often retained the petition's style

85 Zutshi, "The Office of Notary", p. 667.
86 Bock, *Einführung in das Registerwesen*, vol. 31.

(i.e., *stylus curiae*), before sending the document to its second point of call.[87] In the second office, the minute would be engrossed and taxed by scribes, who could wrote their names on the letter.[88] The process of engrossing involved ensuring the letter conformed to yet another set of regulations called the *ars dictaminis* (the art of producing letters, literally 'the art of dictation').[89] Missives followed a rigid structure, comprising five obligatory stages: *salutatio, captatio benivolentie, narratio, petitio, conclusio*.[90] Letters began with the *salutatio* (salutation), which functioned as an introduction of sorts, presenting the sender (i.e., the Pope), noting the recipient's address, and finally issuing the customary apostolic blessing. In the second part of the letter, the request itself was laid out. In the *captatio* (preamble), the Pope developed the subject of the missive in an abstract manner that was nevertheless tailored to the circumstances at hand, integrating relevant biblical quotations and religious generalities. Thereafter, in the *narratio* (exposition) and the *petitio* (request), the letter recapitulated elements supplied in the original petition.[91] The letter then came to a close, revealing the Pope's decision on the matter in a sentence, and offering the fixed phrases of the *conclusio*. Then, even the Pope's 'personal' response was standardized. Once rewritten, the now-finalized letter was transferred to a third office. Here, it could be copied into the register according to its category, and a date was appended after the *conclusio* (Fig. 0.2: § 2).

Apostolic letters were generally divided into two categories for registration, according to their legal function: mandates (i.e., letters of justice, which may contain a measure of grace), and titles (i.e., letters granting grace, including privileges, concessions, dispensations, absolutions, indulgences, donations, benefices, and so on). However, from the twelfth century onwards, a further distinction was made, based on letters' importance. Secret and curial letters were those with diplomatic significance, around 15% of extant documents during the Avignon period (1305–1378), for example.[92] The remainder, comprising 85% of the archive, were communal letters, written in response to a petition regarding the routine management of clerical affairs. Registration entailed recopying the letter, and it is these copies to which we have access today. Scribes had to be meticulous to avoid distorting the text of a letter

87 Rabikauskas, "La cancelleria", p. 228.

88 Barbiche, "Le personnel de la chancellerie", p. 123.

89 Vulliez, "L'*ars dictaminis*", p. 89.

90 Giry, *Manuel de diplomatique*, p. 490; Grévin (ed.), *Le "dictamen" dans tous ses états*.

91 The Pope recalls, writing in the first-person plural, the details that weighed in the decision to grant or not to grant pontifical grace. Thus, not all the ideas developed in the petitions necessarily appear here.

92 Kuras and Sulkowska-Kuras, "Suppliques, brouillons, lettres et registres", p. 724.

approved by the Pope himself. There is little available information regarding the practical logistics of recording petitions and papal letters. However, we do know that registration of these documents was subject to the supplicants' payment of an extra fee. Paid to the Curia as the tax, this fee was added to the initial price of the missive. Registration was neither free nor automatic, but rather 'à la carte': petitioners could choose to have their petition and/or letter copied so that it was kept in perpetuity by the Papal Chancery, guaranteeing its authenticity.[93] It is estimated that between 25% and 50% of acts were registered by the Curia, calculated from the number of original letters kept 'on file' but not recorded in registers.[94] Subsequent to registration (if applicable), Chancery staff affixed the papal bull to the document, as a means of authenticating it, and it was finally ready to be sent.[95]

Chancery staff had to follow strict procedures, set out in official style and form guides, in the process of drawing up a papal letter, one which compelled the standardization of petitioners' original text and testimony.[96] The Apostolic See strengthened its political and administrative power not just by centralizing religious affairs, but by acting, in effect, as an administrative archive for the whole of Christendom. Moreover, the requirement for correspondents to use standard forms, supported by the provision of style guides and formularies, established a homogeneous political language, a common discourse that clergy and laity across Europe were encouraged, if not outright compelled, to adopt.[97] Such standardization was also a necessity for the Papal Chancery in practical terms. On the one hand, clear guidelines meant that individuals could create the requisite original documentation essential to centralization efforts. At the same time, standardized forms helped the Chancery deal more efficiently with the high number of requests it received.[98] In this way, the Apostolic See educated supplicants on its practices in order to streamline the entire process, and thereby to meet petitioners' expectations with more success.

Quid Pro Quo

This book analyses the petition process in its totality, from its logistical practicalities to its ideological function and the power dynamics at play

93 Montaubin, "L'administration pontificale de la grâce", p. 328.
94 Barbiche, *Les actes pontificaux originaux*, pp. ciii–civ.
95 Jamme, "Écrire pour le pape", p. 14.
96 See Barraclough, *Public Notaries*, p. 9.
97 Grévin, *Rhétorique du pouvoir*, p. 21.
98 Grévin, "Les mystères rhétoriques", p. 273.

at every stage. In its most basic iteration, a petition is defined as a humble prayer in order to obtain a privilege or special grace from a sovereign. More than a simple request, a petition must contain acknowledgment of the petitioner's own incapacity, impotence, and/or poverty.[99] In this way, the petition process is a hegemonic cultural practice articulating the power differential between a petitioner and the petitioned individual or institution. The petition establishes a relationship between the parties, one based on an exchange of favours: each benefit from the petition in their own way.[100] The petitioner directly appeals to the recipient's authority, and so doing, further legitimizes it. Indeed, the petitioner becomes even more subservient to this authority, especially if their request is granted: the vocabulary of lament, almost a requirement for such documents, reinforces the notion of the supplicant's inferiority, and their obligatory submission. For powerful donors, then, supplication facilitated a privileged bond with their subjects which concretized their prestige and further entrenched their elevated status, even if petitions were concerned with banalities.[101] This book demonstrates that, for disabled clerics, entering the supplication process entailed submission to the Pope's authority. Nevertheless, petitioners were not rendered completely passive in, and through, the process.

The petition process served to increase supplicants' agency in certain ways. For a start, these documents effectively made individual petitioners visible to the Chancery, and so doing subjectivized them in terms of the institutional apparatus. Following established guidelines, petitioners were able to construct narratives of their own lives and circumstances, and make precise requests of those in power. Petitions preserve the discourse of impaired individuals, albeit couched as appeals to authority. This discourse reflects petitioners' shared desire to remain socially useful, full members of their community. For this desire to be satisfied, petitioners negotiated for papal grace by consciously playing the institutional game of petitions, in turn both passive victims and dynamic actors. In this way, petitions allowed disabled clerics to accede to an active role in negotiating the Church's internal power structures, at least to some degree. Whilst it was impossible for supplicants to liberate themselves from normative regulatory frameworks entirely, petitions gave them room to manoeuvre. Disabled petitioners were agents, in a fundamental sense: subjects with the capacity, means, and

99 Cerutti and Vallerani, "Suppliques"; Nubola and Würgler, *Suppliche e "gravamina"*, p. 10.

100 Whiting, *Women and Petitioning*, p. 2.

101 Thompson, *Customs in Common*.

desire to act in a given situation, according to their own circumstances.[102] By taking advantage of the privilege of applying for a papal exemption, petitioners could decisively influence their own situation. Similarly, such applications could influence the development of normative standards more generally – as some pontifical letters were added in formularies – thereby helping future supplicants.[103]

Petitioners used grants of pontifical grace to serve their own interests, carving out space for themselves in the Church and their community. At the same time, however, letters of grace reinforced the authority of ecclesiastical law and the Church as an institution over society as a whole. The Church followed a juridical logic above all, and it developed specialized skills in order to ensure its own functioning and solidify its authority.[104] Here we find the purpose, and the power, of grace, an asset of divine origin dispensed by the Pope and to which only he had access. This papal prerogative was then integrated into, and mobilized by, a discursive apparatus (or Foucauldian 'dispositif'), which enabled the Church to keep abreast of happenings across Europe, as reported in petitions, and to disseminate its decisions.[105] Thus, the Papal Chancery established a 'dialogue' with Christians similar to an exchange between a prince and his subject, facilitating a quasi-personal relationship.[106] The petition process created a certain intimacy between the parties, as popes personally authorized individuals to pursue practices that were otherwise prohibited, through the case-by-case granting of graces. This provided a mechanism to engender flexibility in the otherwise rigid normative system.[107] Equally, this interventionist policy was motivated by another logic, archival this time: the Church was, to a large extent, defined by its role as a producer and curator of government records.

Timing was a key factor in the petition process, with supplicants and the Chancery alike seeking the 'right moment'.[108] Petitioners had to make careful calculations as to the best time to submit their documentation. They often

102 "Agency" with this meaning can first be found in Thompson, "Socialist Humanism", p. 113.

103 The petitioners show agency in asking for help and become agents of recognition of their status, just as those seeking the intermission of a saint are agents of their miraculous healings. See Lee, "Disability".

104 Revel, "L'institution et le social", p. 88.

105 Foucault, *L'ordre du discours*. "Apparatus" describes any institutional, physical, or administrative mechanism where discourse is a tool of power over the social body.

106 Millet, "Introduction", p. 8.

107 Van Voss (ed.), *Petitions in Social History*, p. 1.

108 Baumgartner and Harf-Lancner (eds.), *Dire et penser le temps*.

chose administratively or practically profitable moments to submit their appeals, such as the beginning of the pontificate, an advantageous papal journey that would come near them, or acquaintances' trips to the Curia. Alternatively, their decision was motivated by their worsening situation, when an impairment had become unbearable and thus necessitated some kind of accommodation. At times, though, the decision was taken out of petitioners' hands, as in the case of petitions compelled by denunciations, compulsory examinations, and the political and epidemiological contexts in which the clerics found themselves. For the pontifical institution, the 'right moment' for petitioners to seek grace was their entrance into orders, accession to the priesthood, or promotion to the highest ecclesiastical offices. More generally, the temporal rhythm of the Church's administrative schedule – pastoral visits, ordination ceremonies, pontifical elections, and so on – shaped the temporality of sending the petitions. Such focus on finding a 'favourable' moment in which to lodge, and deal with, a petition demonstrates that the canonical rules could be bent, but only at the 'right' time and in the 'right' circumstances.[109] The petition process amounts to a conscious strategy to find, or create, this opportune moment, an endeavour instigated by petitioners and then pursued by the pontifical institution. Petitioners' disclosures of their impairment(s), alongside their existing relationship with the Church, were central to judging whether these were, indeed, the 'right' circumstances.

The Status of Disabled Petitioners

Grants of grace could authorize petitioners to contravene existing regulations. Yet it was not clear, even at the end of the medieval period, who precisely was responsible for distributing such divine privileges.[110] The eleventh-century Gregorian Reforms determined that derogation was a right exclusive to the Pope, in theory at least. Adherence to this ruling was shaky at best in the twelfth to the fourteenth centuries. In reality, bishops continued to grant graces to the clergy in their dioceses. Impaired clerics thus appealed to the Apostolic See in two cases: either when their bishop had explicitly deferred to the Pope on the matter, or when the clerics themselves wished to go 'over the head' of their bishop and leverage the Pope's supreme authority. Circumventing the local ecclesiastical hierarchy

109 Le Goff, "Le temps du travail", p. 74.
110 Stöhr, *Körpermakel – Arbeits(un)fähigkeit – Kirchenrecht.*

voluntarily was a strategy with which clerics could protect themselves from disadvantageous episcopal distribution. Issued by the Pope himself, any gracious exemptions they received were essentially immune to objection or modification. In such cases, supplicants took part in a dialogue with the Papal Chancery because they shared its codes. They were mostly rich, powerful, and often impressively connected (Fig. 0.3). Some were masters in the art of intercession, a process which enabled them to activate their networks: bypassing local hierarchies and petitioning the pontiff directly meant that they could position themselves favourably on the chessboard of papal power.

Figure 0.3 Status of supplicants identified in petitions and papal letters in the corpus

Papal letters

Secular orders	
Cardinal	5
Archbishop	32
Bishop	194
Archpriest	5
Priest	39
Archdeacon	18
Deacon	16
Subdeacon	3
Canon	57
Rector	24
Simple cleric	44
Elector	7
Master	0
Scholar	7
Treasurer	4
Other	16
Total	471

Regular orders	
Abbot	99
Abbess	11
Monk	67
Nun	23
Prior/esses	38
Professor	16
Canon	9
Prevost	5
Other	14
Total	282

Petitions

Secular orders	
Cardinal	3
Archbishop	3
Bishop	16
Archpriest	0
Priest	14
Archdeacon	3
Deacon	6
Subdeacon	4
Canon	10
Rector	3
Simple cleric	9
Elector	0
Master	3
Scholar	4
Treasurer	0
Other	9
Total	87

Regular orders	
Abbot	10
Abbess	4
Monk	26
Nun	4
Prior/esses	3
Professor	4
Canon	2
Prevost	1
Other	6
Total	59

Pontifical Interference in Clerical Affairs: Secular vs. Regular Orders

Members of the clergy represented around only 2–3% of the European population in the Middle Ages. In a general sense, then, the lack of practical sources about the lived experiences of clerics, not to mention disabled clerics, explains why they are not the subject of specific studies in the literature on medieval disability.[111] A minority in the population as a whole, the clergy nevertheless occupied a privileged place in the Christian hierarchy, and were directly subject to the pontifical institution that employed them. Hence, sources documenting the interactions between clerics and the Church apparatus offer particularly fruitful insights, heretofore neglected in scholarship. It bears repeating that the petition process began with the decision of an impaired cleric to apply for papal grace, whether his hand was forced or he took the matter in his own hands. As such, petitions bear traces of clerics 'authentic' experiences and desires, however modulated they may have become through the process. Altogether, pontifical letters witnessed of the Curia's interference in clerical affairs, first clearly within secular orders, then increasingly within secular orders (Fig. 0.4).

Figure 0.4 Petitioners identified in pontifical letters: secular vs. regular clerics (one point every fifty letters)

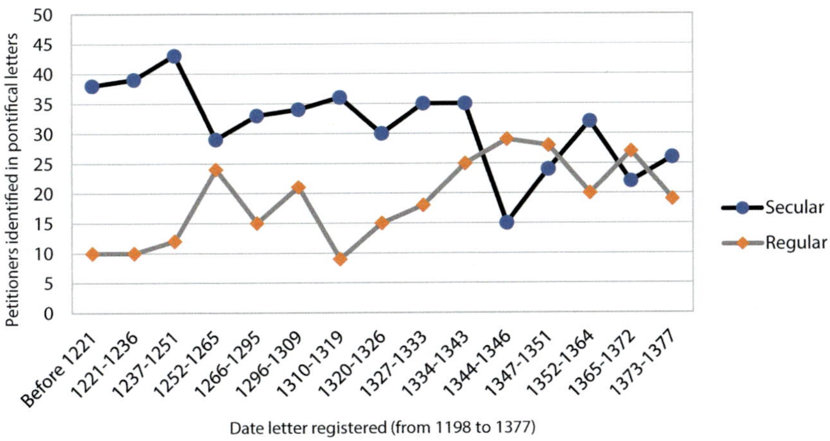

Most supplicants in the corpus of disabled clerics, spanning the twelfth to the fourteenth centuries, are from secular orders. Secular clerics account for 60% (=87) of individuals identified in supplications (from 1342 to 1370), and 63% in letters (=471; 182 in letters dating to the twelfth and thirteenth century, with a further 289 in fourteenth-century missives). In the twelfth century, clerics from the top of the ecclesiastical hierarchy – archbishops and bishops – submitted the majority of petitions, though their junior

111 For example, on the clerics see Metzler, *A Social History of Disability*, p. 55, and p. 144 on their great age.

colleagues began to take greater advantage of the petition process in the fourteenth century (Fig. 0.5).

Figure 0.5 Status of secular clerics identified in pontifical letters (one point every fifty letters)

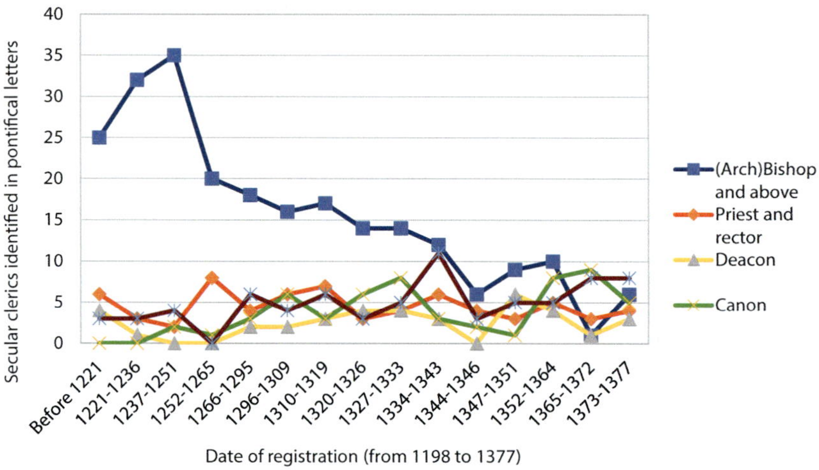

This disparity can be explained, at least in part, by the differences in expectations of individuals for different ranks in the ecclesiastic hierarchy. High-ranking clerics were in direct contact with the faithful and tasked with the most important sacramental duties. For this reason, they were subject to more stringent standards than junior clerics, and specifically the obligation of physical and mental perfection, as will be discussed in depth in Chapter 1. Furthermore, contemporary studies of disability evidence that people of high social status are more likely to suffer profound psychological distress and difficulty in coping after the onset of impairment than those of lower status, particularly when the impairment is visible.[112] Archbishops and bishops belonged to the medieval elite: they were typically part of the royal entourage, well-known and respected locally, and had high levels of administrative responsibility. Whether rural or urban, these elite clerics enjoyed an elevated social position, and profited from the regional and/or supra-local power structures to which they belonged.[113] Due to their prominence, we can trace their career progression, and the sources demonstrate that they benefited from access to wealth and kinship alliances, were fluent

112 Garland, *The Eye of the Beholder*, p. 6.

113 Le Jan, *L'historiographie des élites*, pp. 1–2.

ecclesiastical cultural norms, and secured a certain level of renown. These individuals wrote to the Pope directly because they were representatives of his authority, and as such his direct subordinates. They sought grace to remain in office, as their physical and/or mental impairments compromised their existing roles and privileges in the *ecclesia* (Church). The petition process, and thus the pontifical institution, provided secular clerics at the highest ranks with a framework to strengthen their position within the Church.

In the fourteenth century, there was a shift in the supplicant pool as the petition process opened up to less powerful members of the clergy (see again Fig. 0.5). This correlates with the weakening of regional hierarchies in the face of papal power. The popes seized control of several prerogatives hitherto reserved for local ecclesiastical prelates, archbishops, and bishops. At the same time, the number of priests, deacons, and rectors increased, whilst the proportion of archbishops and bishops decreased. New recruits typically hailed from the rural or urban aristocracy, or were even of noble blood. Even after entrance into the orders, they maintained their aristocratic lifestyle and relationships thanks to the receipt of substantial income.[114] Petitions lodged by these clerics could potentially count on support not just from their local ecclesiastical hierarchy, but from their powerful families, and even the faithful in their community more generally. Their clerical role and attendant duties, especially the *cura animarum* (care of souls), elevated these men above the rest of the faithful, concretizing their status as local elites.[115] Alongside such privileged figures, secular clerics of decidedly lesser status – such as students, singers, or treasurers – were also increasingly represented in supplications. More and more, clerics with limited authority in their local context(s) eschewed their direct superiors in favour of sending their petitions directly to the Pope, thereby becoming more visible to the Church apparatus. This preference is certainly a result of the introduction of letters *in forma pauperum* in the fourteenth century. This allowed cash-strapped secular and regular clergy without prebend to obtain the free dispatch of their petitions.[116] The petition process facilitated the papacy's intrusion into the management of clerical affairs typically handled by bishops, local authorities in a given diocese, whilst simultaneously permitting individuals to stray from the strictures of canon law: it reinforced the authority of the Church's head over its subordinate members. In this way, the popes did not just claim the full extent of their

114 Morsel, *L'aristocratie médiévale*, pp. 130–134.

115 Bougard, Feller and Le Jan (eds.), *Les élites*, p. 361.

116 Meyer, "Les '*littere in forma pauperum*'".

power but expanded it, to the detriment of both the secular elites and regional ecclesiastical hierarchies.

From the middle of the thirteenth century, the petition process evidently further opened to another clergy members, the regular orders. Regular clerics account for 40% (=59) of individuals identified in petitions, and 37% (=282) of supplicants mentioned in papal letters (Figs. 1.3 and 1.4). Their representation in papal letters tripled from the twelfth to the fourteenth century (71 clerics in the twelfth and thirteenth centuries; 211 in the fourteenth century) (Fig. 0.4). This tracks with the popes' increasing interference in monastic affairs. During the eleventh century, the papacy relieved certain religious orders of their dependence on bishops through the 'privilege of exemption'. Thus, the popes removed them from the hierarchical relationship they previously had with local ecclesiastical representatives. Beyond such strategic reorganization, the papacy created other orders directly and explicitly under its power.[117] The Apostolic See became the spiritual and institutional authority for the approval, correction, and interpretation of regular religious life.[118]

The majority of disabled regular clerics who contacted the Papal Chancery during the thirteenth century occupied elevated positions in the hierarchy of their order or monastery: about 39% (=110) of those identified in the corpus were abbots and abbesses, and a further 13.5% (=38) were priors and prioresses (Fig. 0.6).

Initially, regulars with less power, who were subject to local authorities, feature in smaller numbers: some 32% (=90) were monks or nuns, and 15.5% (=44) of petitions were sent by professors and others. The proportion of petitions submitted by regulars of lower rank sharply increased over the decades. After 1330, they accounted for more than 50% of regular petitioners (Fig. 0.6). Regular clerics were obliged to direct requests for any exemptions relating to the rule or customs of their institution to their abbot, or the superior of their order, or in certain cases, the bishop.[119] However, for very specific questions, such as those concerning 'defects' of body, mind, and spirit, regulars had to appeal to the Pope, which could actually be to their advantage. This route was undoubtedly desirable for regular clerics in the fourteenth century, as they had become part of the medieval elite. From

117 For example, Innocent III and his successor Honorius III allowed the foundation of mendicant orders in exchange for their help in preaching the Crusades and in preaching against heretics. See Garcia-Serrano, "Friars and Royal Authority".

118 Bagliani, *Il trono di Pietro*, p. 119.

119 See Falkenstein, "Monachisme et pouvoir hiérarchique", p. 389; Besson, "Dispensation".

the twelfth century onwards, the monastic milieu became increasingly aristocratized. Regulars with the financial and logistical resources to petition the Curia were likely part of the rural and urban elite, or nobility.

Figure 0.6 Status of regular clerics identified in pontifical letters (one point every fifty letters)

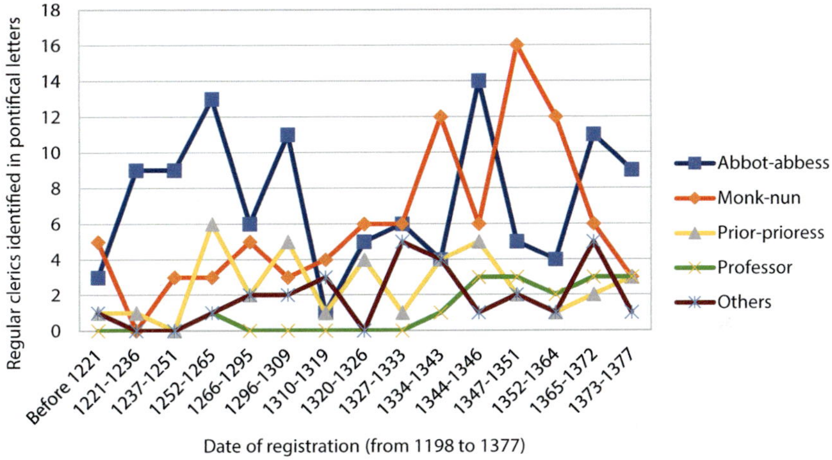

There was no 'one-size-fits-all' kind of relationship between the regular orders and the papacy; the nature of the relationship varied.[120] This is evident in the papal responses to petitions from religious who follow different types of community life. Three monastic types predominate in the petitions, with supplications mainly from: those following the rule of St. Benedict (Cassinians and Clunisians) who were thoroughly subjugated to pontifical power; those following the rule of St. Francis of Assisi (Franciscans and Poor Clares) who had a close, but less subservient, relationship with the Apostolic See, which included the papal appointment of their minister;[121] and those following the Rule of St. Augustine (Hospitallers and Dominicans), who had more independence from papal oversight. Though the Hospitallers were directly subject to the Apostolic See, they were near autonomous, which likely explains their minimal presence in the archive.[122] Similarly, the Dominicans had always maintained a certain distance from the Curia and guarded their sovereignty.[123] The uptick in petitions from monastics clearly indicates the

120 Melville, *The World of Medieval Monasticism*, p. 298.
121 Robson, *The Franciscans in the Middle Ages*, pp. 69–71.
122 Claverie, "Les relations du Siège apostolique".
123 Wirtz, Paulus and Charlier, "La gouvernance des Dominicains".

increased authority exercised by the Pope over monastic communities – especially over traditional, as opposed to mendicant, orders – even though some orders managed to retain their independence. The monastic lifestyle was diverse, with monks and friars living according to the varied precepts of their particular order. As such, the Papal Chancery had to master various coenobitic legislations and monastic customs to craft a response suitable for the petitioner's specific circumstances when replying to a supplication. Skilful administration, incorporating the gathering of all relevant information, was thus key to the Chancery's success in the mission to centralize papal authority. This formed a bureaucratic complement to another essential manoeuvre: progressively transferring power to grant graces from bishops and abbots to the Pope, leveraging the pontiff's exclusive right to deliver grace. As disabled regular clerics bypassed their local power structures to address Rome or Avignon directly, they reinforced pontifical authority.

The policy of channelling all grievances to a single figure, the Pope, strengthened the logic of centralization already at play, with Rome and then, for a time, Avignon as the seat of all Christian authority. This led to a spatial convergence of correspondence, with letters pouring into Rome and Avignon from supplicants across the whole of Christendom, an area that was rapidly developing and reached its apogee, in both size and population, in this period.[124] The efficacy of the centralizing logic that accompanies the Church's mission to subjugate the Christian world to the papal monarchy (at least in theory) is evidenced in the multitude of places from which petitioners hail, an expansive geography that ultimately converges in Rome and Avignon.[125]

The establishment of the papal monarchy in the eleventh century led to the concentration of the popes' authority in and around Rome. The corpus demonstrates, however, that pontifical power spread far beyond a single city. In the thirteenth and fourteenth centuries, for example, we see an over-representation of supplicants who originate from the richest, largest, and therefore most powerful ecclesiastical provinces or dioceses across Europe – those located near urban centres, where power was concentrated. From 1099 to 1309, most supplicants came from France (c. 40%), Italy (c. 20%), or the Holy Roman Empire (c. 15%), with other geographical areas accounting for the remainder (25%). This geographical distribution can be explained by the strategic rationale for lodging a petition, since petitioners often sought to improve their endowment or acquire a more desirable benefice under

124 *Christianitas* consists of the obedience in Rome and the Latin rite. See Bartlett, *The Making of Europe*, p. 243.

125 Morris, *The Papal Monarchy*, p. 178.

the pretext of obtaining an indulgence.[126] Every Christian subject following Roman obedience had the right to petition the Pope. This confirmed the authority of the Church across all Christian territories, even if it remained largely theoretical.

The magnetic pull of the pontiff was reinforced during the fourteenth century as the Curia moved into French territory. With the relocation of the ecclesiastical institution from Rome to Avignon from 1309 to 1378, Christianity's centre of gravity shifted, geographically and figuratively. The move to Avignon engendered a shift in the locations from which petitioners wrote, revealing the influence of the popes' location on the petition process, but also the French monarchy's immense influence over the papacy.[127] About half of all supplicants during this period came from France (c. 55%), with most concentrated along the Paris–Avignon axis, showing that local petitioners took the opportunity to make their appeals because the Pope was close by. Christians from Italy (c. 15%), the Holy Roman Empire (c. 11%) and the British Isles (c. 7%) sent fewer letters than in the preceding era, with the countries of the Iberian Peninsula (around 6%) and Central and Northern Europe significantly under-represented (less than 6%). In addition to the obvious issue of the geographical remoteness of these regions, fierce papal interventionism in 'national' churches was highly unpopular, explaining the resistance of some clerics to further submit to papal authority by engaging with the petition process.[128] Nevertheless, a concerted policy of interference in the affairs of secular and regular clerics meant that the Church wielded greater influence than ever before in the lives of the richest and most powerful medieval elites. As intercessors, they became crucial to the petition process, since they could be entrusted with relaying petitions to the Papal Chancery.

The Role of Intercessors and Intermediaries

In theory, supplicants engaged in dialogue with the popes directly. It entailed meeting them face-to-face for a formal audience when the petition was

126 The thesis of the invocation of impairment as a pretext in no way undermines, in my opinion, the truthfulness of the supplicant's discourse. It is developed in particular by Baix, "De la valeur historique", p. 61.

127 According to Jacques Le Goff, Gregory X and the popes who followed realised that it was in their interest to have a capital that was less outlying than Rome following the Council of Lyon II of 1274. See Le Goff, "1274, année charnière".

128 Hayez, "Les demandes de bénéfices présentées à Urbain V"; Hayez, "Un aperçu de la politique bénéficiale de Grégoire XI".

adjudicated. Indeed, in the twelfth and thirteenth centuries, most papal letters mentioned the possible transfer of the petitioners to the Curia. The increasing centralization of ecclesiastical power, and concomitant increase in the number of letters received by the Papal Chancery, enacted a shift in how favours were requested and formulated stylistically. Over the course of the fourteenth century, details of petitioners' potential visits to the Curia appear less and less frequently: papal letters placed more emphasis on the active role of the supplicant in drafting the initial petition, and less on the request being delivered orally by the petitioner in person.

In about 60% of cases, supplicants sent a request directly to the Papal Chancery, illustrating their ability to obtain grace without the help of contacts in the ecclesiastical hierarchy and/or in powerful secular circles acting as intercessors. Such cases, in which petitioners did not rely on third parties, suggests that some supplicants were excluded from solidarity networks, or were acting in opposition to their superiors' will. Nevertheless, clerics were not legally obliged to use intercessors when filing a petition. And yet, intercessors supported petitioners in about 40% of cases. Intercession does not constitute a single social practice, but rather equates to a multitude of practices, which vary according to each intercessor, in terms of their capacities and also their interests.[129] Instances of intercession in the petition process testifies to the hierarchy's control and/or support of subordinates, as well as revealing a particular petitioner's inclusion or exclusion from solidarity networks. In this way, it reveals a chain of interdependent relationships: those between supplicants and the influential personalities to whom they appealed for help; and those between powerful intercessors and the Pope, with whom they must maintain privileged links in order for the intercession to be effective.

The use of an intercessor had one clear benefit: it allowed less fortunate clerics to obtain grace without any financial outlay, since the petition was paid for by the intercessor. Influential intercessors could submit a single petition or combine a batch into a *rotulus* (roll), which would be sent to the Chancery all in one go.[130] About 10–15% of all requests were submitted in *rotuli*, which typically gathered requests that dealt with related issues, those that were geographically proximate, or gathered by one person or one institution.[131] Furthermore, major clerics in the secular clergy were typically well-connected, and benefited from elevated social status. For this reason,

129 Moeglin, *L'intercession du Moyen Âge à l'époque modern*, notably p. 67.
130 Hayez, "Les *rotuli* présentés au pape Urbain V", p. 328.
131 Hayez, Mathieu, and Yvan, "De la supplique à la lettre", p. 176.

their networks tended to be both broad and deep, and they thus had access to powerful intercessors and could themselves act as effective intercessors. The options for monastic petitioners, by contrast, were much more limited, as they operated in a fairly closed circuit. Indeed, intercessors acting on behalf of regular clerics were mainly authority figures in monastic life, and they in turn requested letters almost exclusively from other regular clerics. Both in the secular and regular orders, hierarchical superiors interceded on behalf of their subordinates because they belonged to the same clerical order, whether local or provincial. Then, the intercession in the supplication illustrates the networking and often local strategies put in place in order to receive the requested grace.

The petitioners had to know their intercessor(s) personally, whilst the latter needed to possess sufficient notability to be able to positively sway or accelerate the pontifical decision.[132] When the supplicants were not themselves in a position of power, it was often their direct superior who took care to intercede for them before the Apostolic See. An abbot might intercede for a monk, for instance, or a bishop for a priest. If, on the other hand, petitioners were high up in the hierarchy, their subordinates could act as intercessors. A suffragan bishop might intercede for an archbishop, or a canon for his bishop, for example. In such cases, appealing to an intercessory could give a subordinate the chance to denounce their superior. Individuals occupying a position of secular authority were also likely to appear as intercessors for secular, and regular. Asking someone to act in an intercessory capacity was arguably an act of flattery, as it entailed a recognition of the would-be intercessor's influence and power. By paying close attention to the minutiae of intercession, it is possible to discern networks and/or relationships of power and influence coalesce around individual petitioners on a case-by-case basis.

Scrutinizing the address to which papal letters were dispatched enables us to shed light on the role of intermediaries, a process parallel to intercession. In approximately 70% of thirteenth-century cases, the Chancery sent their response to a different address than the one initially provided by the supplicant, a figure that declines to around 40% of cases in the fourteenth century (Fig. 0.2: § 3B).[133] This demonstrates the extent to which the pontifical institution relied on trusted middle-men as intermediaries in the petition process. Called the *Reskripttechnik* by German scholars,

132 Gorochov, "Le recours aux intercesseurs", p. 158.

133 On the *si est ita* clause, which assumes that the act is worthless if the supplicant has lied, see Chapter 3.

this system of government mandated that petitioners passed tests to validate the claims made in their letters before grace was actually granted.[134] Intermediate recipients, typically powerful figures of significant local influence, thus played a central role in granting graces. They were endowed with the authority and responsibility to subject petitioners to additional examinations, to ensure they had been fully honest in their appeal – as shown in the case studies presented in Chapter 3. During the thirteenth century, intermediary recipients often served as relays of papal authority, helping the centralized Church apparatus to manage local affairs.[135] In this way, intermediaries strengthened the ecclesiastical hierarchy, which was organized in parallel with the vassalage of the lay lords. The intervention of the ecclesiastical hierarchy was not always necessary, however, for granting graces, nor was there any requirement for them even to be notified of such grants. Whilst papal letters of grace were sent directly to petitioners in only 30% of cases in the thirteenth century, things changed dramatically in the fourteenth century, with 60% of petitioners now receiving letters direct. This increase highlights the success of the fourteenth-century mission to centralize pontifical authority, since such letters offered the Pope the ability to manage local clergy directly, bypassing the usual ecclesiastical supervisory hierarchy.

Conclusion

The petition process established a 'dialogue' between the Pope and individual clerics, one in which all parties acted in line with a shared code. With grants of papal grace, disabled supplicants gained room to manoeuvre within the strictures of canonical regulation, as long as they submitted themselves to the protocols established by the Papal Chancery.[136] Formalization of requests led to the creation of categories according to which supplicants were classified, based on the rationale underlying their petition. The recognition of disability as an organizational category allowed the Chancery to standardize and streamline the way in which they handled the increasing volume of requests that were being submitted by clerics from all over Christendom. Whilst increasing efficiency, the formal standardization of petitions served to flatten the messiness of human experiences into

134 Zutshi, "Petitioners, Popes, Proctors", p. 266, quoting Pitz, *Papstreskript und Kaiserreskript*.

135 Jamme, "Écrire pour le pape", p. 4.

136 Fassin, "La supplique", p. 961.

bureaucratic and administrative order. The popes' growing interference in clerical affairs explains, above all, the growing heterogeneity of supplicants, alongside the overall increase in correspondence, from the twelfth to the fourteenth century. The pontificate wrested power from all levels of the Church, with intermediary ecclesiastical authorities forced to cede control in the face of the centralizing zeal of Rome and Avignon. This book focuses on disabled clerics' life experiences, interrogating medieval ecclesiastical norms to reveal how disabled clerics could be, and indeed were, included within the Church. It is organised in five chapters, highlighting the legal and cultural aspects of impairment in petitions and papal letters, by following the consequences of disability during a clerical career.

Chapter 1 investigates the legal origins of the prohibition against impaired clerics. Petitions and letters helped to define 'invalidity' as a legal category, since they contributed directly to medieval canon law's statues regarding so-called 'defects' of body and mind. This institutional construction of disability allowed the Apostolic See to set a standard for bodies and minds, in order to distinguish the normatively able-bodied from those deemed 'abnormal', impaired. The Papal Chancery thus defined a physical standard in which a body diverging from the norm was considered 'defective', and thereby unfit for clerical office, according to two criteria: its capacity and its image. They were only two mitigating factors for disabled clerics: their innocence and their 'ignorance', that is, their lack of 'culpability' in relation to the existence of their impairment. During the petition process, supplicants defined their impairments through dialogue with the Papal Chancery, as shown in Chapter 2. They drew on medical and religious culture, evident in the specific words deployed in letters, to present the causes of their impairments and to relate their ongoing experiences. Letters from the Chancery, in response, make use of similar terminology and frameworks, highlighting that petitioners' conceptualizations of disability was shared by the Curia's staff and vice-versa. The legal, cultural, and linguistic frameworks provided by Chapters 1 and 2 allow us to develop argumentative strands in the later chapters.

Chapter 3 interrogates the tests used by the Church to determine disability. These were required at several stages of the clerical profession: canon law stipulates that all candidates applying for admission to the secular and regular orders, and all clerics wishing to receive a promotion, must be examined before their appointment. Supposedly a 'quality-control' measure to guarantee the uniformity of the clerical condition at all levels, this evaluation was required from a cleric's first tonsure to his entrance into the priesthood, up until his election as bishop or abbot, when the Pope himself, in theory at least, conducted the examination. Chapter 4 moves on to examine the consequences of the 'failure' of such disability tests and of clerics' disclosures of impairment in petitions. In such cases, gracious papal letters sometimes allowed for the relaxation of ecclesiastical regulations to accommodate the disabled cleric's conditions, if he himself desired to remain in the clergy and was deemed capable enough. The process of supplication was used to improve clerics' lives by adapting existing statutes to their personal situations. Chapter 5 probes the fate of the disabled men who were less fortunate, those who had to leave the clergy entirely, either of their own volition or due to the severity of their disability. At times, poor health or impairment forced clerics to resign from their positions as they became unable to perform their rights and duties. Often, they were forced to find care and support outside of their clerical community. Case studies demonstrate, however, that petitions and pontifical letters sometimes allowed for the adaptation, even contravention, of existing rules so that the disabled former clerics could see out the remainder of their lives with dignity.

Documents in the corpus bear witness to the blurry bounds between clerical impairment as bio-medical fact and disability as a category constructed by Church authorities. Obliged to follow the directives of the Chancery when formulating their petitions, supplicants adhered to the representation of physical and/or mental impairment mandated by the papacy. This served to suppress any traces of disagreement between the papally authorized conceptualization of disability and petitioners' own. At the same time, the process of supplication could erase the negative institutional effects of disability by actively including the disabled cleric within the ecclesial and Christian body. With this process, the Apostolic See thus created a metaphorical space conducive to negotiation, where disabled clerics could disclose their physical and/or mental difference in order to advocate for themselves, requesting – and often benefiting from – accommodations from the institutional Church.

Bibliography

Primary Sources

AD CLARAS AQUAS (ed.), *Opera omnia*, PP. Collegii a S. Bonaventura, 1882.

FRIEDBERG (ed.), *Corpus iuris canonici*, Akademische Druck- u. Verlagsanstalt, 1959.

Robert DIGARD, Antoine FAWTIER, Maurice FAUCON and Antoine THOMAS (eds.), *Les registres de Boniface VIII: recueil des bulles de ce Pape publiées ou analysées d'après les manuscrits originaux des Archives du Vatican*, Bibliothèque des Écoles françaises d'Athènes et de Rome, 1884.

Antonio GARCÌA Y GARCÌA (ed.), *Constitutiones Concilii quarti Lateranensis una cum Commentariis glossatorum*, Biblioteca apostolica vaticana, 1981.

Jacques Paul MIGNE (ed.), *Patrologiae Cursus Completus, Series Latina*, Migne, 1844–1855.

Oxford *Cantigas de Santa Maria* Database (http://csm.mml.ox.ac.uk/index.php?p=poemdata_view&rec=206).

Giulio SILANO (ed.), *The Sentences*, Pontifical Institute of Mediaeval Studies, 2007–2010.

José RIUS SERRA (ed.), *Summa iuris*, Barcelone, López, 1945.

THOMAS AQUINAS, *Summa theologiae*, and *Summe contra gentiles*, ed. By The Aquinas Institute and transl. by Fr. Laurence SHAPCOTE, URL consulted on 31 July 2021: https://aquinas.cc/.

Secondary Sources

Agostino P. BAGLIANI, *Il trono di Pietro: l'universalità del papato da Alessandro III a Bonifacio VIII*, Carocci, 1996.

François BAIX, "De la valeur historique des actes pontificaux de collation des bénéfices", *in Hommage à Ursmer Berlière*, H. Lamertin, 1931, pp. 57–66.

Patricia BAKER, Han NIJDAM and Karine van't LAND (eds.), *Medicine and Space: Body, Surroundings and Borders in Antiquity and the Middle Ages*, Brill, 2012.

Bernard BARBICHE, *Les actes pontificaux originaux des archives nationales de Paris 1, 1198–1261*, Biblioteca Apostolica Vaticana, 1975.

Bernard BARBICHE, "Le personnel de la chancellerie pontificale aux XIIIe et XIVe siècles", *in* Françoise AUTRAND (ed.), *Prosopographie et genèse de l'État moderne*, ENSJF, 1986, pp. 117–130.

Colin BARNES (eds.), *Implementing the Social Model of Disability: Theory and Research*, Disability Press, 2004.

Geoffrey BARRACLOUGH, *Public Notaries and the Papal Curia; A Calendar and a Study of a Formularium Notariorum Curie from the Early Years of the Fourteenth Century*, Macmillan and Co., 1934.

Geoffrey BARRACLOUGH, "Formulare für Suppliken aus der ersten Hälfte des 13. Jahrhunderts", *Archiv für katholisches Kirchenrecht*, 115 (1935), pp. 435–456.

Robert BARTLETT, *The Making of Europe: Conquest, Colonization and Cultural Change 950–1350*, Princeton University Press, 2015.

Emmanuèle BAUMGARTNER and Laurence HARF-LANCNER (eds.), *Dire et penser le temps au Moyen Âge: frontières de l'histoire et du roman*, Presses Sorbonne Nouvelle, 2005.

Pierre–Marie BERTHE, *Les procureurs français à la cour pontificale d'Avignon (1309–1376)*, École des chartes, 2014.

Jules BESSON, "Dispensation", *The Catholic Encyclopedia*. Vol. 5, Robert Appleton Company, 1909 (URL consulted on 31 July 2021: http://www.newadvent.org/cathen/05041a.htm).

Friedrich BOCK, *Einführung in das Registerwesen des Avignonesischen Papsttums; Textt. u. Tafelbeil.*, Regenberg, 1941.

François BOUGARD, Laurent FELLER and Régine LE JAN (eds.), *Les élites au haut Moyen Âge, crises et renouvellements*, Brepols, 2006.

Leonard E. BOYLE, *A Survey of the Vatican Archives and of Its Medieval Holdings*, Revised ed., Pontifical Institute of Mediaeval studies, 2001.

Scott Campbell BROWN, "Methodological Paradigms that Shapes Disability Research", *in* Gary L. ALBRECHT, Katherine D. SEELMAN and Michael BURY (eds.), *Handbook of Disability Studies*, Sage, 2001, pp. 145–170.

James A. BRUNDAGE, *The Medieval Origins of the Legal Profession: Canonists, Civilians, and Courts*, University of Chicago Press, 2008.

Madeline BURGHARDT, "The Human Bottom of Non-human Things: on Critical Theory and its Contributions to Critical Disability Studies", *Critical Disability Discourses*, 3-0 (2011), pp. 1–16.

Caroline BYNUM, *Christian Materiality an Essay on Religion in Late Medieval Europe*, Zone Books, 2011.

Marcel CALVEZ, "Le handicap comme situation de seuil: éléments pour une sociologie de la liminalité", *Sciences sociales et santé*, 12.1 (1994), pp. 61–88.

Fiona K. CAMPBELL, *Contours of Ableism: The Production of Disability and Abledness*, Palgrave Macmillan, 2009.

Simona CERUTTI, "Normes et pratiques, ou de la légitimité de leur opposition", *in* Bernard LEPETIT (ed.), *Les Formes de l'expérience: une autre histoire sociale*, Albin Michel, 1995, pp. 161–186.

Simona CERUTTI and Massimo VALLERANI, "Suppliques. Lois et cas dans la normativité de l'époque moderne. Introduction", *L'Atelier du Centre de recherches historiques. Revue électronique du CRH*, 13 (2015) online: https://doi.org/10.4000/acrh.6545.

Christopher R. CHENEY, *Notaries Public in England in the 13th and 14th Centuries*, Clarendon Press, 1972.

Julie CLAUSTRE, "La grâce et la norme. Les cas des lettres de répit (royaume de France, XIVe et XVe siècles)", *in* Véronique BEAULANDE, Julie CLAUSTRE and Elsa MARMURSZTEJN (eds.), *La fabrique de la norme: lieux et modes de production des normes au Moyen Âge et à l'époque moderne*, Presses universitaires de Rennes, 2012, pp. 161–176.

Pierre-Vincent CLAVERIE, "Les relations du Siège apostolique avec les ordres militaires sous le pontificat d'Honorius III (1216–1227)", *in* Damien CARRAZ, Philippe JOSSERAND and Luís Filipe OLIVEIRA (eds.), *Élites et ordres militaires au Moyen Âge*, Casa de Velázquez, 2017, pp. 277–292.

Franck COLLARD and Evelyne SAMAMA (eds.), *Handicaps et sociétés dans l'histoire: L'estropié, l'aveugle et le paralytique de l'Antiquité aux temps modernes*, L'Harmattan, 2010.

Leonard A. COOMBS, Elizabeth YAKEL, Claudia CARLEN and Katherine J. GILL, *Vatican Archives: An Inventory and Guide to Historical Documents of the Holy See*, Oxford University Press, 1998.

Léo DELAUNE, "Le handicap dans les *exempla* médiévaux", Master thesis, University of Strasbourg, 2019.

Mikee C. DELONY, "Alisoun's Aging, Hearing-Impaired Female Body. Gazing at the Wife of Bath in Chaucer's Canterbury Tales", *in* Wendy J. TURNER and Tory V. PEARMAN (eds.), *The Treatment of Disabled Persons in Medieval Europe: Examining Disability in the Historical, Legal, Literary, Medical, and Religious Discourses of the Middle Ages*, Edwin Mellen Press, 2010, pp. 313–346.

Antoine DONDAINE, "Barthélemy de Trente O.P," *Archivum Fratrum Praedicatorum*, 45 (1975), pp. 79–105.

Ninon DUBOURG, "European Medieval Disability History: An Overview", in Marcia RIOUX and Renu ADDLAKHA (eds.), *Handbook of Critical Disability Studies*, Springer, 2022, https://doi.org/10.1007/978-981-16-1278-7_2-1.

Pierre-Toussaint DURAND DE MAILLANE, *Dictionnaire de droit canonique et de pratique bénéficiale*, Saillant et Nyon, 1770.

Georg ERLER, *Der Liber cancellariae apostolicae vom Jahre 1380; und, Der Stilus palatii abbreviatus*, Scientia Verlag, 1971.

Joshua EYLER (ed.), *Disability in the Middle Ages: Reconsiderations and Reverberations*, Ashgate, 2010.

Ludwig FALKENSTEIN, "Monachisme et pouvoir hiérarchique à travers les textes pontificaux (x^e, xiie siècle)", *in* Jean-Loup LEMAÎTRE and Pierre GONNEAU (eds.), *Moines et monastères dans les sociétés de rite grec et latin*, Genève, Droz, 1996, pp. 389–418.

Didier FASSIN, "La supplique. Stratégies rhétoriques et constructions identitaires dans les demandes d'aide d'urgence", *Annales. Histoire, Sciences Sociales*, 55.5 (2000), pp. 955–981.

Michel FOUCAULT, *L'ordre du discours*, Gallimard, 1971.

Michel FOUCAULT, *Surveiller et punir: naissance de la prison*, Gallimard, 1975.

Bianca FROHNE and Klaus P. HORN, "On the Fluidity of "Disability" in Medieval and Early Modern Societies", *in* Sebastian BARSCH, Anne KLEIN and Pieter

VERSTRAETE (eds.), *The Imperfect Historian: Disability Histories in Europe*, Peter Lang, 2013, pp. 17–40.

Louis Prosper GACHARD, "Les archives du Vatican", *in Compte rendu de la Commission royale d'histoire de l'Académie royale de Belgique, ou recueil de ses bulletins*, F. Hayez, 1873, fourth series, pp. 211–386.

Francisco GARCIA-SERRANO, "Friars and Royal Authority in the Thirteenth-century Castillian Frontier", *in* Yuen-Gen LIANG and Jarbel RODRIGUEZ (eds.), *Authority and Spectacle in Medieval and Early Modern Europe*, Routledge, 2017, pp. 104–117.

Robert GARLAND, *The Eye of the Beholder: Deformity and Disability in the Graeco-Roman World*, Ithaca, Cornell University Press, 1995.

Pierre GASNAULT, "Une supplique originale de l'abbaye de Cluny approuvée par Martin V", *Revue Mabillon*, 51 (1961), pp. 325–328.

Jennifer GIANFALLA, "Discours of Disability in Pierce Plowman", *in* Joshua EYLER (ed.), *Disability in the Middle Ages: Reconsiderations and Reverberations*, Ashgate, 2010, pp. 119–134.

Arthur GIRY, *Manuel de diplomatique*, Hachette, 1894.

Barney G. GLASER and Anselm L. STRAUSS, *The Discovery of Grounded Theory: Strategies for Qualitative Research*, Aldine Pub. Co., 1967.

Brendan J. GLEESON, *Geographies of Disability*, Routledge, 1999.

Richard H. GODDEN, "Prosthetic Ecologies: Vulnerable Bodies and the Dismodern Subject in Sir Gawain and the Green Knight", *Textual Practice*, 30.7 (2016), pp. 1273–1290.

Dan GOODLEY, *Disability Studies: an Interdisciplinary Introduction*, Sage Publications, 2011.

Nathalie GOROCHOV, "Le recours aux intercesseurs, l'exemple des universitaires parisien en quête de bénéfices ecclésiastiques (vers 1340–vers 1420) », *in* Hélène MILLET (ed.), *Suppliques et requêtes: le gouvernement par la grâce en Occident, XIIe–XVe siècle*, École française de Rome, 2003, pp. 151–164.

Benoît GRÉVIN (ed.), *Le "dictamen" dans tous ses états: perspectives de recherche sur la théorie et la pratique de l'"ars dictaminis" (XIe–XVe siècles)*, Brepols, 2015.

Benoît GRÉVIN, *Rhétorique du pouvoir médiéval: les lettres de Pierre de la Vigne et la formation du langage politique européen (XIIIe–XVe siècles)*, École française de Rome, 2013.

Benoît GRÉVIN, "Les mystères rhétoriques de l'État médiéval", *Annales. Histoire, Sciences Sociales*, 63.2 (2008), pp. 271–300.

Jussi HANSKA and Kirsi SALONEN, *Entering a Clerical Career at the Roman Curia, 1458–1471*, Ashgate, 2013.

Wilfried HARTMANN and Kenneth PENNINGTON, *The History of Medieval Canon Law in the Classical Period, 1140–1234 from Gratian to the Decretals of Pope Gregory IX*, Catholic University of America Press, 2008.

Anne-Marie HAYEZ, "Les *rotuli* présentés au pape Urbain V durant la première année de son pontificat (6 nov. 1362, 5 nov. 1363)", *Mélanges de l'École française de Rome*, 96.1 (1984), pp. 327–394.

Anne-Marie HAYEZ, Janine MATHIEU and Marie-France YVAN, "De la supplique à la lettre: le parcours des grâces en cour de Rome sous Urbain V (1362–1366)", *in Aux origines de l'État moderne. Le fonctionnement administratif de la papauté d'Avignon*, École française de Rome, 1991, pp. 171–205.

Anne-Marie HAYEZ, "Un aperçu de la politique bénéficiale de Grégoire XI: première moitié du pontificat (1371–1375)", *in FS Peter Herde* (*Reich*), 2 (1998), pp. 685–698.

Anne-Marie HAYEZ, "Les demandes de bénéfices présentées à Urbain V, une approche géographico-politique", *in* Hélène MILLET (ed.), *Suppliques et requêtes: le gouvernement par la grâce en Occident, XIIe–XVe siècle*, École française de Rome, 2003, pp. 121–150.

Rudolf von HECKEL, "Das Aufkommen der ständigen Prokuratoren an der päpstlichen Kurie im 13. Jahrhundert", *Miscellanea Francesco Ehrle*, 2 (1924), pp. 290–321.

Paul HEROLD (eds.), *Vom Nutzen des Schreibens*, Österreichische Akademie der Wissenschaften, 2002, pp. 225–236.

Jacqueline HOAREAU-DODINAU, *Le pardon*, Presses Universitaires de Limoges, 1999.

Jonathan HSY, *The Open Access Companion to the Canterbury Tales*, online publication, 2017 (URL consulted on 31 July 2021: https://opencanterburytales.dsl.lsu.edu/).

Jonathan HSY, Tory V. PEARMAN, and Joshua EYLER (eds.), *A Cultural History of Disability in the Middle Ages*, Bloomsbury, 2020.

Bill HUGHES and Kevin PATERSON, "The Social Model of Disability and the Disappearing Body: Towards a Sociology of Impairment", *Disability and Society*, 12.3 (1997), pp. 25–34.

Nichola HUTCHINSON, "Disabling Beliefs? Impaired Embodiment in the Religious Tradition of the West", *Body & Society*, 12.4 (2006), pp. 1–23.

Marie-Céline ISAÏA and Thomas GRANIER (eds.), *Normes et hagiographie dans l'Occident (VIe–XVIe siècle)*, Brepols, 2014.

Armand JAMME, "Écrire pour le pape du XIe au XIVe siècle. Formes et problèmes", *Mélanges de l'École française de Rome – Moyen Âge*, 128.1 (2016) online: https://doi.org/10.4000/mefrm.3121.

Jean-René KIEDI KIONGA, *Dispenses en droit canonique*, Cerf, 2020.

Christian KRÖTZL, Katariina MUSTAKALLIO, and Jenni KUULIALA (eds.), *Infirmity in Antiquity and the Middle Ages: Social and Cultural Approaches to Health, Weakness and Care*, Ashgate, 2015.

Christian KRÖTZL, Katariina MUSTAKALLIO and Jenni KUULIALA, "Introduction: *Infirmitas* in Antiquity and the Middle Ages", in KRÖTZL, MUSTAKALLIO and

Kuuliala (eds.), *Infirmity in Antiquity and the Middle Ages: Social and Cultural Approaches to Health, Weakness and Care*, Ashgate, 2015, pp. 1–11.

Catherine J. Kudlick, "Disability History, Power, and Rethinking the Idea of "The Other"", *PMLA*, 120.2 (2005), pp. 557–561.

Stefanie Künzel and Erin Connelly (eds.), *New Approaches to Disease, Disability, and Medicine in Medieval Europe*, Archaeopress, 2018.

Stanislaw Kuras and Irena Sulkowska-Kuras, "Suppliques, brouillons, lettres et registres de la Chancellerie apostolique relatifs à la Pologne à l'époque d'Avignon (1305–1378)", *Mélanges de l'École française de Rome. Moyen-Âge – Temps modernes*, 96.2 (1984), pp. 719–725.

Jenni Kuuliala, *Childhood Disability and Social Integration in the Middle Ages: Constructions of Impairments in Thirteenth and Fourteenth-Century Canonization Processes*, Brepols, 2016.

Jenni Kuuliala, Rose-Marie Peake, and Päivi Räisänen-Schröder (eds.), *Lived Religion and Everyday Life in Early Modern Hagiographic Material*, Palgrave McMillan, 2019.

Christina Lee, "Disability", *in* Jacqueline Stodnick and Renée R. Trilling (eds.), *A Handbook of Anglo-Saxon Studies*, John Wiley & Sons, 2012, pp. 27–29.

Jacques Le Goff, "1274, année charnière: mutations et continuités", *in Actes du colloque international du Centre national de la recherche scientifique 1974*, Édition du CNRS, 1977, pp. 481–489.

Jacques Le Goff, *L'Europe est-elle née au Moyen Âge?*, Seuil, 2013.

Jacques Le Goff, "Le temps du travail dans la "crise" du xive siècle: du temps médiéval au temps moderne", *in Pour un autre Moyen Âge: temps, travail et culture en Occident: 18 essais*, Gallimard, 2013, pp. 66–79.

Régine Le Jan, *L'historiographie des élites dans le haut Moyen Âge*, Universités de Marnes-la-Vallée et de Paris I, 2005 (URL consulted on 31 July 2021: https://lamop.univ-paris1.fr/fileadmin/lamop/publications/Haut-MoyenAge_Elites/HMA_elites_introduction_LeJan_2003.pdf>).

Didier Lett, "Des compilateurs au travail. Groupe et identité des *statutari* dans les Marches centro-méridionales du xve siècle", *in* Lett (ed.), *La confection des statuts dans les sociétés méditerranéennes de l'Occident (xiie–xve siècle)*, Publications de la Sorbonne-CERM, 2017, pp. 197–224.

Corinne Leveleux-Teixeira, "Fabrique et réception de la norme. Brèves remarques sur l'effectivité en droit médiéval", *in* Véronique Beaulande, Julie Claustre and Elsa Marmursztejn (eds.), *La fabrique de la norme: lieux et modes de production des normes au Moyen Âge et à l'époque moderne*, Presses universitaires de Rennes, 2012, pp. 17–30.

Simi Linton, "What Is Disability Studies?", *PMLA*, 120.2 (2005), pp. 518–522.

Elizabeth M. MAKOWSKI, *English Nuns and the Law in the Middle Ages: Cloistered Nuns and Their Lawyers, 1293–1540*, Boydell Press, 2012.

Carmelo MASALA and Donatella R. PETRETTO, "From Disablement to Enablement: Conceptual Models of Disability in the 20th Century", *Disability and Rehabilitation*, 30.17 (2008), pp. 1233–1244.

Teresa MEADE and David SERLIN, "Editors' Introduction", *Radical History Review*, 94 (2006), pp. 1–8.

Helen MEEKOSHA and Russell SHUTTLEWORTH, "What's so "Critical" about Critical Disability Studies?", *Australian Journal of Human Rights*, 15.1 (2009), pp. 47–75.

Gert MELVILLE, *The World of Medieval Monasticism: Its History and Forms of Life*, Liturgical Press, 2016.

Irina METZLER, *Disability in Medieval Europe. Thinking about Physical Impairment in the High Middle Ages, c.1100–c.1400*, Routledge, 2006.

Irina METZLER, *A Social History of Disability in the Middle Ages: Cultural Considerations of Physical Impairment*, Routledge, 2013.

Irina METZLER, "Then and Now: Canon Law on Disabilities", in Christian LAES (ed.), *Disabilities in Roman Antiquity: Disparate Bodies, a capite ad calcem*, Brill, 2013, pp. 455–467.

Irina METZLER, *Fools and Idiots? Intellectual Disability in the Middle Ages*, Manchester University Press, 2016.

Andreas MEYER, "Les "*littere in forma pauperum*" aspects socio-historiques des provisions pontificales", *in Le fonctionnement administratif de la Papauté d'Avignon*, École française de Rome, 1991, pp. 315–327.

Hélène MILLET, *Suppliques et requêtes: le gouvernement par la grâce en Occident, XIIe–XVe siècle*, École française de Rome, 2003.

Hélène MILLET, "Introduction", *in* Hélène MILLET (ed.), *Suppliques et requêtes: le gouvernement par la grâce en Occident, XIIe–XVe siècle*, École Française de Rome, 2003, pp. 1–18.

Charles De MIRAMON, "L'invention de la Réforme grégorienne: Grégoire VII au XIXe siècle. Entre pouvoir spirituel et bureaucratisation de l'Église", Revue de l'histoire des religions, 2 (2019), pp. 283–315.

Jean-Marie MOEGLIN, *L'intercession du Moyen Âge à l'époque moderne: autour d'une pratique sociale*, Droz, 2004.

Pascal MONTAUBIN, "L'administration pontificale de la grâce au XIIIe siècle, l'exemple de la politique bénéficiale", *in* Hélène MILLET (ed.), *Suppliques et requêtes: le gouvernement par la grâce en Occident, XIIe–XVe siècle*, École française de Rome, 2003, pp. 321–342.

Neville MORLEY, *Theories, Models, and Concepts in Ancient History*, Routledge, 2004.

Colin MORRIS, *The Papal Monarchy: The Western Church from 1050 to 1250*, Oxford University Press, 1989.

Joseph MORSEL, *L'aristocratie médiévale: v^e–xve siècle*, Armand Colin, 2004.

Cordula NOLTE (ed.), *Homo debilis: Behinderte, Kranke, Versehrte in der Gesellschaft des Mittelalters*, Didymos, 2009.

Cecilia NUBOLA and Andreas WÜRGLER, *Suppliche e "gravamina": politica, amministrazione, giustizia in Europa: secoli xive–xviiie*, Il mulino, 2002.

Brandon PARLOPIANO, '*Propter Deformitatem*: Towards a Concept of Disability in Medieval Canon Law', *Canadian Journal of Disability Studies*, 4.3 (2015), pp. 72–102.

Jean-Claude PASSERON and Jacques REVEL (eds.), *Penser par cas*, Éditions de l'EHESS, 2005.

Ernst PITZ, *Papstreskript und Kaiserreskript im Mittelalter*, Max Niemeyer, 1971.

Paulis RABIKAUSKAS, "La cancelleria e le concessioni papali delle grazie", *in Aux origines de l'État moderne. Le fonctionnement administratif de la papauté d'Avignon*, École française de Rome, 1991, pp. 223–236.

Jacques REVEL, "L'institution et le social", *in* Bernard LEPETIT (ed.), *Les Formes de l'expérience: une autre histoire sociale*, Albin Michel, 1995, pp. 85–113.

Michael ROBSON, *The Franciscans in the Middle Ages*, Boydell, 2006.

Connie L. SCARBOROUGH, *Viewing Disability in Medieval Spanish Texts*, Amsterdam University Press, 2018.

Tom SHAKESPEARE, "Cultural Representation of Disabled People: Dustbins for Disavowal?", *Disability & Society*, 9.3 (1994), pp. 283–299.

Selina SCHUSTER, *Der Dictatus Papae. Eine historische Einordnung*, GRIN Verlag, 2010.

Brigide SCHWARZ, "The Roman Curia", *in* Wilfried HARTMANN and Kenneth PENNINGTON (eds.), *The History of Courts and Procedure in Medieval Canon Law*, CUA Press, 2016, pp. 160–228.

Margrit SHILDRICK and Janet PRICE, "Uncertain Thoughts on the Dis/abled Body", *in* SHILDRICK and PRICE, *Vital Signs: Feminist Reconfigurations of the Bio/logical Body*, Edinburgh University Press, 1998, pp. 224–249.

Margrit SHILDRICK, "Critical Disability Studies, Rethinking the Conventions for the Age of Postmodernity", in Nick WATSON, Alan ROULSTONE, and Carol THOMAS (eds.), *Routledge Handbook of Disability Studies*, Routledge, 2012, pp. 30–41.

Tobin SIEBERS, "Disability in Theory: From Social Constructionism to the New Realism of the Body", *American Literary History*, 13.4 (2001), pp. 737–754.

Henri-Jacques STIKER, Jean-François RAVAUD, and Gary L. ALBRECHT, "L'émergence des disability studies: état des lieux et perspectives", *Sciences sociales et santé*, 19.4 (2001), pp. 43–73.

Friederike STÖHR, *Körpermakel – Arbeits(un)fähigkeit – Kirchenrecht: Körperlich versehrte, kranke und alte Geistliche im spätmittelalterlichen Deutschen Reich und in Skandinavien*, Didymos-Verlag, 2020.

Michael TANGL, *Die päpstlichen Kanzleiordnungen: von 1200–1500*, Scientia Verlag, 1959.

Carol THOMAS, "Disability Theory: Key Ideas, Issues and Thinkers", in Colin BARNES, Michael OLIVER and Len BARTON (eds.), *Disability Studies Today*, Blackwell Publishers, 2002, pp. 38–57.

Edward P. THOMPSON, "Socialist Humanism, an Epistle to the Philistines", *The New Reasoner. A Quaterly Journal of Socialist Humanism*, 1 (1957), pp. 105–143.

Edward P. THOMPSON, *Customs in Common*, The Merlin Press, 1991.

Rosemarie G. THOMSON, *Extraordinary Bodies: Figuring Physical Disability in American Culture and Literature*, Columbia University Press, 1997.

Tanya TITCHKOSKY, "Disability Studies: The Old and the New", *The Canadian Journal of Sociology*, 25.2 (2000), pp. 197–224.

Benoît-Michel TOCK, "Auteur ou impétrant? Réflexions sur les chartes des évêques d'Arras au XIIe siècle", *Bibliothèque de l'école des chartes*, 149.2 (1991), pp. 215–248.

Wendy TURNER and Tory V. PEARMAN (eds.), *The Treatment of Disabled Persons in Medieval Europe: Examining Disability in the Historical, Legal, Literary, Medical, and Religious Discourses of the Middle Ages*, Edwin Mellen Press, 2010.

Wendy TURNER and Sarah BUTLER (eds.), *Medicine and the Law in the Middle Ages*, Brill, 2014.

Wendy TURNER and Christina LEE (eds.), *Trauma in Medieval Society*, Brill, 2018.

Walter ULLMANN, *The Growth of Papal Government in the Middle Ages*, Routledge, 2012.

Massimo VALLERANI, *Medieval Public Justice*, Catholic University of America Press, 2012.

Émile-A. Van MOÉ, "Suppliques originales adressées à Jean XXII, Clément VI et Innocent VI", *Bibliothèque de l'école des chartes*, 92.1 (1931), pp. 253–276.

Paul VAN TRIGT, Dominik GROSS and Iva SÖDERFELDT, "Historicizing the Social Model: Some Preliminary Thoughts about the History of Disability, Science, and Politics in Postwar Britain and the Netherlands", *in "Disability Studies" meets "History of Science" körperliche Differenz und soziokulturelle Konstruktion von Behinderung aus der Perspektive der Medizin-, Technik- und Wissenschaftsgeschichte*, Kassel University Press, 2017, pp. 93–103.

Lex H. VAN VOSS (ed.), *Petitions in Social History*, Cambridge University Press, 2001.

Charles VULLIEZ, "L'*ars dictaminis* et sa place dans la "préhistoire" médiévale de la requête écrite", *in* Hélène MILLET (ed.), *Suppliques et requêtes: le gouvernement par la grâce en Occident, XIIe–XVe siècle*, École française de Rome, 2003, pp. 89–102.

Anne WALDSCHMIDT, "Warum und wozu brauchen die Disability Studies die Disability History?", in Elsbeth BÖSL, Anne KLEIN and Anne WALDSCHMIDT (eds.), *Disability History: Konstruktionen von Behinderung in der Geschichte. Eine Einführung*, Transcript, 2010, pp. 13–27.

Max WEBER, *Rechtssoziologie* (sociology of law), Luchterhand, 1967.

Brett E. WHALEN, *Dominion of God*, Harvard University Press, 2010.

Amanda J. WHITING, *Women and Petitioning in the Seventeenth-Century English Revolution: Deference, Difference, and Dissent*, Brepols Publishers, 2015.

Jeffrey WILLETT and MaryJo DEEGAN, "Liminality and Disability: Rites of Passage and Community in Hypermodern Society", *Disability Studies Quarterly*, 21.3 (2001).

Peter WIRTZ, Odile PAULUS and Patrice CHARLIER, "La gouvernance des Dominicains au-delà des théories établies", *in Conférence Internationale de Gouvernance 2012*, online: https://halshs.archives-ouvertes.fr/halshs-00691233, 2012.

Patrick N. R. ZUTSHI, "Proctors Acting for English Petitioners in the Chancery of the Avignon Popes (1305–1378)", *The Journal of Ecclesiastical History*, 35.1 (1984), pp. 15–29.

Patrick N. R. ZUTSHI, "The Office of Notary in the Papal Chancery in the Mid-fourteenth Century", *in* Enno BÜNZ, Karl BORCHHARDT and Peter HERD (eds.), *Forschungen zur Reichs-, Papst- und Landesgeschichte*, Hiersemann, 1998, vol. 2, pp. 665–683.

Patrick N. R. ZUTSHI, "The Personal Role of the Pope in the Production of Papal Letters in the Thirteenth and Fourteenth Centuries", *in* Walter POHL and Paul HEROLD (eds.), *Vom Nutzen des Schreibens*, Österreichische Akademie der Wissenschaften, 2002, pp. 225–236.

Patrick N. R. ZUTSHI, "The Origins of the Registration of Petitions in the Papal Chancery in the First Half of the Fourteenth Century", *in* Hélène MILLET (ed.), *Suppliques et requêtes: le gouvernement par la grâce en Occident, XIIe–XVe siècle*, École française de Rome, 2003, pp. 177–191.

Patrick N. R. ZUTSHI, "Petitioners, Popes, Proctors: the Development of Curial Institutions, c. 1150–1250", *in Pensiero e sperimentazioni istituzionali nella societas Christiana (1046–1250)*, Vita e Pensiero, 2007, pp. 265–293.

1 Legal Origins of the Prohibition on Clerical Disability

Abstract

This chapter investigates the legal origins of the prohibition against impaired clerics. Petitions and letters helped to define 'invalidity' as a legal category, since they contributed directly to medieval canon law's statutes regarding so-called 'defects' of body and mind. This institutional construction of disability allowed the Apostolic See to set a standard for bodies and minds, in order to distinguish the normatively able-bodied from those deemed 'abnormal', impaired. The Papal Chancery thus defined a physical standard in which a body diverging from the norm was considered 'defective', and thereby unfit for clerical office, according to two criteria: its capacity and its image. They were only two mitigating factors for disabled clerics: their innocence and their 'ignorance' (i.e., their lack of 'culpability') in relation to the existence of their impairment.

Keywords: Canon Law; Default; Irregularity; Normality; Circumstances

To the eternal memory of the fact. The bishop, the prioress and the canon's assembly of the aforementioned monastery [the Augustinian monastery of Saint-Saturnin in Toulouse, France] beg us devoutly to consent to prevent more firmly, through our authority, the abbot of the aforementioned monastery of Saint-Saturnin from receiving as a canon a person who is one-eyed (*monoculus*), lame (*claudus*), one-armed (*mancus*), or in any other way unfit (*inhabilis*) for divine service.[1]

1 RV 83, f. 163 R (RA 27, f. 152) – John XXII to the abbot of the Augustinian monastery of Saint-Saturnin in Toulouse, 1 March 1327. Text analysed by Mollat (ed.), *Jean XXII*, n° 28 051, for which I give the transcription according to the register: '*Ad perpetuam rei memoriam.* [...] *Episcopi, priorisse et conventus canonicorum devotis supplicationibus annuentes, auctoritate predicta districtius inhibemus ne abbas dicti monasterio sancti Saturnini qui est et pro tempore fuerit aliquam monoculam,*

Dubourg, N., *Disabled Clerics in the Late Middle Ages. Un/suitable for Divine Service?*
Taylor & Francis Group, 2023
DOI: 10.5117/9789463721561_CH01

The prospect of a wholly undesirable – an impaired – cleric serving in their midst was simply too much for the Augustinian community of Saint-Saturnin (Toulouse) to countenance. They were compelled to appeal to the very top of the Church hierarchy, the Pope himself. With this letter to Saint-Saturnin's abbot, Pope John XXII acceded to the wider community's wishes and recalled the prohibition of such improper clerical appointments, presumably much to their relief. So doing, John lent papal authority to the characterization of impaired men as unfit for clerical office, further concretizing statutes set out in canon law. Physical, sensory, and/or intellectual 'defects' disqualified men from clerical office, not the least because such impairments were often, though not always, considered to reflect the individual's moral defect.[2] Alongside stipulating specific impairments, the Chancery's response is productively expansive, with an effusive prohibition on any condition, physical or mental, which rendered a cleric 'in any other way unfit' for the role. In canon law, such conditions were grouped similarly broadly under the categories of 'defects of body' (*defectus corporis*) or 'defects of mind' (*defectus mentis*). From the fifth to the twentieth century, men with such 'defects' were thus blocked from joining the ranks of the clergy, unless they were in receipt of pontifical grace. Likewise, clerics who had acquired an impairment after embarking upon an ecclesiastical career were obliged to obtain papal favour if they wished to maintain their previous religious and social functions within the Church.[3]

Any study of disability necessitates the interrogation of the institutional processes that produce the category of disability itself. More specifically, it is essential to examine the ways in which a given institution determines the eligibility criteria for inclusion in the category of 'the disabled', the specific rights that may be granted following such classification, and the manner in which the institution acts when extending those rights.[4] The implementation of laws that recognize the status of disabled persons may be affirmative, for example by offering specific legal protections to the disability community. At the same time, however, such laws exert a stigmatizing

claudam, mancam, vel alias ad obsequium divinum inhabilem canonicare sive in canonicam recipi facere'. All English translations throughout are my own, unless otherwise stated.

2 *Inhabilitas* as a noun, from the thirteenth century onwards, meant incapacity, or, in the modern sense, can mean disability. See Niermeyer (ed.), *Mediae latinitatis lexicon*, article "*inhabilitas*".

3 This prohibition for recipients to join orders despite a defect in the body and for ordinands to remain there without grace was lifted only belatedly, by the Code of Canon Law of 1983, see Conclusion.

4 Revillard and Baudot, "Introduction", p. 12.

effect in general terms: disability is established as a sub-category split off from the normative population.[5] Today, public policy tends to take a universalist view of disability (i.e., everyone should have access to the same opportunities), rather than the categorical approach to disability (i.e., seeking to determine whether, and to what extent, individuals are disabled) which historically prevailed. The medieval pontificate's approach to impairment corresponds closely to the categorical model as the Church/ Canon Law sets out a specific category of impairment. A third approach, founded upon a more subject-specific conceptualization of disability – with disability produced in, and modulated by, the interaction between an individual and their environment – predominates in disability activism and academic scholarship: the social model. The medieval pontificate's approach to disability corresponds most closely to this third approach.[6] The coexistence of this categorical approach with the social model, then, shows that the law can be surprisingly flexible – allowing for impaired people to carve out space, not be disabled by their impairments. In fact, analysis of petitions and pontifical letters shows that the Chancery recognized, and legitimized, the agency of impaired individuals who, within the limits of the law, wished to adapt their functions or duties to their abilities. As in all legal systems, the presence of physical impairment did not necessarily equate to the presence of disability, according to the medieval Church.[7]

It appears, then, that law is the best framework in which to comprehensively examine disability. A well-constituted legislative system, such as the one operating in medieval society, deals with both theory and practice: rules are prescribed, alongside the extent to which those rules will be applied. Whilst legal statutes construct specific subject categories, the individuals in those categories, and the categories themselves, become that much more visible when law is actually put into practice, on a case-by-case basis. Using the framework of canon law, the Chancery examined whether a specific petitioner's impairment constituted an 'irredeemable' irregularity, or not. In the twelfth century, the pontificate and the Chancery adjudicated cases by relying on criteria of 'purity' and 'impurity' attached to conditions and impairments that had prevailed among the first decretists, such as Yvo of Chartres (1140–1115). The criteria for determining clerical irregularity as a result of impairment was not fixed, however, and steadily evolved in the works of later commentators of the Gregory IX's *Decretals* (1234) and other decretists.

5 Legros, *Les processus discriminatoires*, p. 10.

6 See for example Hahn, "Toward a politics of disability".

7 Garland, *The Eye of the Beholder*, p. 5.

Jurists were no longer bound to, or seemingly particularly bothered by, the notion of impurity. Other criteria to determine irregularity were introduced in its stead: the extent to which an impairment might cause *laesio* (damage) to the Church, a concept borrowed from Roman law; the potential *scandalum* an impairment might generate in parishioners; and, the level of responsibility, or 'fault', an individual bore in terms of the onset of their impairment.

Irregularity: *Ex Defectu Corporis* and *Ex Defectu Mentis*

This chapter examines the relationship between supplicants and the ecclesiastical authority instantiated by the notion of irregularity, a canonical category produced by 'defects' of body or mind – or rather, papal adjudications as to whether a given cleric's impairment should be classified as such. Disability, as a construct, was not just defined in canon law, but also in its practical application, which established precedents that then fed back into legal statutes. In this way, the pontifical institution both imposed normative standards on the clerical community *and* had a direct hand in the formulation of norms, demonstrating its substantial power. Notwithstanding the significant influence wielded by the Chancery and its administrative regime upon the law and its evolution, it is essential to understand the general legal framework in which the Church operated, the legalistic source material that it sought to modify. Crucially, this source material was, itself, neither static nor monolithic. As a juridical object, 'irregularity' gradually gained currency over the course of the twelfth, thirteenth, and fourteenth centuries to the point of becoming a special condition for the granting of apostolic favours.

Idoneity and Irregularity

Men who applied for entrance into clerical orders faced an uphill struggle if they were impaired. Impairment and illness directly contravened the canonical prescription for clerical idoneity, that is, suitability to receive ecclesiastical office. Applicants who could not meet the requisite standards were prohibited from admission to the clergy. Numerous canonical statutes governed idoneity, construed as the satisfactory fulfilment of detailed criteria. Canon 16 of the Fourth Lateran Council (1215), for example, sets out regulations on clerics' grooming and apparel:

> They [the clerics] must have a becoming crown and tonsure and apply themselves diligently to the study of the divine offices and other useful

> subjects. Their garments must be worn clasped at the top and neither too short nor too long. They are not to use red or green garments or curiously sewed together gloves, or beak-shaped shoes or gilded bridles, saddles, pectoral ornaments (for horses), spurs, or anything else indicative of superfluity. At the divine office in the church, they are not to wear cappas with long sleeves, and priests and dignitaries may not wear them elsewhere except in case of danger when circumstances should require a change of outer garments. Buckles may under no condition be worn, nor sashes having ornaments of gold or silver, nor rings, unless it be in keeping with the dignity of their office. All bishops must use in public and in the church outer garments made of linen, except those who are monks, in which case they must wear the habit of their order; in public they must not appear with open mantles, but these must be clasped either on the back of the neck or on the bosom.[8]

Two attributes in particular manifested the cleric's renunciation of the world, the tonsure and the habit. Clerics' group identity cohered around a variety of shared characteristics: they were Christians, male, and members of the clergy (regular or secular). Rigid standards for personal grooming and dress further reinforced this shared identity by ensuring visual uniformity. This served to underscore that clerics were set apart from other dominant groups; they were 'those who pray[ed]', as opposed to 'those who [fought]' (secular elites, knights).[9] Ecclesiastical supplicants all received the tonsure, whether they were members of the secular or regular orders, as a physical marker of their status, and the acquisition of a new identity.[10] The tonsure served as a multi-faceted symbol. It denoted chastity, and visually testified to an applicant's uptake of the religious life or the end of the candidate's selection period. Clothing similarly distinguished clerics from the laity. In general terms, the clerical uniform comprised long robes that were dark, sober, and plain. Despite its lack of adornment, clerical apparel was not a simple matter: the specifics of the uniform varied according to the function fulfilled by the wearer in the ecclesial body and/or their religious order, marking the position and rank he occupied in the social space.[11] Alongside such appearance-based requirements, clerics had to be literate and capable

8 Schroeder, *Disciplinary Decrees*, pp. 236–296. Fourth Lateran Council, canon 16. This rule applies until the 1917 code.

9 Murray, "Masculinizing Religious Life", p. 27.

10 Bock, "Tonsure monastique", p. 389 and following.

11 Bourdieu, *La distinction*, p. 61.

of serving as models for the lay community, as humble and forgiving as they were chaste and measured.[12] Religious men and women alike were recognizable as such thanks to their adoption of ecclesiastical norms, which marked them out as a group apart from lay society, and indeed one considered to be of superior character.[13]

Alexander III (1159–1181) offers an explicit definition of idoneity in an undated letter addressed to the Bishop of Canterbury and his suffragans, compiled in Gregory IX's *Decretals*:

> No one shall be appointed to the administration of the church if he has proven to be unworthy in his knowledge of science, his morals, or his age or who has two churches: if so, he shall resign of the first one, unless there is a hidden reason.[14]

The Pope sets out the qualities of a good cleric: education (*scientia*), good morals (*moribus*), and the necessary age (*aetate*), which varied according to the clerical role for which one applied.[15] His statements were anything but theoretical. The bishop had intended, it seems, to ordain an 'unworthy' individual; Alexander writes to block this egregious act. For this reason, the first part of the letter refers expressly to some provisions of the Fourth Lateran Council concerning the election of priests by bishops. Canon 30, in fact, introduced criteria governing candidates' suitability, permitting their classification as *idoneus* (suitable) or *indignus* (unworthy). Only those deemed 'suitable' were worthy of receiving a benefice. Canon 27 similarly focused on idoneity, in the context of ecclesiastical offices and major orders.[16] The Council also added another layer of protection, by enacting clauses to allow for the correction of errors of appointment, in case a successful candidate was later discovered to be unsuitable for office.

Canonical prescriptions of bodily and spiritual perfection governed all clergy. Clerics were obliged to follow papal regulations, which included

12 Destemberg and Kouamé, "Aux origines de l'*homo academicus*", p. 50.

13 From this perspective, male and female religious inhabited a 'third gender', beyond the binary gender system of lay culture. See Murray, "One Flesh, Two Sexes, Three Genders?".

14 *Decretales Gregorii IX*, edited in Friedberg (ed.), *Corpus iuris canonici,* book I, title 14: '*De aetate et qualitate et ordine praeficiendorum*' ('on the age, quality and rank of the applicants'), chapter 4.

15 Dohar, "*Sufficienter litteratus*", pp. 309–311.

16 Schroeder, *Disciplinary Decrees*, pp. 236–296. Fourth Lateran Council, canon 30: 'on the suitability instituted within the Church'; canon 27: 'incompetent persons must not be promoted to the priesthood or given the direction of souls'.

examinations. Such tests allowed for the detection not only of the specific bodily defects or invisible conditions discussed in canon law, but any and all abnormalities, physical and otherwise.[17] In a letter sent to Lucanian and Bruttian bishops, compiled by Gratian, Pope Gelasius expounds on characteristics which rendered a candidate unsuitable for holding divine office:

> Someone cannot [access to monastic discipline or clerical office] if he [has been] infected by crime, [is] illiterate, remarried, barely out of adolescence, bodily vitiated, servile or of servile origin, involved in public or curial affairs, known to have undergone public penance or [is] sometimes unable to hold a proper discussion.[18]

Thus, in order to be admitted to offices and receive a benefice, the candidate must satisfy various conditions. He must be: at least eighteen years old, in good health, well-educated, unmarried, free-born, without debt nor involved with another religious order, and, above all, have obtained the clericate. Any deviation from these standards was considered to be a 'defect' which meant an individual did not fulfil the requirement of idoneity. For example, an applicant's illegitimate origins were considered to be a defect of birth.[19] An applicant who was too young was determined to have an age defect.[20] A supplicant living with physical or mental impairment was judged to have a defect of body or mind.[21]

Strictly speaking, clerics judged to be physically 'defective' were not allowed to enter the orders nor to obtain the tonsure. Bodily defect rendered the cleric *irregular*, that is, subject to 'a canonical and perpetual disqualification from receiving or lawfully exercising holy orders and tonsure'.[22] From as early as the eleventh century, a list (or canon) was compiled of ordained clerics, grouped under the heading of *regulares*. The term 'irregular', then, refers to individuals who cannot be entered in this register, or must be removed from it, due to their defect(s) and their inability to fulfil the role

17 Mulchahey, *'First the Bow is Bent in Study'*, chapter 2. According to the author, these provisions are part of the first constitutions of 1225 and 1231.

18 *Decretum Gratiani*, edited in Friedberg (ed.), *Corpus iuris canonici,* distinctio 55, canon 1: 'that the lay person who wishes to accede to monastic discipline and clerical office should have his or her life examined beforehand'.

19 Fossier, "A propos du *defectus natalium*".

20 Barrow, *The Clergy in the Medieval World*, p. 38.

21 Ullmann, *A Short History of the Papacy*, p. 154.

22 Naz, *Dictionnaire de droit canonique*, "irrégularités", tome VI, p. 43.

at hand.[23] The irregularities *ex defectu corporis* and *ex defectu mentis* were effective measures to ensure that only those who could adequately exercise most, if not all, ecclesiastic functions were 'on the list', ordained members of the orders. Nevertheless, the candidacy of 'irregular' clerics was not entirely impossible.

A pontifical letter, granted by the Chancery, could permit the flexibility of canonical regulations and thereby support clerics' entrance, or continued presence, in the orders. This is demonstrated, for example, in a letter by Boniface IX, dated 4 December 1397, regarding the case of Wenceslaus Duberman, canon of the cathedral church of Vyšehrad in the Prague diocese. The Pope explicitly describes Wenceslaus' illness as an impediment (*impedimentus*) and defect (*defectus*):

> It has been brought to our attention by your supplication that, although you are suffering from a serious illness called 'apoplexy' and you suffer immoderately from an impediment and a defect in your left arm and leg, you can still walk and ride a horse to move around, less than before however, and you still take part in divine services at opportune times.[24]

The use of the term 'defect' (*defectum*) here suggests an impairment, and indeed, the letter confirms Wenceslaus' diagnosis of apoplexy, alongside emphasizing its gravity. Although he can still walk, ride horses, and take part in divine services, he can no longer fulfil all his ecclesiastical duties as before. This includes visiting his rather meagre second benefice, at the chapel of St. Clement in the same diocese, which was worth less than 40 silver marks. Nevertheless, Wenceslaus asks to retain all privileges and income associated with the benefice, a request which was granted to him by pontifical grace, expressly despite his impediment and defect.

Irregularity, as a concept, was nuanced in canon law, differentiated according to the varying consequences of stipulated conditions. The condition of irregularity could, for example, be absolute (i.e., a permanent condition) or time-limited (i.e., corresponding to the duration of the illness). Whilst

23 Hollweck, *Die Kirchlichen*, quoted in Naz, *Dictionnaire de droit canonique*, '*defectus*', tome III, p. 1068.

24 RL 52, f. 23 V – Boniface IX to Wenceslaus Duberman, canon of the cathedral church of Vyšehrad (diocese of Prague), on 4 December 1397. Text edited by Krofta (ed.), *Monumenta vaticana*, n° 1238, tome 5, p. 669: '*Exhibita nobis nuper pro parte tua peticio continebat, quod tu quadam infirmitate 'apoplexia' nuncupata adeo gravatus existis, quod, licet ambulare ac ire et equitare possis, non tamen sicut prius, et divinis officiis interesse temporibus oportunis, quodque in tuis brachio et crure sinistris impedimentum et defectum non modicum paciaris*'.

technically rendering an individual 'irregular' in terms of idoneity, cases of temporary 'defects' were more properly known as 'simple impediments'.[25] Hence, the description of Wenceslaus Duberman's condition as an impediment (*impedimentum*) is significant. Wenceslaus suffered from apoplexy. Typically the result of a violent blow, this condition causes sudden haemorrhages which can cause the patient to suffocate, though it can be cured.[26] As such, Wenceslaus' defect may not be permanent: after some period of time, he may well be once more able to take care of his second benefice. For this reason, Wenceslaus' condition is labelled an impediment, and not an irregularity per se. An irregularity was inherently permanent, and is thus distinct from an impediment, which can disappear.[27] In the strictest sense, then, only permanent conditions, alongside incurable or chronic illnesses, could lead to irregularity.

The Apostolic See created the juridical categories of 'defects' of body and mind as an administrative boon in order to more easily classify supplicants according to the type of grace they requested, and thereby streamline the petition process. At the same time, such classifications enabled the ecclesiastical institution to define the capacity required of its clerics, and enforce quality-control measures on clergymen in office. They thus operated in practical and ideological terms: facilitating the work of the Chancery while also supporting the theoretical construction of physical and mental suitability for clerics, and deficits thereof. The Chancery considered a cleric's condition from a variety of angles – including its form, its curability, and its typical duration – with the aim of offering adaptations to suit a cleric's given circumstances. Such adaptations set precedents which were then incorporated into canon law. From this perspective, the evolution of canon law from the twelfth to the fourteenth century is therefore not just logical, but inevitable.

Defectus Corporis in Early Christianity

The notion of *defectus corporis* has been a part of canon law since the Christianity's earliest days. Its longevity as a legal precept does not equate to conceptual stasis, however. Indeed, in the run-up to the fourteenth century, the definition of such bodily defects steadily evolved in three distinct stages.

25 Guaydier, *Les irrégularités*, p. 97.

26 This is the definition proposed by Guillaume Le Talleur, *Dictionarius familiaris*: '*est subita sanguinis effusio qua suffocati intereunt, sic dicta quia ex tali percussione repentinus casus fiat*'.

27 Naz, *Dictionnaire de droit canonique*, 'irrégularités', tome VI, p. 43.

Whilst physical perfection was initially viewed as synonymous with moral purity, the former became progressively distinguished from the latter, until the linkage between bodily and moral integrity disintegrated entirely. The prohibition on clerical disability was, as ever, rooted in protecting the Church from the 'impurity' of clergymen with bodily defects, yet the defects themselves were no longer understood in terms of moral corruption. Such developments, as espoused by generations of decretists and decretalists, led to an evolution in thinking on the nature of impairment and clerical irregularity, especially in terms of which impairments rendered a cleric irregular.

In early Christian texts, a simple equation ruled: bodily deficiency directly illustrated moral vice.[28] For this reason, impaired people were excluded from leading worship, a prohibition in operation in numerous ancient cultures and explicitly stated in the Old Testament.[29] In this text, disability is equated to spiritual impurity, with impaired individuals therefore ineligible to perform divine services.[30] According to Leviticus 21:16–24, clerics must possess a perfect body in the image of Christ, to avoid desecrating holy places with the 'corruption' of an impairment:

> And the Lord spake unto Moses, saying, Speak unto Aaron, saying, Whosoever he be of thy seed in their generations that hath any blemish, let him not approach to offer the bread of his God. For whatsoever man he be that hath a blemish, he shall not approach: a blind man, or a lame, or he that hath a flat nose, or any thing superfluous, Or a man that is brokenfooted, or brokenhanded, Or crookbackt, or a dwarf, or that hath a blemish in his eye, or be scurvy, or scabbed, or hath his stones broken; No man that hath a blemish of the seed of Aaron the priest shall come nigh to offer the offerings of the Lord made by fire: he hath a blemish; he shall not come nigh to offer the bread of his God. He shall eat the bread of his God, both of the most holy, and of the holy. Only he shall not go in unto the vail, nor come nigh unto the altar, because he hath a blemish; that he profane not my sanctuaries: for I the Lord do sanctify them.[31]

Similar restrictions deprived impaired persons of an active role in worship in many other religious systems, as their presence risks desecrating the

28 Barnes, "A Legacy of Oppression", p. 16.

29 Hentrich, "Being Disabled in the Ancient Near East".

30 Raphael, *Biblical Corpora*, pp. 31–40.

31 *The New King James Version*, 2020, Leviticus 21:16–24.

sanctity and purity of the shrine. Sanctity, since the impaired body is neither perfect nor whole, and is therefore ineligible for admission to the holy space.[32] Purity, since the 'defective' impaired body of the priest threatens to defile divine perfection.[33]

In his *Pastoral Rule* (composed c. 590), Gregory the Great recapitulates the relevant section of Leviticus to further elaborate on the link between moral vice and physical impairment of the servant:

> Let each one therefore measures himself carefully: so that he will not have the audacity to assume the function of governing if the vice still reigns within him, condemning him; if a serious personal fault disfigures him, let him not seek to be an intercessor for the faults of others.[34]

Corporal and moral vices coincide to such a degree that an impure man cannot intercede for another person before God. Gregory supports his arguments further by drawing on material in the New Testament, in which a parallel between spiritual and bodily corruption is emphasized in the depiction of Jesus, as a healer, absolving men's sins.[35] Indeed, Timothy, 3:2 underscores that priests are subject to the same spiritual requirements that God makes of bishops: 'The bishop must therefore be blameless, the husband of one wife, sober, moderate, orderly in his conduct, hospitable, fit for teaching'.[36] It is not a question here of their physical perfection, but of their moral purity.[37]

By contrast, the first canonical legislations, promulgated between the fourth and ninth centuries, differentiated between two defects: moral and physical. It is only the former that made an individual fundamentally unworthy of service, although the latter could prevent ordination on the grounds of incapacity. For example, the Apostolic Constitutions, dating from the second half of the fourth century, proposed that only the moral qualities of an applicant were relevant when determining his suitability for

32 Douglas, *Purity and Danger*, p. 76.

33 See for example Wilgaux, "'Υγιὴς καὶ ὁλόκλαρος'"; Downer, "The Coptic and Ethiopic Traditions". The author notes, for example, four accounts of miracles that attest to the obligation of physical perfection for the priests.

34 Judic, Rommel, and Morel (eds.), *Règle pastorale*, p. 165, chapter 11, my translation.

35 *The New King James Version*, 2020, Matthew 9:2: And, behold, they brought to him a man sick of the palsy, lying on a bed: and Jesus seeing their faith said unto the sick of the palsy; Son, be of good cheer; thy sins be forgiven thee'.

36 Judic, Rommel, and Morel (eds.), *Règle pastorale*, see Pauline epistles 1; Timothy 3:2.

37 Stamps and Wesley (eds.), *Fire Bible – KJV*, p. 191.

entrance into office, explicitly admonishing consideration of his physical state:

> In order to establish a priestly tribe made up of each best person with a view to being elected priest, one does not dwell on his vices of the body (*corporum vitia*), but on his piety and his life.[38]

At this time, the Church was engaged in a violent struggle to spread the Christian religion across the globe. As such, this permissible stance is likely rooted in the need to avoid discouraging Christians from participating in the righteous fight, which exposed them to the very real danger of martyrdom and mutilation.[39] Similarly, men who had taken up arms for their faith, who were more likely to have become impaired, were those who had clearly demonstrated the strength of their piety and were, in theory, some of the best candidates for ordination. Hence, it seems, the appointment of particularly suitable impaired priests was encouraged. Indeed, canon 76 of the Constitutions authorized one-eyed or mobility-impaired men to receive the sacrament of Holy Orders, if the man in question proved himself to be otherwise worthy:

> If someone who is deprived of sight, or wounded in the thigh, is worthy of being a bishop, let him be a bishop. The question is not whether his body is defiled by this injury, but the defilement of his soul.[40]

As justification for this position, the text further noted that it is the impurities of the soul, not the defilements of the body, that make a man unworthy of orders. Consequently, physical defects do not reflect moral defects; in the eyes of the Church, the former are far less serious than the latter.

The question of impaired clerics and bishops was first explicitly considered in canon law at the end of the fifth century by Pope Gelasius (492–496), with further detail added by subsequent pontiffs up to the end of Eugene II's tenure (824–827) and later compiled in Gratian's *Decree* (c. 1140). The examples used in canon law refer exclusively to situations of fixed impairment (such as cases of leprosy) and mutilation (such as cases of limb loss). This illustrates the distinction made between fixed conditions, understood to cause irregularity, and variable, or time-limited diseases that cause

38 Metzger, *Les constitutions apostoliques*, book 6, chapter 23, n° 5, my translation.

39 Guaydier, *Les irrégularités*, p. 31.

40 Metzger, *Les constitutions apostoliques*, book 8, chapter 47, n° 77, my translation.

impediment. Gelasius was the first to legislate the prohibition on ordination for individuals deemed to possesses bodily defect(s). Later pontiffs followed his lead closely, fleshing out his earlier regulation in more detail but adding little, if any, direction of their own to the statutes at hand.[41] For example, the Third Council of Orléans, held in 538, stipulated the sanctions to be levied against individuals who contravened the prohibition on the ordination of men with a bodily defect first formulated by Gelasius.[42] The Fourth Council of Toledo in 633 expanded the punitive scope. As before, men with bodily defect were blocked from ordination, and subject to disciplinary action if they sought to be ordained. But now, any clerics that helped them, including ordaining them, were to be punished similarly, and themselves removed from office.[43] Gradually between the fifth and the twelfth century, physical defects and moral vices became two distinct legal categories, yet their application had the same effect: the prohibition on ordination for impaired men.

The collections of decrees used in the twelfth and thirteenth centuries highlight the distinction between moral and physical vices. The texts chosen by jurists to illustrate certain points of canon law bear witness to the ever-widening gap between the two kinds of defect in the construction of clerical irregularity.[44] Gratian opens Distinction 49 of his *Decree* with a quotation from Gregory the Great (590–604). Individuals possessing a 'weakness of body' (*imbecillitatem corpus*), or a 'repulsive mind' (*repugnat spiritus*) cannot, Gregory proclaims, be considered worthy of leading worship.[45] Bodily vices and defects of morality (*infamis*) constitute irregularities of equal importance with similar consequences, he maintains, though they form two distinct legal categories. Indeed, Gregory had earlier written a letter to John, Bishop of Squilace in Calabria, in which he clearly drew a parallel between bodily vice (*parte corporis uitiatum*) and the eight deficiencies that give rise to a *defectus mentis* irregularity, including illiteracy.[46] Yet Gratian,

41 Guaydier, *Les irrégularités*, p. 25. These precepts are notably found in canonical collections such as the *Decretum Gratiani* and the *Decretales Gregorii IX*.

42 Hardouin, *Conciliorum collectio*, tome II, p. 1424. The council recommends punishing both the person who would have been ordained despite an imperfection of the body (*semus corporeum*), which is then deposited, and the bishop who performed the ordination, which is suspended for six months.

43 *Decretum Gratiani*, edited in Friedberg (ed.), *Corpus iuris canonici*, distinctio 51, canon 5.

44 The list of irregularities was not updated until 1917 by the Apostolic See; only the canonists would update it during our period of study.

45 *Liber pastoralis*, chapter 10. See *Decretum Gratiani*, edited in Friedberg (ed.), *Corpus iuris canonici*, distinctio 49, prelude.

46 *Decretum Gratiani*, edited in Friedberg (ed.), *Corpus iuris canonici*, distinctio 34, canon 10. Other conditions causing irregularity *ex defectu* are failure to follow the vow of chastity

in his analysis of Gregory's missive, provides an alternative explanation for the prohibition. According to established legal precepts, a bodily defect prevents an ordained man from giving the sacraments because it evidences his vice, whereas illiteracy is simply prohibited on pragmatic grounds:

> The illiterate and any other person who lacks a part of the body, let no one think of promoting them as a priest, for whoever cannot read the sacred letters is not fit for the office, and whoever is vitiated cannot offer anything to God as forbidden by the precepts of the law.[47]

From the twelfth to the fourteenth centuries, the detrimental moral dimension of physical deficiency was de-emphasized, and steadily faded. Incapacity, whether physical or intellectual, was no longer synonymous with moral turpitude, and thus impairment became subject to pontifical pardon. The petitions and letters in the corpus reflect the conception of bodily defects as developed in thirteenth-century compilations of canon law, insofar as impairment is never linked to a *moral* defect. Jurists no longer depended upon vice as a framework in which to orient the ecclesiastical response to impairment. Instead, they turned to other concepts to adjudicate cases, namely: *laesio* and *utilitas* from Roman law; *scandalum*; and individual fault. Notwithstanding shifts in the precise delineation of the legal precepts of *defectus corporis* and *mentis*, such categories remained invaluable, especially in the thirteenth century. At this time, they allowed the Chancery to classify supplicants and thereby to automate, to some degree, the processing of petitions.

Canonical Standards of Normality: Capacity and Image

During the supplication process, the Papal Chancery evaluated petitioners' impairment according to two standards of normality: capacity and image. On the one hand, members of the Curia considered the petitioner as an individual, and more precisely his capacity to undertake essential ministerial acts, such as leading Mass, and to fulfil religious obligations, such as Lenten

(*bigamus*), penance, criminal guilt (*curiae obnoxius*, lack of gentleness) or servile condition (*conditioni obnoxius*, lack of liberty).

47 Op. cit., distinctio 36, canon 1, my translation. In it, Gratian takes up a letter written by Pope Gelasius in which the vice of body, defined by the lack of a part of the body, forbids access to the clericature in the same way as illiteracy. This passage is also present in Yvo of Chartres' *Panormia*, book 3, chapter 47.

fasting, giving penance, and so on. On the other hand, they evaluated the broader impact of an individual's impairment in terms of its potentially detrimental social impact, or *scandalum*: the effect that it might have on the Christians around him, potentially leading to the cleric's marginalization, alongside a loss of faith in his congregation.[48] Taken together, these two criteria reflect the cleric's *integritas*, as defined by Thomas Aquinas. Entrance into the orders, according to Aquinas, requires that an ordinand possess *claritas* (i.e., a good reputation), and that the performance of his duties be unimpeded by physical impairment:

> To the fourth question, it should be said that, as is clear from what has been said, someone becomes unsuitable for the reception of holy orders either because of an impediment to the act or because of an impediment to the person's prominence (*claritas*). And therefore those suffering a defect (*defectus*) in their members are impeded from the reception of holy orders, if there were such a defect that it left a noticeable mark (*macula*) by which the prominence of the person would be obscured, like having one's nose cut off, or if it could endanger the exercise of holy orders; otherwise, they would not be impeded. But this integrity (*integritas*) is required from the necessity of precept, not as necessary to the sacrament.[49]

The problem is not impairment per se, it is both the visible impairment which may negatively affect the man's *claritas*, and which interferes with the cleric's fulfilment of duties. This allows ordination for a whole range of impaired men, insofar as it this is more of a canonical law matter than a sacramental issue. Then, it also allows an opening up a space for more 'disabled' men, as the sense we understand it today, to be involved in the Church. Anyhow, the Church, as an institution, was responsible for ensuring that the men applying to become members of its highest ranks, and especially those serving on its front lines with the care of souls, were up to the task. They must possess integrity, and the demonstrate the capacity to fulfil their core functions.

Capacity: Ability and Functionality

It is hard to overstate the importance of capacity – understood as a cleric's ability to perform the functions of their office – in discussions to determine

48 See also Stöhr, *Körpermakel – Arbeits(un)fähigkeit – Kirchenrecht*.

49 Thomas Aquinas, *Commentary on the Sentences*, book IV, distinctio 25, question 2, article 2.

supplicants' bodily and mental defects in the corpus.[50] Drawing from Galenic medicine, the documents testify to a functional approach to impairment. In the Galenic model, illness equates to a state in which 'one can no longer freely go about one's business, through a total or partial impediment'.[51] Such an emphasis on the practical consequences of physical incapacity is equally evident in the writings of Thomas Aquinas, who offer a definition of the medieval 'invalidity' when discussing the issue of 'bodily impairment':

> I answer that, the cause of sin is on the part of the soul, in which, chiefly, sin resides. Now weakness may be applied to the soul by way of likeness to weakness of the body (*infirmitatis corporis*). Accordingly, man's body is said to be weak (*infirmus*), when it is disabled (*debilitare*) or hindered (*impedere*) in the execution of its proper action, through some disorder of the body's parts, so that the humors (*humores*) and members of the human body cease to be subject (*non subdere*) to its governing and motive power (*virtus*). Hence a member is said to be weak (*infirmus*), when it cannot do the work of a healthy (*sanus*) member, the eye, for instance, when it cannot see clearly, as the Philosopher [Aristotle] states (*De Hist. Animal.* x, 1).[52]

The theologian proposes a functionalist definition of physical weakness and invalidity that is connotative of the social model's concept of bodily impairment. In this context, disability is clearly linked to an individual's ability, or lack thereof, to perform various social and professional functions. It is thus construed as a deviation from the norm, with the latter defined both by assumptions as to the capacity of healthy, able-bodied members of society and by the expectations of the pontifical institution. By characterizing impairment as an obstacle to the accomplishment of certain activities, Aquinas addresses the first social consequence of medieval impairment, according to canon law and the papal letters: the (in)ability to undertake work. Is this the first way in which an impairment may become a disability.

Gregory IX's *Decretals*, compiled by Raymond de Peñafort in 1234, questioned the ordination of applicants with bodily impairments, leveraging

50 Disability historians commonly admit that this medical approach appeared with the emergence of industrialization and capitalism at the end of the nineteenth century. See Finkelstein, *Attitudes and Disabled People*, p. 37.

51 Gourevitch, "La conception galénique", p. 1999, quoting the chapter 4 of the *Ars medica* by Galen.

52 Thomas Aquinas, *Summa Theologiae I–II*, q. 77, article 3, 'Whether a sin committed through passion should be called a sin of weakness?'

bulls written by a series of pontiffs spanning the reigns of Alexander III (1159–1181) and Honorius III (1216–1227). Title 20, *De corpore vitiatis ordinandis vel non* ('whether persons with bodily imperfection should be ordained or not'), emphasizes that issues relating to capacity and reputation are of grave importance, and serve to disqualify men from the clerical profession for a number of reasons.[53] In this context, jurists distinguish two types of irregularity produced by *defectus corporis*: total and partial. Total irregularity makes it impossible to exercise the ecclesiastical function.[54] This would be the case, for example, for a bishop who permanently lost the ability to say Mass due to a glossal injury. On the other hand, partial irregularity – more precisely termed, an impediment – necessitates only the reduction in a clergyman's activities commensurate to his capacity, as he is still able to fulfil certain functions of the office. A lack of capacity explains, then, the prohibition on the ordination of the 'dumb, deaf, and blind' that has existed in canon law from its earliest formulation. Men with these kinds of sensory impairments were in a state of total irregularity: they were unable to read aloud, and therefore cannot exercise the office properly.[55] By contrast, a bishop who became blind after ordination would not necessarily be removed from his post. Whilst he could no longer read the sacred texts to say Mass, he might very well retain the ability to confess the laity, for example.[56] In other words, his blindness could be considered only a *partial* irregularity. Irregularity related to *defectus mentis* was less nuanced, in theory at least. It was impossible to gauge with confidence whether a mentally impaired applicant's stated desire to be baptized, to marry, or to enter holy orders truly reflected their wishes, or if they were of sound mind. As such, *defectus mentis* represented total irregularity. However, if the individual experienced intervals of lucidity – that is, moments when their impairment had no discernible consequences – the *defectus mentis* could be considered only a partial irregularity, that is, an impediment. The granularity of such legal distinctions meant that the ecclesiastical authority was obliged to judge

53 *Decretales Gregorii IX*, edited in Friedberg (ed.), *Corpus iuris canonici,* book I, title 20: '*De corpore vitiatis ordinandis vel non*'.

54 In the context of the sale of slaves during antiquity, the author Aulu-Gelle (123–180) distinguishes *morbus* (disease) from *vicium* (body defect), taking into account the ability to work and not the temporary or permanent nature of the symptoms. See Laes, Goodey, and Rose, "Approaching Disabilities", p. 7.

55 See for example Bidez et al. (eds.), *Histoire ecclésiastique*, book 6, chapter 30. Sozomen developed the famous example of Ammonius who mutilated his ear to prevent him from becoming a bishop in the fifth century, and then threatened to cut out his tongue to prevent him from speaking if his voters tried to force him again.

56 Naz, *Dictionnaire de droit canonique*, 'irrégularités', tome VI, p. 48.

cases 'according to the nature and gravity' of the applicant's condition, especially the extent to which an illness impacted the '[optimal] exercise of priestly functions'.[57] The pontifical institution thus required in-depth knowledge of the specificities of physical and mental conditions, alongside the theological dangers they might pose. The Chancery's expertise in this arena is demonstrated throughout the corpus.

Whilst theologians described the consequences of impairment in detail, they did not dwell on its causes.[58] The only thing that mattered was the issue of capacity, since it was on this question that the Chancery had to rule during the petition process. In the *Summa Aurea*, for example, the canonist Henry of Segusio (1200–1271) delineates several criteria for irregularity *ex defectu corporis* that rendered an individual unfit for divine service, without any mention of the moral valency of such conditions:

> Debility (*debilitas*) occurs when one has a limb that cannot function as expected (*inefficax*). Deformity (*deformitas*) occurs when one has a spot in the eye, when one is hunchbacked or bent, if one has six fingers in one hand or other unnatural features. Impotence (*impotentia*) appears when one is mutilated.[59]

Such functionalist characterization of impairment, which we equally find in the petitions and letters, clearly breaks with earlier conceptualizations of bodily imperfection as moral impurity, and vice versa. For example, canon 47 of the Apostolic Constitutions, written in the fourth century, insists that incapacity, and not moral corruption, is the reason for barring individuals with certain impairments from the episcopate: 'The deaf (*surdus*) or the blind (*caecus*) will not become a bishop; not because he is defiled (*pollutus*), but so that the affairs of the Church do not suffer (*impediantur*)'.[60]

Chief amongst the pontifical institution's responsibilities was the management of ecclesiastical goods and affairs. Its willingness to grant pardons according to a supplicant's capacity, or lack thereof, was directly related to its strategic managerial mission.[61] Incapacity had to be adjudicated on a case-by-case basis: measurements of normative capacity were tied to the

57 Tinel, "Étude de quelques maladies", p. 72.

58 Parlopiano, "*Propter deformitatem*", p. 88.

59 Wahrmund (ed.), *Summa Aurea*, tome I, p. 20, my translation.

60 Hardouin (ed.), *Conciliorum collectio*, tome I, p. 27.

61 The idea of functionality of the disabled persons are found in other religious traditions, notably in the Koran, where the disabled person is exempted from going into battle for example. Stiker, *A History of Disability*, quoting the Koran, suras 24 and 48.

requirements and expectations of a given role. In this way, an individual's capacity was defined by the community's sense of the missions with which the cleric was tasked, and by the individual's subjective ability to succeed on those terms.[62] A letter from Gregory XI to the Bishop of Palencia on 3 January 1376, regarding Abbot Lupus of the Benedictine monastery of San Salvatore de Oña (diocese of Burgos), is particularly illustrative on this topic:

> The request sent to us by the dear brothers Petrus Fernandus de Castellanos, prior of the cloister and the convent of the Benedictine monastery of Onia, immediately submitted to the Holy See, in the diocese of Burgos, contains that in order to provide for the dear son Lupus, abbot of the said monastery, who about three years ago contracted a serious illness leading to continuous mental insanity, so much so that he has become useless to administer anything, [to the extent that] the properties of the said monastery are a little more in ruins every day, but, wishing that the said monastery be managed in a healthy way, they elected dear brother Garsius Fernandi, sacristan of the said monastery, as coadjutor[.][63]

Some three years after its initial onset, Lupus' mental dysregulation remains grave. It seems this is not a condition from which he will ever recover, nor is it compatible with the smooth running of the monastery for which the abbot is responsible. It is for this reason that Prior Petrus Fernandus de Castellanos and the entire monastic community at Oñia wrote to the Pope. After setting out their complaint about the inefficiency of their 'useless' abbot, they informed the Chancery that they had voted for the installation of a coadjutor. Gregory concurs with the community's decision, eventually ruling that Lupus' incapacity contributed to the progressive ruin of the monastery, as he could no longer perform any administrative tasks attached to his office. The Pope thus endorsed the appointment of a coadjutor to assist Lupus, which dealt with the problem at hand without the need to remove

62 Edwards Rose, "Constructions of Physical Disability", p. 35.

63 RA 198, f. 24 R – Gregory XI to the Bishop of Palencia, 3 January 1376. Text analysed by Hayez, Mathieu, and Yvan (eds.), *Grégoire XI*, n° 41 460, for which I give the transcription according to the register: '*Sane petitio pro parte dilectorum filiorum Petri Fernandi de Castellanos, prioris claustralis, et conventus monasterio de Onia, ad eandem Romanam ecclesiam nullo medio pertinentis, O.S.B., Burgensis diocesis, nobis nuper exhibita continebat quod dudum ipsi providere, accedentes quod dilectus filius Luppus abbas eiusdem monasterii qui gravem infirmitatem continuam insanae mentis a tribus annis citra contraxerat, adeo inutilis factus erat administrator in omnibus quod bona dicti monasterio cotidie perdebantur, ac cupientes eidem monasterii salubriter promoveri dilectum filium Garsiam Fernandi, sacristam dicti monasterii eundem, in coadiutorem elegerunt quamvis de facto*'.

Lupus from his prestigious office.[64] In the interchange, no mention is made of the moral dimension of the abbot's condition, nor is it explained in terms of moral corruption. All parties involved in the case concentrate instead on the consequences of Lupus' impairment in terms of his capacity. This reflects the focus in canon law on the cleric's impairment in terms of their functional ability in a given set of circumstances. In discussions of defects of body and mind, canonical texts offer fuzzy, imprecise explanations for the cause of impairment, whilst attending meticulously to the minutiae of its associated effects.[65]

Canonical texts and petitions dating to the thirteenth century demonstrate a rather tolerant attitude in terms of accommodating impairment, as evidenced by material relating to prebends and dignities in Gregory IX's *Decretals*. Drawing from a letter from Alexander III to the clerk and the chapter of Lille, canon law stated that a priest must celebrate Mass every day, unless he was prevented from doing so by 'bodily infirmity'.[66] As will be discussed in depth in Chapter 4, from a canonical perspective, neither physical nor mental impairment prohibited an officiant from retaining his benefice. Nevertheless, an impaired cleric might well be stripped of some of his functions and benefices owing to the effect of the condition on their capacity. Such subtleties come into focus, for example, in the case of supernumerary fingers. The canonist Goffredo da Trani maintains that the presence of additional digits does not de facto constitute an impediment. Henry of Segusio is in agreement, adding the provision that the defect must not lead to *scandalum* and thereby negatively impact the cleric's ability to fulfil the duties of his role.[67] Once more, the question of functionality becomes central.

Image: Scandalum and Suitability

Discussion of capacity centres the impaired cleric as an individual. This is of critical importance, yet it provides only half the story. The development of a comprehensive understanding of medieval disability demands the consideration of another, parallel perspective: the opinion of those around the impaired individual, understood in the present context as the

64 See Chapter 4 on the appointment of coadjutors.

65 See Metzler, "Then and Now".

66 *Decretales Gregorii IX*, edited in Friedberg (ed.), *Corpus iuris canonici*, book III, title 5 – *De praebendis et dignitatibus*, chapter 11.

67 On this debate, see Parlopiano, "*Propter deformitatem*", p. 94.

Christian worshippers who comprised the impaired cleric's community and congregation. Disability enacts not just physical change, but also a shift in an individual's social identity. Whether or not an impairment practically prevented a cleric from performing their duties adequately, their condition affected their reputation. Not all impairments are equally visible, and thus the social impact of an impairment depends on how visible, how 'intelligible', a cleric's condition was to those around them.[68] Called a *stigma* when visible, this marks a disfavour or disgrace and reveals a person's virtual social identity.[69]

Canon 27 of the Fourth Lateran Council insisted on the obligation to recruit only ministers genuinely worthy of divine office:

> Since the direction of souls is the art of arts, we strictly command that bishops, either themselves or through other qualified men, diligently prepare and instruct those to be elevated to the priesthood in the divine offices and in the proper administration of the sacraments of the Church. If in the future they presume to ordain ignorant and unformed men (a defect that can easily be discovered), we decree that both those ordaining and those ordained be subject to severe punishment. In the ordination of priests especially, it is better to have a few good ministers than many who are no good, for if the blind lead the blind both will fall into the pit (Matt. 15:14).[70]

Priests were not just representatives of the Church, but of Christianity itself – and they were tasked with the most important work of all, the care of souls. It follows, then, that the papacy evinced a particular interest in the exemplarity, or representative-ness, of all aspects of the clerical subject, including his body, mind, and social identity. By dint of its authority over Christian bodies, the Church defined the level and type of stigma generated by impairments, and whether stigmatized applicants could enter the clericate.[71] Those ecclesiastical precepts could partly be integrated in medieval society, which marginalized individuals according to the relative visibility of their impairment.[72] In this way, both cultural norms were reproduced and concretized with the rejection or integration of impaired people.

68 Shaking hands or stuttering, for example, could be visible signs of mental disorders.

69 See Link and Phelan, "Conceptualizing Stigma".

70 Schroeder, *Disciplinary Decrees*, pp. 236–296. Fourth Lateran Council, canon 16.

71 Ostinelli, "I chierici e il '*defectus corporis*'", p. 11.

72 Abberley, "Disabled People", p. 53.

For the medieval Church, *scandalum* (which we can more or less translate as 'scandal' – the disapproval of the public knowledge of a fact), including negative responses to a cleric's impairment, should be avoided at all costs. The question of the attribution of the sacraments – and therefore of access to major orders – loomed especially large, concentrating institutional fears more generally on the issue of clerical disability.[73] The ecclesiastical authority was apprehensive, lest a cleric administering the sacraments were perceived to be 'impure' due to the presence of an impairment. This would inevitably taint the purity of the sacraments, tarnish the holiness of the place of worship, and besmirch the image of the Church itself amongst the faithful. The more visible the impairment, and the more it was a matter of public knowledge, the greater the risk it posed. Broadly speaking, jurists characterized *scandalum* as the incitement of another to mortally sin, achieved through an act or sign, including the presence of a visible impairment.[74] An individual committing a scandalous act damages the *caritas*, that is, the cohesion, of the Christian community.[75] Canon law, and especially Gregory IX's *Decretals*, defined scandal in detail within the ecclesiastical framework, explaining that impairment – as stigma – constituted an impediment to the ministry.

A letter composed by Pope Eugene, compiled in the *Decretals*, features an illustrative example of the practical application of legal statutes:

> We will not allow the celebration of Mass to a priest whose two fingers in the centre of his hand are known to have been cut off by a brigand, for fear of his illness and the scandal caused by his deformation which we are convinced will result. We do not in any way prohibit him from performing any other priestly offices he may perform.[76]

The anonymous priest is no longer eligible to celebrate Mass, due to his digital amputations. Yet he is explicitly permitted to continue carrying out all other priestly functions. Indeed, as Eugene's ruling demonstrates, the issue of *scandalum* could be managed to a certain degree. If in receipt of papal grace, clerics in a state of *partial* irregularity could continue to meaningfully fulfil clerical role, in which the visibility of their impairment would not cause

73 See Dubourg, "Un/Acceptable Disability?".

74 Helmholz, "*Scandalum* in the Medieval Canon Law", p. 260.

75 Fossier, "*Propter vitandum scandalum*", p. 319.

76 *Decretales Gregorii IX*, edited in Friedberg (ed.), *Corpus iuris canonici*, book III, title 6, chapter 2.

public outcry. However, to justify the ban from the celebration of the Mass, Eugene admits to being concerned about the priest's physical capacity to officiate, alongside the scandal that his highly visible manual deformation would likely generate. In canon law, total or partial irregularity caused by a defect of body or mind renders a cleric unsuitable for sacramental service.[77] If ordained without *integritas*, an irregular cleric finds himself in a scandalous position, owing to the detrimental impact of such improper events on the laity.

The nature and extent of the supplicant's impairment conditioned the dispensation of pontifical grace.[78] This is amply demonstrated in a letter sent by Alexander IV (1199–1261) on 18 January 1260. In this missive, the pope confirmed the authorization given by special mandate by Hugh of Saint-Cher, cardinal of Santa Sabina and Major Penitentiary of the pope from 1256 to 1263, to Matheo of Gusencia, deacon and monk of the Benedictine monastery of Saint Médard (diocese of Soissons) to stay and be promoted in the orders despite a sensory impairment affecting the vision in his left eye.

> It has been brought to our attention by your [Matheo] supplication, that, insofar as you suffer from a defect of light in your left eye as a result of an illness, neither so important nor so serious as to be likely to cause a scandal, you received the authorization of our dear son Hugo de San Caro, priest cardinal of Santa Sabina at the moment, who dispensed you with mercy on our special mandate, by letters fortified by the seal of the cardinal himself, so that you may be promoted to the service of the aforementioned orders and to the priestly order as well as to the administration of the priory of your order on condition that you maintain good health.[79]

Hugh does not think that Matheo's relatively minor impairment, or the illness that caused it, will cause any scandal. It seems that the Pope also

77 See for example the manuscript of Galvanus de Bononia, *De presbytero irregularitati*, compiled between 1361 and 1385.

78 Shinners and Dohar, *Pastors and the Care of Souls*, p. 52.

79 RV 25, f. 237 V – Alexander IV to Matheo of Gusencia, deacon and monk of the monastery of Saint Médard, 18 January 1260. Text edited by Loye, Cenival, Coulon, and La Roncière (eds.), *Les registres d'Alexandre IV*, n° 3 045: '*Sane exhibita nobis tua petitio continebat quod dilectus filius noster H.[Hugo de San Caro] tituli Sancte Sabine presbiter cardinalis, in cujus eras presentia constitutus, attendens quod licet defectum luminis ex quadam supervenienti infirmitate in sinistro oculo patiaris, non tamen est talis vel tantus quod propter hoc possit scandalum generari, tecum in susceptis ministrare ordinibus ac ad sacerdotii ordinem pr[o]moveri necnon ad administrationes prioratuum tui ordinis dumtaxat assumi valeas de speciali mandato nostro misericorditer dispensavit prout in litteris inde confectis ipsius cardinalis sigillo munitis plenius dicitur contineri*'.

considers him sufficiently able-bodied not only to receive a promotion to the priesthood, but to take over the administration of the Dominican priory. The latter is a particularly good fit for Matheo, given that the position does not require him to make an appearance before the lay faithful, nor act in a representative, or exemplary, capacity for worshippers. Matheo of Gusencia is by no means an isolated case. Similar examples can be found in Gregory IX's *Decretals*. Alexander III, for instance, permits an impaired priest to celebrate Mass, with the proviso that his disfigurement is not too 'excessive' (*excessus*), as that would create a scandal among his parishioners.[80] As in these examples, papal letters paid close attention to the potential impact of an impairment as a cause for *scandalum*. With the power to grant grace, the ecclesiastical institution possessed an invaluable tool to assert its will. Papal letters were a means of pursuing its aims, chief amongst them the preservation of the social status quo, in which the Church operated as the predominant authority. The irregularity of ecclesiastical officials or regular clerics suffering, literally or figuratively, from the stain (*macula*) of impairment, compromised this mission.[81] It was essential, then, for the Church to develop a means to neutralize, or proactively manage, any potential 'scandal' associated with clerical impairment – hence, the strategic utility of the petition process and grants of grace. This required the formulation of metrics by which the relative acceptability of a given impairment could be judged. Indeed, theologians insisted on the need to determine an 'acceptable' degree of deformity, beyond which a cleric would be prohibited to celebrate Mass. Perhaps the most extensive treatment of the issue is found in a chapter on the age and necessary qualities of applicants for ordination in *Pupilla oculi*, a treatise on the sacraments written in 1384 by Jean de Bourg, Chancellor of Cambridge.[82]

From a modern sociological standpoint, an individual's identity depends on the presence, and opinions, of an Other. The latter functions as a 'social mirror', into which an individual gazes in order to perceive their reputation, who they are perceived to be. This feeds directly into who an individual's perception of themselves, and thus becomes part of their internal sense of self. A similar process is at play in the Middle Ages, as evoked in the complex notion of *fama* (reputation).[83] If impaired clerics' physical or mental

80 *Decretales Gregorii IX*, edited in Friedberg (ed.), *Corpus iuris canonici*, book 1, title 20, chapter 1.

81 Fossier, "*Propter vitandum scandalum*", p. 328.

82 Metzler, "Then and Now", p. 456.

83 Leveleux-Teixeira, "*Fama* et mémoire", p. 45.

defects were visible, they might suffer from *mala fama* (bad reputation). Then, *mala fama* can be understood as the negative external perception of an individual, whilst *scandalum* is the effect of that perception, in terms of negative *reactions* to the person. In such instances, impaired priests 'become a scandal for those to whom they were supposed to show themselves exemplary'.[84] This is demonstrated, for example, in another case found in Gregory IX's *Decretals* regarding a leprous priest. The afflicted cleric can no longer administer the divine office, the Pope rules, because of his *mala fama*, the scandal his condition would certainly generate, rooted in the widespread belief that leprosy was an abomination.[85] As illustrated in this case, the Church authority explicitly took into account the broader Christian community's views on clerical eligibility when adjudicating on supplications. From the beginning of the thirteenth century onwards, conceptualizations of impairment relied less and less on the notion of purity, with ever greater weight placed on *scandalum* and *fama* in canon law and in letters issued by the Apostolic See.[86] These paired concepts became central in the investigative procedures used by the Chancery to determine the relative acceptability of a given cleric's impairment, triggering individual investigations in the cases of scandalous clergymen and providing metrics by which cases could be judged.

The Chancery's attribution of *defectus corporis* and *mentis* depended on two factors: the physical and/or mental capacity of the impaired supplicant, and the image that they presented to other Christians. Ecclesiastical authorities defined normative standards of impairment and reputation, grounded in its construction of a baseline of capacity deemed to be necessary for the fulfilment of clerical duties. In canon law and papal letters, then, the essential nature of clerical work, especially the care of souls, is revealed. The pontifical institution determined who belonged in the clergy and who, emphatically, did not, alongside staking out its domain and its authority over the laity thanks to the juridical categories of *defectus corporis* and *mentis*. The capacity to grant grace supported the pontificate in these aims, providing a flexible framework in which the Church could most effectively react to the specific circumstances of individual supplicants. When granting pardons, the Chancery recognized, and thus affirmed, petitioners' capacity (i.e., what abilities they retained), rather than exclusively focusing on incapacity, or assigning impairment a moral value. The Curia's emphasis on the concrete

84 Fossier, "*Propter vitandum scandalum*", p. 325 (my translation).

85 See Dubourg, "Being a Leprous Cleric", and *Decretales Gregorii IX*, edited in Friedberg (ed.), *Corpus iuris canonici,* book III, title 6, chapters 3–4.

86 See Eichbauer, "Legal Authorities and their Legislative Priorities".

consequences of impairment can be understood as pragmatic. Above all, the letters issued by the Apostolic See were practical in nature, written to resolve specific problems. With the granting of grace, the Chancery's goal was not to intervene in the treatment of an impairment, but rather to find a workable solution to the troubles the condition caused, whether theological, ecclesiastical, or logistical in nature.

Personal Responsibility and Mitigating Circumstances

One final factor was critical in the pontifical institution's response to petitions: the extent to which a supplicant could be considered to be responsible for the onset, and ongoing circumstances, of their impairment. The irregularity caused by an impairment was classified as *ex defectu*, originating in a 'defect' and thus handled, in theory, on the assumption that the supplicant was not morally at fault. By contrast, the condition of irregularity *ex delicto* was a direct result of an individual's sin (as murder for example).[87] Even if a supplicant's physical or mental condition was classed as *ex defectu*, however, the question of their 'guilt' in producing their impairment remained central. The supplicant's liability was judged on their intent, rather than the nature of their 'crime', the moral fault which led to their condition. This approach was inspired by Roman law and the logic of punishment it enshrined, as exemplified in the *Digest*.[88] At the same time, the Chancery's conceptual framework reflected the institution's broader preoccupations. From the twelfth century onwards, the question of the morality of intention (an individual's choices) had become a crucial issue.[89] Religious men who engage in self-mutilation of any kind are, thus, typically excluded from clerical office and subjected to vehement condemnation.[90] Indeed, in a letter to Felix, Bishop of Nucere Umbria, Innocent I (401–417) stated unequivocally that an individual who injures themselves but is otherwise healthy should not be admitted to the clerical office.[91] If the individual in question were already a cleric, Innocent maintained, they should be summarily expelled from the Church. Petitioners were thus obliged to demonstrate the presence

87 Naz, *Dictionnaire de droit canonique*, tome VI, p. 48.

88 See Le Goff, "Métier et profession".

89 See Wilks, "Moral Intention".

90 Caspar, *Le peuple des silencieux*, p. 59.

91 *Decretum Gratiani*, edited in Friedberg (ed.), *Corpus iuris canonici*, distinctio 55, canons 6–7. Also quoted in *Decree* of Yvo of Chartres, edited in Migne (ed.), *Patrologia Latina*, vol. 161, book 6, chapter 58.

of 'mitigating factors' – genuine or, at the very least, plausible – in the circumstances of their own impairment in order to qualify for pontifical grace. Individuals either claimed no fault whatsoever for their condition, or admitted to partial liability. Latter cases could be excused, it was argued, if the cleric were ignorant of relevant laws. The explanations provided emphasize that, in their opinion at least, petitioners' impairment was not related to any moral corruption (thus reinforcing the idea that the two were clearly distinct impediments). Indeed, clerics skilfully mobilized rhetorical devices to attest that, though they are physically and/or mentally impaired, their morals were fully intact.

'Faultless' Impairment

Historically, protocols for dealing with bodily defects amongst the clergy were harsh and inflexible. Canon law, however, offered the means to soften such regulations, on the proviso that a cleric bore no 'fault' for his impairment. Such legislation profoundly shaped the Chancery's approach, as is clearly shown in the papal letters. Alongside conforming to stipulations found in canonical compilations, the correspondence underlines that supplicants' potential liability is nullified if any of three conditions are met: if the impairment were congenital, or if it were acquired as a result of self-defence or necessary medical intervention. Petitioners were therefore classified as entirely 'innocent' if their physical incapacity was caused by a third party. Whether an impairment was inflicted by a master (*dominus*), a doctor, or a pagan, the impaired individual was himself blameless without possible doubt, and no further explanation was required. The first canon of the First Council of Nicaea (325), preserved in Gratian's *Decree*, was a touchstone for popes on this subject:

> If anyone due to sickness has undergone a surgical operation, or if he has been castrated by barbarians, he is allowed to remain among the clergy. But if anyone enrolled among the clergy has castrated himself when in perfect health, it is good for him to leave the ministry. From now on, no such person should be promoted to the clergy. But since this applies only to those who willfully castrate themselves, if anyone has been made a eunuch by barbarians, or by his master, and is otherwise fit for office, church law admits him to the clergy.[92]

92 Schaff (ed.), *Nicene/Post-Nicene Fathers*, volume 14, pp. 8–42. See also *Decretum Gratiani*, edited in Friedberg (ed.), *Corpus iuris canonici*, distinctio 55, canons 7–9. This provision can be

Even if caused by a third party, impairment could even be presented as 'no fault'. The madness of an assailant, for example, is an argument often used in petitions to attract pontifical grace.[93]

A letter written by Innocent III (1160–1216) to the Bishop of Odense, Sweden, concerning the impairment of O., a priest of the same diocese, highlights the way in which mental impairment could exculpate the avowedly guilty party:

> Having reached our presence, the priest O. warned us with a humble notification that, while some men were quarrelling in front of his house and he had left that house accidentally, without having committed any fault, one of them, throwing himself on him, excited by the devil (*diabolo instigante*), tore a finger from his left hand. The priest O. then humbly begged us to judge him worthy to continue his divine office. We therefore command your brotherhood [the Bishop of Odense] by apostolic writings to allow this priest, if it is proved, to serve freely in his order, the obstacle having been removed of any objection and appeal, for there are things that sometimes prevent one from being promoted but should not cause the rejection of those who are already promoted.[94]

In this instance, O. is faultless, as is his attacker. The injury was accidental: O. was in the wrong place at the wrong time, and his assailant was out of his senses. Innocent III deploys the classic legal formula of a criminal act *diabolo instigante* (instigated by the devil) to signify that the situation could lead to a great scandal, according to the medieval 'moral code'.[95] The Latin expression makes it possible to describe the intensity of the violence inflicted upon the priest, not just physical but moral. Moreover, it proves

found in the *Decree* of Yvo of Chartres, edited in Migne (ed.), *Patrologia Latina*, vol. 161, book 6, chapter 34. This passage is attributed to the collection of Greek decrees kept by Martin, Bishop of Braga.

93 Craig, "The History of Madness", p. 732.

94 Migne (ed.), *Patrologia Latina*, vol. 215, lettre 124, col. 1222 – Innocent III to the Bishop of Odense, 19 September 1207: '*Veniens ad praesentiam nostram O. presbyter humili nobis insinuatione monstravit quod cum ante domum suam quidam homines invicem rixarentur, et ipse casu domum exivisset eamdem, unus de rixantibus, nulla ejusdem presbyteri praecedente culpa, irruens in eumdem, diabolo instigante, sinistrae manus digitum amputavit eidem. Unde nobis humiliter supplicavit ut exsequendi suum officium ei licentiam concedere dignaremur. Quocirca fraternitati tuae per apostolica scripta mandamus quatenus, si est ita, presbyterum ipsum in ordine suo, sublato cujuslibet contradictionis et appellationis obstaculo, libere ministrare permittas, quaedam enim interdum impediunt promovendum quae non deiiciunt iam promotum*'.

95 See Turlan, "*Instigante diabolo*".

O.'s innocence in this brawl: the layman who attacked him was explicitly incited by the devil. More generally, this legal formula served to minimize the role, or responsibility, of an aggressor in the perpetration of a crime. If the guilty party later returned to health, here by 'regaining his senses', he would face a lesser punishment.[96] At times, then, this legal precept functioned to mitigate the consequences of certain criminal actions. In Innocent's letter, it functions to demonstrate O.'s innocence, whilst simultaneously mitigating the fault ascribed to his assailant. It seems unlikely, though, that O. really did leave his home entirely by chance, ignorant of the noisy row taking place outside his front door. Even if O.'s curiosity had compelled him to leave his residence, that would not necessarily make him wholly 'guilty' of his impairment. Yet it was customary for supplicants to proactively neutralize any presumption of their fault. Indeed, such narrative strategizing was essential: only if O. is considered faultless will he obtain a dispensation to continue to serve.

In canonical statues, exemptions were made for clerics who had undergone medically necessary amputations. For example, canon 22 of the Council of Lleida of 524 states that 'if a cleric, having fallen ill, is rendered lame by an operation which would have healed him, he may nevertheless be promoted to Holy Orders'.[97] Innocent III offers a similar ruling, in a letter addressed to the Bishop of Paris dated 12 February 1198, in the case of Michael, a leprous priest. The supplicant had been castrated, a condition which would normally disqualify him from office. However, he is allowed to keep his position as the castration was a medical intervention, with the express purpose of managing his leprosy.[98] Cases of childhood amputation were handled similarly. Childhood was the age of life characterized above all by innocence; a child could not knowingly commit a fault, nor were they responsible for acts done to them. This is illustrated, for instance, in a letter written by Clement III (1130–1191) and copied in Gregory IX's *Decretals*, regarding Bartholomew, a eunuch applicant for clerical office. Bartholomew was castrated as a baby, and thus bears no fault for his condition. Clement emphasizes the integral purity of the newborn by allowing Bartholomew

96 *Decretum Gratiani*, edited in Friedberg (ed.), *Corpus iuris canonici*, second part, cause 15, question 1, canon 12.

97 See op.cit., distinctio 55, canon 10 and the *Decree* of Yvo of Chartres, edited in Migne (ed.), *Patrologia Latina*, vol. 161, book 6, chapter 34.

98 Migne (ed.), *Patrologia Latina*, vol. 214, col. 15 D – Innocent III to the Bishop of Paris, 12 February 1198, also quoted in *Decretales Gregorii IX*, edited in Friedberg (ed.), *Corpus iuris canonici*, book I, title 20.

to enter the Church and become a priest.[99] If the supplicant could not demonstrate their innocence outright, however, they had one final avenue to pursue: an exculpatory plea of ignorance.

Partial Liability: Ignorance of the Law

The notion of personal liability for impairment allowed the Apostolic See to categorize supplicants as either 'guilty' or 'innocent', an efficient means by which to determine who qualified for papal grace. In canon law, this debate takes shape around the notion of *culpa precedens* (previous fault), which prompted canonists to question an individual's guilt.[100] However, this binary framework was not sufficient to handle cases in which supplicants were neither wholly guilty nor innocent, but rather *partially* liable: if they were, technically, responsible for their condition but there were substantive mitigating factors at play, such as in cases of self-injury. On this issue, canon law, theological texts, and pontifical letters were concerned above all with the intentions of the individual at the heart of the case, what motivated their self-mutilation.

In the Middle Ages, people with mental illness were not held responsible for their actions in civil, criminal, or canon law. Gratian's *Decree* explains, for example, that the deaf (*surdus*) and the mad (*prorsus*) cannot bring a case before a judge, as they do not have the faculty to hear or to understand what is happening to them.[101] Insanity could thus be invoked as an exculpatory factor in cases of self-injury. Legally speaking, an individual with madness cannot commit a criminal act. Similarly, Thomas Aquinas maintains that a madman cannot be blamed for his sins, if he lacks awareness that he is transgressing religious prohibitions:

> If the ignorance be such as to exclude the use of reason entirely, it excuses from sin altogether, as is the case with madmen (*furiosus*) and fools (*amentis*): but such is not always the ignorance that causes the sin; and so, it does not always excuse from sin altogether.[102]

99 *Decretales Gregorii IX*, op. cit., book I, title 20, chapter 3; see also *Decretum Gratiani*, op. cit. distinctio 55, canon 8.

100 On the concept of *culpa precendens*, see Parlopiano, "*Propter deformitatem*", p. 90.

101 *Decretum Gratiani*, edited in Friedberg (ed.), *Corpus iuris canonici*, second part, cause 3, question 7, chapter 1.

102 Thomas Aquinas, *Summa Theologiae I–II*, q. 76, article 3. On the vocabulary, see Gourevitch, "Les mots pour dire la folie".

Ignorance of a given law or regulation could, in certain circumstances, excuse its contravention.[103] The Church faced a particularly tricky set of cases: clergymen who had castrated themselves. On the one hand, this course of action was an explicit violation of ecclesiastical law. Yet clerics took the decision to castrate themselves, in some sense, to obey theological stricture more closely, and specifically to more easily resist temptations of the flesh.[104] In this, they followed the famous example of Origen (185–253), an early Christian theologian who proclaimed that he would castrate himself to guard against the sin of fornication.[105] Sinful sexual desire was such a problem for these clerics that the struggle for chastity became the primary means to demonstrate their piety and willingness to serve God. Their self-mutilation, then, is explained as a means to control their lust, and thereby to show their exemplary devotion to the Lord.[106] Indeed, clerics castrated by their own hand in the corpus explicitly distinguish themselves as more devout than their peers: rather than following their own desires, they serve God alone. This supports claims that they were ignorant that their actions would endanger their position in the orders. Owing to such ignorance, the supplicants are functionally blameless in their impairment. Such claims were not entirely spurious. After all, the Bible legitimizes self-castration in order to serve God more perfectly in Matthew 19:12:

> For there are some eunuchs, which were so born from their mother's womb: and there are some eunuchs, which were made eunuchs of men: and there be eunuchs, which have made themselves eunuchs for the kingdom of heaven's sake. He that is able to receive it, let him receive it.[107]

Correspondence in the case of the cleric Jacobus Bertrandi emblematizes the way in which cases of auto-castration were tackled. Jacobus had castrated himself in a fit of youthful zeal. Nevertheless, in a letter dated 7 March 1318, John XXII (1244–1334) grants him the right of full participation in the Church:

> The petition you have sent us contains that, while you were in your sixteenth year, seeking to extinguish the stimulating sting of the flesh

103 Thomas Aquinas, *Summa Theologiae I–II*, q. 88, article 6 or, on the same subject, *II–II*, q. 154, article 5.

104 On this see Dubourg, "Émasculations cléricales".

105 See Collins, "Appropriation and Development of Castration".

106 Karras, *Sexuality in Medieval Europe*, p. 39.

107 *The New King James Version*, Matthew 19:12.

> and wishing to serve God better, you committed the abominable crime of amputating your testicles with your own hand, and therefore, coming in pain towards the apostolic seat, you humbly beg us to judge you worthy in this matter with mercy. Therefore, we dispense you with our apostolic authority, inclined with compassionate affection to your supplications, so that, notwithstanding the above, you may be promoted in all orders and enter all religious orders.[108]

Here, Jacobus is cast as misguided, but not malign. He commits the sacrilege of self-castration, thereby risking his life, in an effort to prove his virtue and obedience to God by converting his desires into devotion. It is noteworthy that the mutilation occurred during his adolescence, a period in which it was widely acknowledged that temptations of the flesh multiplied.[109] Aged sixteen, Jacobus was two short years away from becoming eligible for the role of subdeacon, a rank with the requirements of both sufficient age and chastity. Locked in a ceaseless battle to control his sinful desires, his impulses finally took precedence over his reason.[110] Jacobus' intention was pure, even if his actions were ill-advised, to say the least. This provides sufficient grounds to exculpate him in the eyes of the Chancery, a decision supported by canonical precedent. In canon law, the precise issue of self-castration is discussed in a letter by Clement III, incorporated in the Gregory IX's *Decretals*. Clement reiterates the testimony of Archpriest Robert of Ravenna, who had appealed to the pontiff on behalf of one of his priests. Staunch in the belief that it would please God, the anonymous cleric had had his genitalia (*virilia*) amputated. Given the mitigating circumstances, Clement permits the cleric to continue to celebrate Mass.[111] Yet the Apostolic Constitutions prohibit the ordination of any individual with a bodily defect

108 RV 67, f. 224 V – John XXII to Jacobus Bertrandi, a schoolboy from Burgos, on 7 March 1318. Text analysed by Mollat (ed.), *Jean XXII*, n° 6 477, for which I give the transcription according to the register: '*Directa nobis ex parte petitio continebat quod cum tu olim in sextodecimo etatis tue anno constitutus existeres affectans extinguere carnis stimulos incentivos ut Deo acceptus servire valeres, ausu nephario tibi vasa seminaria propriis manibus amputasti propter quod ad apostolicam sedem laborans nobis fecisti humiliter supplicari, ut providere tibi super hoc de oportuno remedio misericorditer dignaremus. Nos igitur pro tibi super hoc compatientes affectu tuis supplicationibus inclinati, tecum ut premissis nequaquam obstantibus possis ad omnes ordines te facere promoveri et aliqua intrare religionem de ordinibus approbatis auctoritate apostolica dispensamus*'.

109 McGuire, "Jean Gerson and Traumas", p. 85.

110 Thibodeaux, "From Boys to Priest", p. 143.

111 *Decretales Gregorii IX*, edited in Friedberg (ed.), *Corpus iuris canonici,* book I, title 20, chapter 4.

for which they are directly liable.[112] Letters of papal grace, such as those issued by Clement III to the anonymous cleric and by John XXII to Jacobus Bertrandi, countermand such ordinances and allowed for the inclusion of impaired clerics in the Church, even those with personal responsibility for their condition.

In its adjudication of petitioners' personal liability, the pontifical administration exhibited a very narrow scope of interest. If a petitioner satisfied basic conditions, or if they could provide a plausible narrative that established their lack of blame, then their impairment could be classed as 'faultless'. In more complex cases, intention was everything. The Chancery's role, in cases of self-injury or partial liability, was to determine whether an individual had expressly intended to transgress the relevant laws. In the period spanning the twelfth to the fourteenth century, the moral integrity of clerics with mental illness or those responsible for their own injuries was not a relevant topic – as long as such petitioners' claims of impairment-related 'innocence' were upheld. In the petitions and letters, we find traces of the personal experiences of disabled clerics. But such testimonies are modulated due to the nature of the purpose they served. Supplicants supplied biographical narratives with the aim of fulfilling criteria established by the Church to regulate the recognition of disability. In this way, the petitions shed light on the way in which the Apostolic See constructed disability, and the way in which clerics practically responded to the institution's demands.

Conclusion

Comparative analysis of relevant texts – petitions and papal letters, canon law, and theological works – demonstrates that the pontifical institution had more leeway than one might first expect when responding to supplicants. The Chancery had grounds to expel an impaired cleric from the Church, or alternatively to implement or relax canonical regulation and permit their continued presence in the clerical community. Whilst defects of body and mind were serious issues, in legal terms, they did not present insurmountable obstacles for clerics. Petitioners had several avenues at their disposal to mitigate the gravity of defects or to neutralize their negative ramifications outright. Firstly, applicants had to establish their moral purity, and precisely delineate the effects of their condition, in terms of

112 Metzger, *Les constitutions apostoliques*, VIII, 47. 22–24 and *Decretum Gratiani*, edited in Friedberg (ed.), *Corpus iuris canonici*, distinctio 55, chapter 4.

any associated incapacity. Secondly, petitioners had to demonstrate that their presence would not generate *scandalum* in the community, even if they were unable to perform their duties as usual. Finally, they had to convince the Apostolic See that they bore no liability for their impairment, or if they did, then there were mitigating circumstances that exculpated them. This was achieved by tailoring their petitions to the expectations of the Chancery, by providing 'acceptable' explanations. If these three criteria were met, petitioners were eligible to receive a pontifical grace, an outcome explored in depth in Chapters 3 and 4. If, however, petitioners failed any of these criteria, their fate was rather grim. This left the Apostolic See little, if any, room to manoeuvre in terms of flexing canonical prohibitions: clerics who failed in their petitions could be dismissed from their office, as in the cases discussed in Chapter 5.

The framework of canon law that emerged in the period between the fourth and sixth centuries distinguishes moral and bodily defects, both of which lead to prohibition. The development of contemporary pontifical theocracy closely followed the legal trajectory. From the eleventh century onwards, however, doctrine gradually evolved: 'bodily defect' become less serious than moral 'defect' and does not have the same consequences. The Gregorian reforms further advanced legal thinking, instantiating the notion of the pontificate as an agent of divine law endowed with superior spiritual and temporal.[113] This meant that the Pope could now grant grace, a policy that came into full effect in the thirteenth century, though it had been developed before the second half of the twelfth century. Individuals in receipt of papal grace were permitted to adapt their personal situation to their abilities. Crucially, such grants did not create new legislation, nor did they always dispense with a given law. Rather, they applied or interpreted existing law in specific ways, thereby establishing precedent that led to further developments in doctrine. Above all, papal letters were practical documents, operating as a formal guide for the daily activity of the clergy to whom they were addressed.[114]

The presence of a physical or mental defect constituted an irregularity, a deviation from the standard of moral, physical, and intellectual perfection that all clerics were expected to uphold. The category of defect was integrally diverse, reflecting the wide array of impairments with which clerics lived. A similar flexibility is evident in the notion of incapacity,

113 Robinson, "The Institutions of the Church", p. 373.

114 Gaudemet, *Les sources du droit canonique*, p. 63. These pontifical letters can also be taken as decrees, to be integrated into the scholastic canons according to their degree of applicability.

another crucial concept in the construction of irregularity. There was no singular standard for capacity, against which all clerics were judged. Instead, petitioners' relative (in)capacity was determined in the context of their specific circumstances, and their lived experience of impairment. Chapter 2 analyses the ways in which such determinations were made.

Bibliography

Primary Sources

Joseph BIDEZ et al. (eds.), *Histoire ecclésiastique. Livres V–VI*, Éditions du Cerf, 2005.
FRIEDBERG (ed.), *Corpus iuris canonici*, Akademische Druck- u. Verlagsanstalt, 1959.
GALVANUS DE BONONIA, *De presbytero irregularitati subiecto ob consecratum extra Missam Eucharisticum Panem*, B. A.V., Vat. Lat. 2683.
GUILLAUME LE TALLEUR, *Dictionarius familiaris et compendiosus: dictionnaire latin-français de Guillaume Le Talleur*, ed. Brian MERRILEES, William EDWARDS, Brepols, 2002.
Jean HARDOUIN (ed.), *Conciliorum collectio regia maxima*, Ex Tipographia Regia, 1715.
Anne-Marie HAYEZ, Janine MATHIEU and Marie-France YVAN (eds.), *Grégoire XI (1370–1378): lettres communes analysées d'après les registres dits d'Avignon et du Vatican*, École française de Rome, 1992.
Bruno JUDIC, Floribert ROMMEL and Charles MOREL (eds.), *Règle pastorale*, Éditions du Cerf, 1992.
Ludwig WAHRMUND (ed.), *Summa Aurea*, Scientia Verlag, 1962.
Kamil KROFTA (ed.), *Monumenta vaticana res gestas Bohemicas illustrantia T. 5 – Acta Urbani VI et Bonifatii IX*, Typis Gregerianis, 1903.
Joseph DE LOYE, Pierre DE CENIVAL, Auguste COULON and Charles DE LA RONCIÈRE (eds.), *Les registres d'Alexandre IV: recueil des bulles de ce pape*, Boccard, 1953.
Marcel METZGER (ed.), *Les constitutions apostoliques*, les Éditions du Cerf, 2012.
Jacques Paul MIGNE (ed.), *Patrologiae Cursus Completus, Series Latina*, Paris, Migne, 1844–1855.
Guillaume MOLLAT (ed.), *Jean XXII (1316–1334): Lettres communes analysées d'après les registres dits d'Avignon et du Vatican*, Albert Fontemoing, 1923.
Jan Frederik NIERMEYER (ed.), *Mediae latinitatis lexicon minus*, Brill, 1993.
Philip SCHAFF (ed.), *Nicene/Post-Nicene Fathers*, series 2, ed. By Christian Classics Ethereal Library, transl. by Aaron M. Jensen on fourthcentury.com website.
The New King James Version, Thomas Nelson publishers, 2020.

THOMAS AQUINAS, *Commentary on the Sentences*, ed. By The Aquina Institue and transl. By Beth MORTENSEN, URL consulted on 31 July 2021: https://aquinas.cc/.
THOMAS AQUINAS, *Summa Theologiae I–II*, ed. By The Aquinas Institute and transl. by Fr. Laurence SHAPCOTE, URL consulted on 31 July 2021: https://aquinas.cc/.

Secondary Sources

Paul ABBERLEY, "Disabled People, Normality and Social Work", *in* Len BARTON (ed.), *Disability and Dependency*, Falmer Press, 1989, pp. 53–66.
Colin BARNES, "A Legacy of Oppression: A History of Disability in Western Culture", *in* Len BARTON and Michael OLIVER (eds.), *Disability Studies: Past, Present and Future*, Disability Press, 1997, pp. 3–24.
Julia BARROW, *The Clergy in the Medieval World: Secular Clerics, their Families and Careers in North-Western Europe, c. 800–c. 1200*, Cambridge University Press, 2015.
Columban BOCK, "Tonsure monastique et tonsure cléricale", *Revue de droit canonique*, 2 (1952), pp. 373–406.
Pierre BOURDIEU, *La distinction: critique sociale du jugement*, Éditions de minuit, 1979.
Philippe CASPAR, *Le peuple des silencieux: une histoire du handicap et de la déficience mentale*, Édition Fleurus, 1994.
Jack COLLINS, "Appropriation and Development of Castration as Symbol and Practice in Early Christianity", *in* Larissa TRACY (ed.), *Castration and Culture in the Middle Ages*, D.S. Brewer, 2013, pp. 73–86.
Leigh Ann CRAIG, "The History of Madness and Mental Illness in the Middle Ages: Directions and Questions", *History Compass*, 12.9 (2014), pp. 729–744.
Antoine DESTEMBERG and Thierry KOUAMÉ, "Aux origines de l'*homo academicus*: Les signes de distinction sociale chez les universitaires médiévaux", *in* Jean-Philippe GENET and E. Igor MINEO (eds.), *Marquer la prééminence sociale*, Éditions de la Sorbonne, 2015, pp. 45–55.
William J. DOHAR, "*Sufficienter litteratus*: Clerical Examination and Instruction for the Cure of Souls", *in* Jacqueline BROWN and William P. STONEMAN (eds.), *A Distinct Voice: Medieval Studies in Honor of Leonard E. Boyle*, University of Notre Dame Press, 1997, pp. 305–321.
Mary DOUGLAS, *Purity and Danger: An Analysis of Concepts of Pollution and Taboo*, Routledge & Kegan Paul, 1966.
Carol DOWNER, "The Coptic and Ethiopic Traditions", *in* Christian LAES (ed.), *Disabilities in Roman Antiquity: Disparate Bodies, a Capite ad Calcem*, Brill, 2013, pp. 367–375.
Ninon DUBOURG, "Émasculations cléricales. Itinéraires particuliers pour aborder l'identité du clerc émasculé (XIIe–XVe siècle)", *Encyclo. Revue de l'école doctorale ED 382*, 4 (2014), pp. 89–101.

Ninon DUBOURG, "Being a Leprous Cleric – In/ability to Hold a Benefice (XIIIth and XIVth centuries)", in Erin CONNELLY and Stefanie KÜNZEL (eds), *New Approaches to Disease, Disability and Medicine in Medieval Europe*, collection *Studies in Early Medicine*, Archaeopress, 2018, pp. 62–77.

Ninon DUBOURG, "Un/Acceptable Disability? *Defectus Corporis, Scandalum,* and Pontifical Grace", in Teodora ARTIMON and Andrea ZNOROVSZKY (eds), *Materializing Ugliness and Deformity in the Middle Ages*, Trivent Publishing, (forthcoming).

Martha L. EDWARDS ROSE, "Constructions of Physical Disability in the Ancient Greek World: the Community Concept", *in* David T. MITCHELL and Sharon L. SNYDER (eds.), *The Body and Physical Difference: Discourses of Disability*, University of Michigan Press, 1997, pp. 35–50.

Melodie EICHBAUER, "Legal Authorities and their Legislative Priorities: The Treatment of Leprosy in the Sources of Canon Law", *Zeitschrift der Savigny-Stiftung für Rechtsgeschichte: Kanonistische Abteilung*, 106.1 (2020), pp. 153–195.

Vic FINKELSTEIN, *Attitudes and Disabled People: Issues for Discussion*, International Exchange of Information in Rehabilitation, 1980.

Arnaud FOSSIER, "*Propter vitandum scandalum.* Histoire d'une catégorie juridique (XIIe–XVe siècles)", *Mélanges de l'École française de Rome-Moyen Âge*, 121.2 (2009), pp. 317–348.

Arnaud FOSSIER, "A propos du *defectus natalium.* Un cas paradigmatique du pouvoir pontifical de dispense (XIe–XVe siècle)", *in* Carole AVIGNON (ed.), *Bâtards et bâtardises dans l'Europe médiévale et moderne*, Presses Universitaires de Rennes, 2016, pp. 115–124.

Robert GARLAND, *The Eye of the Beholder: Deformity and Disability in the Graeco-Roman World*, Cornell University Press, 1995.

Jean GAUDEMET, *Les sources du droit canonique, VIIIe–XXe siècle: repères canoniques, sources occidentales*, Cerf, 1993.

Danielle GOUREVITCH, "Les mots pour dire la folie en latin: à propos de passages de Celse et de Célius Aurélien", *L'évolution psychiatrique*, 56.3 (1991), pp. 561–568.

Danielle GOUREVITCH, "La conception galénique de la maladie", *La revue du praticien*, 51.18 (2001), pp. 1995–2000.

Gilbert GUAYDIER, *Les irrégularités* "ex defectu corporis", Société Générale d'Imprimerie et d'Édition, 1933.

Harlan HAHN, "Toward a politics of disability: Definitions, disciplines, and policies", *The Social Science Journal*, 22.4 (1985), pp. 87–105.

Richard HELMHOLZ, "*Scandalum* in the Medieval Canon Law and in the English Ecclesiastical Courts", *Zeitschrift Der Savigny-Stiftung fur Rechtsgeschichte: Kanonistische Abteilung*, 127 (2010), pp. 258–274.

Thomas HENTRICH, "Being Disabled in the Ancient Near East. A Brief Compilation from Mesopotamia to Qumran", *Revue d'Études des Civilisations Anciennes du Proche-Orient*, 13 (2007), pp. 29–35.

Joseph HOLLWECK, *Die Kirchlichen Strafgesetze*, Franz Kirchheim, 1899.

Ruth Mazo KARRAS, *Sexuality in Medieval Europe: Doing unto Others*, Routledge, 2005.

Christian LAES, Chris F. GOODEY and Martha Lynn ROSE, "Approaching Disabilities a Capite ad Calcem: Hidden Themes in Roman Antiquity", *in* Christian LAES, Chris F. GOODEY and Martha Lynn ROSE (ed.), *Disabilities in Roman Antiquity: Disparate Bodies, a Capite ad Calcem*, Brill, 2013, pp. 1–15.

Jacques LE GOFF, "Métier et profession d'après les manuels de confesseurs au Moyen Âge", *Miscellanea Mediaevalia*, III: Beiträge zum Berufsbewufitsem des mittelaterlichen Menschen (1964), pp. 44–60.

Patrick LEGROS, *Les processus discriminatoires des politiques du handicap*, Presses universitaires de Grenoble, 2014.

Corinne LEVELEUX-TEIXEIRA, "*Fama* et mémoire de la peine dans la doctrine romano-canonique (XIIIe–XVIe siècle)", *in* Jacqueline HOAREAU-DODINAU and Pascal TEXIER (eds.), *La peine: discours, pratiques, représentations*, Presses Universitaires de Limoges, 2005, pp. 45–61.

Bruce LINK and Jo PHELAN, "Conceptualizing Stigma", *Annual Review of Sociology*, 27 (2001), pp. 363–385.

Brian Patrick MCGUIRE, "Jean Gerson and Traumas of Masculine Affectivity and Sexuality", *in* Jacqueline MURRAY (ed.), *Conflicted Identities and Multiple Masculinities: Men in the Medieval West*, Garland, 1999, pp. 45–72.

Irina METZLER, "Then and Now: Canon Law on Disabilities", *in* Christian LAES, Chris F. GOODEY and Martha Lynn ROSE (eds.), *Disabilities in Roman Antiquity: Disparate Bodies, a capite ad calcem*, Brill, 2013, pp. 455–467.

Michèle MULCHAHEY, *'First the Bow is Bent in Study…': Dominican Education Before 1350*, Pontifical Institute for Medieval Studies, 2000.

Jacqueline MURRAY, "Masculinizing Religious Life: Sexual Prowess, the Battle for Chastity and Monastic Identity", *in* Katherine Jane LEWIS and Patricia H. CULLUM (eds.), *Holiness and Masculinity in the Middle Ages*, University of Wales press, 2004, pp. 24–42.

Jacqueline MURRAY, "One Flesh, Two Sexes, Three Genders ?", *in* Lisa M. BITEL and Felice LIFSHITZ (eds.), *Gender and Christianity in Medieval Europe: New Perspectives*, University of Pennsylvania Press, 2008, pp. 34–51.

Raoul NAZ, *Dictionnaire de droit canonique*, Letouzey et Ané, 1935.

Paolo OSTINELLI, "I chierici e il "*defectus corporis*": Definizioni canonistiche, suppliche, dispense", *in* Gian Maria VARANINI (ed.), *Deformità fisica e identità della persona tra medioevo ed età moderna*, Firenze University Press, 2015, pp. 3–30.

Brandon PARLOPIANO, "*Propter deformitatem*: Towards a Concept of Disability in Medieval Canon Law", *Canadian Journal of Disability Studies*, 4.3 (2015), pp. 72–102.

Rebecca RAPHAEL, *Biblical Corpora: Representations of Disability in Hebrew Biblical Literature*, Bloomsbury, 2008.

Anne REVILLARD and Pierre-Yves BAUDOT, "Introduction: une sociologique de l'état par les droits", *in* Pierre-Yves BAUDOT and Anne REVILLARD (eds), *L'État des droits: politique des droits et pratiques des institutions*, SciencePo. Les presses, 2015, pp. 11–58.

Ian S. ROBINSON, "The Institutions of the Church, 1073–1216", *in* David LUSCOMBE and Jonathan RILEY-SMITH (eds.), *The New Cambridge Medieval History*, Cambridge University Press, 2004, pp. 368–460.

Henry Joseph SCHROEDER, *Disciplinary Decrees of the General Councils: Text, Translation and Commentary*, B. Herder, 1937.

John R. SHINNERS and William J. DOHAR, *Pastors and the Care of Souls in Medieval England*, University of Notre Dame Press, 1998.

Donald STAMPS and Adams J. WESLEY (eds.), *Fire Bible – KJV: A Study Bible for Spirit-Led Living*, Hendrickson Publishers, 2012.

Henri-Jacques STIKER, *A History of Disability*, The University of Michigan Press, 2020 (revised edition).

Friederike STÖHR, *Körpermakel – Arbeits(un)fähigkeit – Kirchenrecht: Körperlich versehrte, kranke und alte Geistliche im spätmittelalterlichen Deutschen Reich und in Skandinavien*, Didymos-Verlag, 2020.

Jennifer D. THIBODEAUX, "From Boys to Priest: Adolescence, Masculinity and the Parish Clergy in Medieval Normandy", *in* Jennifer THIBODEAUX (ed.), *Negotiating Clerical Identities: Priests, Monks and Masculinity in the Middle Ages*, Palgrave Macmillan, 2010, pp. 136–158.

J. TINEL, "Étude de quelques maladies nerveuses et mentales au point de vue de l'admission au sacerdoce", *Bulletin de la société médicale de Saint Luc, Saint Côme et Saint Damien*, 1929, pp. 66–77.

Juliette M. TURLAN, "*Instigante diabolo*", *in Mélanges offerts a Jean Dauvillier*, Centre d'histoire juridique méridionale, 1979, pp. 803–808.

Walter ULLMANN, *A Short History of the Papacy in the Middle Ages*, Taylor & Francis, 2004.

Jérôme WILGAUX, "Ὑγιὴς καὶ ὁλόκλαρος. Le corps du prêtre en Grèce ancienne", in Pierre BRULÉ (ed.), *La norme en matière religieuse en Grèce ancienne*, Presses universitaires de Liège, 2013, pp. 231–242.

Ian WILKS, "Moral Intention", in John MARENBON (ed.), *The Oxford Handbook of Medieval Philosophy*, Oxford University Press, 2012, pp. 588–604.

2 Aetiologies of Impairment: Congenital, Geriatric, and Acquired Conditions

Abstract

As presented in this chapter, during the petition process, supplicants defined their impairments through dialogue with the Papal Chancery. They drew on medical and religious culture, evident in the specific words deployed in letters, to present the causes of their impairments and to relate their ongoing experiences. Letters from the Chancery in response make use of similar terminology and frameworks, highlighting that petitioners' conceptualizations of disability was shared by the Curia's staff and vice versa. The legal, cultural, and linguistic frameworks provided by Chapters 1 and 2 allow us to develop argumentative strands in the later chapters.

Keywords: Discourses; Aetiology; Medicine; Religion

All applicants to the orders were subject to vetting to ensure their suitability. Yet men hoping to become responsible for the care of souls (*cura animarum*) were under even more intense scrutiny. The care of souls was perhaps the single most important task in the clerical portfolio; clerics with such benefices must be above reproach, and thus were held to higher standards of idoneity than the rank-and-file clergy. This is exemplified in a letter from Urban VI (1318–1389) to the Franciscan leadership, written at some point after 1381 and collected by the convent S. Francesco di Conegliano, now preserved in the Archivio Status Tervisii. The Pope addresses Ludovicus de Venetiis, Minister General of the Order of Friars Minor, and Marcus de Conegliano, professor of the same Order, on an urgent matter: ensuring that sufficient checks have been undertaken on a candidate pursuing the role of master in the order, Brother Franciscus Belluni. Beyond illuminating this specific case, the letter reveals how the popes continued to resolve the tricky question of access to the sacred orders at the beginning of the Great Schism.

Dubourg, N., *Disabled Clerics in the Late Middle Ages. Un/suitable for Divine Service?*
Taylor & Francis Group, 2023
DOI: 10.5117/9789463721561_CH02

Franciscus' request is neither as straightforward nor as simple as it might first appear. Masters in the Franciscan order were permitted to preach, to give sermons and to celebrate the divine offices. Accession to the vaunted rank of master thus obligated scrupulous attention to applicants' suitability, as Urban emphasizes:

> Consequently, having no certainty as to the capacity and idoneity of Franciscus we ask your discretion to inform us of this, in which we have great faith in the Lord, and we undertake and request that you or one of you, verify that Franciscus is indeed thirty years of age, that he is indeed the offspring of a legitimate marriage, that he is not tainted by any criminal infamy or serious and notorious crime, nor of a monstrous body, nor born (*naturaliter*) without one of his limbs, nor mutilated because of an accident (*casualiter*), and that, if this Franciscus studies and reads philosophy and theology for at least eight years, [...] it is conceded by the apostolic authority that he is authorized to teach in the faculty, in the city of Padua and other places of the Veneto in which he has received the title of master.[1]

Here, the Pope sets out the intellectual and practical criteria that Franciscus must fulfil in order to become a master. The cleric must be of appropriate age, of legitimate birth, and without a reputation of criminality. More importantly for the present discussion, his body must not bear any mark of 'mutilation' nor any sign of 'monstrosity'. This prohibition holds even if such deformities originated in 'natural or accidental causes', as long as the applicant himself was deemed 'faultless' for the condition. Fulfilment of such criteria was only the first stage in the process of becoming a master, however. As recounted in the rest of the letter, a roster of witnesses – in this case, all masters of the Order – had to attest to Franciscus' exemplary faith and morality. Once that had been settled, he would embark upon a

1 Cenci, *Supplementum*, n° 34, p. 84. Urban VI to Ludovicus de Venetiis, Minister General of the Order of Friars Minor, and to Marcus de Conegliano, professor of that Order, 12 June 1381. Text edited by Sartori, *Archivio Sartori*, n°4, p. 578: '*Nos igitur de suficientia et idoneitate ipsius Francisci ad hoc certam notitiam non habentes, discretioni tue de qua in iis et aliis gerimus in Domino fiduciam specialem per apostolica scripta committimus et mandamus, quatenus vos vel alter vestrum dicto Francisco si ipsum triginta annos habere, de legitimo matrimonio procreatum, nullaque infamia criminali respersum, aut gravi notatum crimine vel corpore monstruosum, aut membro aliquo naturaliter carere, vel casualiter mutilatum fore, et si eundem Franciscum studuisse et legisse ad minus in Philosophia octo annis, et totidem in Theologia,* [...] *in civitate Paduana vel in dicto loco Venetiarum huiusmodi magistrerii honorem et licentiam docendi in facultate predicta auctoritate apostolica concedatis.*'

long and rigorous course of education.[2] With the enumeration of defects that would block Franciscus' promotion to the role of master, this letter effectively offers a definition of idoneity, or at least the one mobilized by Urban VI and his Chancery. At the same time, this document operates as something of a primer on the causes of impairment typically referred to in papal letters – be they congenital, accidental, disease-, or age-related – as well as to the standard vocabulary used by both supplicants and the Chancery. Analysis of these elements, whether deployed consciously or unconsciously, reveals the writing strategies and goals of the various actors in the supplication process. Indeed, supplicants present the cause(s) and the consequence(s) of their impairment by mobilizing discursive strategies, in order to implement the recognition of their disability. They must then navigate smartly to receive their pontifical grace.

There were two main approaches to the relationship between grace, sin, and impairment in the Middle Ages. In his twelfth-century *Sentences*, Pierre Lombard (c. 1100–1160) offers a useful summary. Quoting Bede the Venerable (c. 672–735), Lombard delineates the five reasons for which individuals receive bodily afflictions:

> For scourges befall (*flagello*) in five ways: either so that the merits of the just be increased by their patience, as with Job; or for the safe-keeping of the virtues, lest pride attack, as in Paul; or to correct sins, as in Mary's leprosy; or to the glory or for the *glory* of God, like the man born blind; or for the beginning of punishment, like Herod, that here may be seen what happens in hell, according to this saying: 'Consume them with double contrition, oh Lord'.[3]

Drawing on biblical exempla, the author elucidates the strong link between personal or parental fault and physical or mental impairment. During her lifetime Mary was punished with leprosy for slandering her brother, Moses; in the afterlife, Herod, the king of Jerusalem, was punished by being eaten alive by worms for his murder of the apostle James.[4] God's chastisement is twofold: individuals are first punished in the earthly world with physical affliction, and then again in the spiritual realm, by the denial of salvation.[5]

2 Clerical education programmes of this kind are discussed in depth in Chapter 3.

3 Silano (ed.), *The Sentences*, vol. 4 (distinctio 15, chapter 2), p. 78. He quotes Matthew 9:4; Job 1:12–22; Corinthians II:12, 7; Numbers 12:10; John 9:3; Acts 12:23.

4 On the link between impairments and sins, see Metzler, *Disability in Medieval Europe*, pp. 38–55.

5 Gianfalla, "'Ther is moore mysshapen'", p. 127.

In other words, impairment occurs at both a physical and spiritual level. This so-called moral model corresponds to the historical interpretation of impairment as a marker of sin, an interpretation that has existed from Antiquity onwards, and is supported by the Bible.[6] The second approach offers a more positive view of impairment, however, and is equally supported by biblical material. Impairment is a test set by God to enable an individual to prove their faith.[7] Man must endure all the calamities that his Creator sends him without questioning his goodness. Here again, Lombard leverages biblical examples to underscore his point. Job endures agony upon agony, yet his faith only keeps growing; Paul embraces sickness in order to safeguard his humility and get closer to the suffering of Christ. Similarly, the healing of unnamed blind men in The New Testament demonstrates God's munificence. Their sensory impairment is an opportunity to manifest divine goodness in the world.

Such a binary cultural conception of impairment echoes anthropological theories, shedding light on the psychic ambivalence we show towards physical and mental disability, vacillating between compassion and rejection.[8] In the Middle Ages, the choice of approach largely depends on the type of documentation at hand.[9] The first paradigm foregrounds and legitimizes societal exclusion, providing that such action complies with the salvation doctrine as established in theology. It presupposes a direct, albeit theoretical, link between sin and impairment, and thus dominates in canon law. The second approach, by contrast, underscores that the inclusion of difference is one of the core characteristics of medieval Christian society.[10] Unsurprisingly, it prevails in petitions, papal letters, and other practical documentation which discusses the societal integration of disabled people. Thus, it appears that the Chancery cares about the clerical consequences of impairment, that is to say, about the cleric's disability and not his impairment (or the specificities thereof).

The Principal Causes of Clerical Impairment

Notwithstanding any moral aetiology, the majority of supplicants in the corpus are disabled by bodily weakness, both congenital and acquired (65%)

6 Kristiansen, Vehmas, and Shakespeare, *Arguing about Disability*, p. 2.

7 Cusack, "*Graciosi*", p. 414.

8 On the continuity of the binary approach between acceptance and exclusion from an anthropological perspective, see Stiker, "Pour une nouvelle théorie".

9 See Scarborough, *Viewing Disability*.

10 Frohne and Horn, "On the Fluidity of 'Disability'", p. 18.

(Fig. 2.1). The next most frequent causes of disability, age-related incapacity (12%) and sensory impairments, both congenital and acquired (10%), trail distantly behind. I gather under the terminology of 'physical weaknesses' undefined infirmities and diseases (referred to by the vague terms *infirmitas* or *debilitas*) in order to respect the imprecision of medieval terms (see the next section, Writing Disability). Collectively, these categories account for more than 87% of the impairment burden of the total cohort. The remainder are ascribed to: mutilation, such as limb loss (6%); physical impairment, such as mobility-limiting conditions both congenital and acquired (5%); leprosy (1%); and mental weakness both congenital and acquired (1%).

Figure 2.1 Main causes of clerical impairment on 1140 cases (twelfth to fourteenth century)

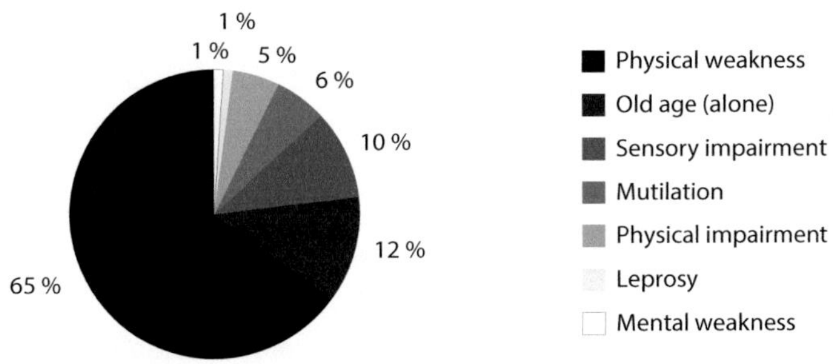

The following sections discuss aetiologies of disability in the corpus, along the life-stage trajectory. At birth, congenital conditions come to light, and later impairments are acquired through disease, in accidents, or as a result of advancing age. This study productively increases our understanding on two intersecting planes.[11] On a micro level, consideration of supplicants' age allows us to discern the specificities of their lived experiences in greater detail. At the macro level, such framing allows us to identify the archetypes of medieval impairment. The transition between childhood and adulthood, and the shift from mid-life to old age, constitute two distinct periods of identity construction. The former marks the beginning of working life, in which the impaired cleric may require certain accommodations for the first time. The latter signifies the end of work, a period in which some clerics may experience impairment for the first time in their lives, and impaired clerics may experience new symptoms or an age-related increase in the severity of their existing condition(s). In all periods, impaired clerics relied on the

11 See Irwin, "Repositioning Disability".

receipt of papal grace in order to facilitate their integration in the Church, and the appropriate adjustment of ecclesiastical regulations.

Congenital Impairment

Today, only 15% of disabilities are congenital.[12] In the corpus of papal letters, we find fourteen cases in which 'proven' birth defects play a role (a little more than 1%). This includes, for example, supplicants living with clubfoot, deafness, and certain types of blindness.[13] The medieval conception of heredity explains the causes of physical impairment in terms of the mixture of both parents' humours during the formation of the foetus. Although this theory has its roots in medical theories inherited from Antiquity, it was significantly developed in the Middle Ages.[14] It became an established medical category from the 1250s onwards, accepted both in intellectual circles and in canon law.[15] Theological discourse adopted, and adapted, medical conceptions of heredity. From a theological perspective, parental sin was a direct cause of physical infirmity in newborns, a conjecture supporting the Church's aim of regulating, or 'normalizing', sexual practices.[16] The formation of the foetus was not a purely biological affair, but intrinsically moral, too. Parents' moral faults *and* humoral qualities were passed on to their offspring, forever marking them in the form of impairment.[17]

Ecclesiastical authorities endorsed the notion of the fundamentally moral dimension of procreation. This supported the widespread dissemination of the theory in canon law and medical texts. As witnessed by examples from the corpus, such ideas filtered into supplications and papal letters, which dealt with matters of heredity in more practical terms. This is evident, for example, in the case of Johannes of Kemnicz, a subdeacon in the diocese of Prague, whose dossier was filed by the Chancery on 20 April 1344. Johannes had asked Pope Clement VI (1291–1352) to be allowed to receive major orders and an ecclesiastical benefice with or without care of souls, despite his ocular birth defect. Clement responds:

12 Siebers, "Disability in Theory", p. 742.

13 There were few birth defects in the medieval period due to the infant mortality rate, which was between 12 and 20 per cent according to experts, and the high rate of chronic illness among children. See Rawcliffe, "Sickness and Health". The numbers were drawn from Sandidge, "Changing Contexts of Infanticide", p. 301.

14 Metzler, "Disabled Children", p. 165.

15 See Lugt and Miramon (eds.), *L'hérédité entre Moyen Âge et époque moderne*.

16 Thomasset, "La représentation de la sexualité", p. 13.

17 Pearman, "'O Sweete Venym Queynte!'", p. 32.

> And so you, who believed yourself to be the product of a legitimate marriage, received minor orders in spite of the birthmark (*macula*) in your left eye, [...] you were elected a canon in the churches of Prague by the chapter of this canonical church and promoted to all sacred orders, but then a certain doctor from Paris, who promised to remove the birthmark from your eye, ended up destroying your eye, and so you were able to be a prebendary canon of the church of Wrocław thanks to our letters.[18]

The letter explicitly establishes a parallel between moral and physical defects of birth, with mention of 'legitimate' parentage (and thus the spectre of *il*legitimate parentage) juxtaposed with the literal stain on Johannes' eye. The two congenital conditions seem to be accorded equal weight.[19] Johannes' ocular stain, a physical birth defect, was not a bar to joining minor orders, when Johannes was unaware of his *defectus natalis* (defect of birth). Indeed, we learn elsewhere in the letter that the cleric's enemies accuse him of a moral defect which would cast his ocular impairment in an altogether different light. They proclaim that he is of illegitimate birth, the product of a clandestine marriage, with his parents living in sin under the same roof for several years.[20] The issue at stake in the letter, however, is not Johannes' parentage per se – even if he also must receive a pontifical grace for it – but rather his own actions. His congenital impairment only became an ecclesiastical problem after Johannes sought medical treatment from a Parisian doctor to remove the stain. Instead, the procedure 'destroyed' his eye. It is for this reason that Johannes appeals to the Pope for a special pardon, both for his *defectus corporis*, owing to the mutilation of his eye, and for his *defectus natalis*, citing his ignorance of any immorality in his parents' union for not having asked for grace before.

In his supplication, which is repeated in its entirety in the Chancery's letter of response, Johannes himself could underscores that the contravention of religious prohibitions during intercourse endangers any children conceived

18 RV 159, f. 414 (RA 76, f. 288) – Clement VI to Johannes of Kemnicz, subdeacon in the diocese of Prague, 20 April 1344. Text edited by Klicman, *Monumenta vaticana*, n° 335, p. 198: '*Tuque postmodum, qui te credebas prout credis fore de legitimo matrimonio procreatum, omnes minores ordines suscepisti et deinde quadam macula in oculo tuo sinistro orta* [...] *per eleccionem dd. ff. capituli eiusdem ecclesie canonicatum fuisti alias canonice assecutus teque fecisti ad omnes sacros ordines promoveri, quodque postmodum quidam medicus existens Parisius, qui tibi promiserat huiusmodi maculam de ipso oculo removere, oculum ipsum destruxit, ac deinde canonicatum sub expectactione prebende ecclesie Wratislaviensis per nostras litteras assecutus fuisti*'.

19 On the notion of a *macula* (stain), see Steinberg, *Une tache au front*, p. 19.

20 On clandestine marriages, see Avignon, "Les mariages clandestins".

from the act.[21] Such unfortunate offspring are marked with impairment, deformity, epilepsy, or leprosy according to Church authorities, including second-century authors Caesarius of Arles and Gregory of Tours, alongside material compiled in Gratian's *Decree*.[22] From the latter anthology, a letter written in the mid-seventh century by Boniface, Archbishop of Mainz, is particularly useful in forwarding Johannes' agenda. In this text, Boniface suggests that corrupt carnal unions produce vitiated children. This idea was frequently repeated in the following centuries, perhaps most notably by Lothair of Segni, who was elected Pope in 1198 and reigned as Innocent III.[23] Johannes' supplication bears witness, thus, to the fact that deviant sexual behaviour was increasingly prohibited and punished by the Church during the thirteenth century, whilst the sacrament of marriage was promoted with ever more fervour.[24]

Accidentally Acquired Impairments

In theory, clerical supplicants are under the aegis of the Church, and as such are protected from the violence of war or private conflict. At the same time, they are still human, and full members of Christian society: they cannot escape the everyday violence of adult life. Around 6% of the letters explicitly refer to impairments caused by accidents occurring between the ages of eleven and sixty. Small children can become disabled in their own homes due to domestic accidents, even in loving families in which neglect and abuse are absent.[25] Once out of infancy, the risk of accidental disability increases and the spaces in which it occurs become more diverse, as children move away from the parental home.[26] For example, Julianus Boysseli, a cleric in Le Mans, was deemed unsuitable by a visual impairment, an ocular condition caused by an accident in his youth:

21 RS 4, f. 302 R – Johannes of Kemnicz, subdeacon in the diocese of Prague, to Clement VI on 20 April 1344 (text edited by Klicman, *Monumenta vaticana*, letter 334, p. 198).

22 Boswell, *The Kindness of Strangers*, p. 260, quoting Krusch (ed.), *Gregorii Turonensis*, book 8, p. 617 and Morin (ed.), *Sancti Caesarii*, p. 199.

23 *Decretum Gratiani*, edited in Friedberg (ed.), *Corpus iuris canonici*, distinctio 56, chapter 10 and Stange, "*Oculi cordis*".

24 Lugt, "Le fœtus", p. 355.

25 Accidents in the home account for 65% of invocations and 59% of French and English miracles of the twelfth and thirteenth centuries. See Lett, *L'enfant des miracles*, p. 60. In cases where injured children become disabled, they are cared for by their families or communities, as revealed in the books of miracles. See Kuuliala, *Childhood Disability*.

26 See Lett, "Les lieux périlleux".

> In view of what has been presented to us in the petition of the dear son Julianus Boysseli, cleric of the diocese of Le Mans, the said Julianus suffers from a defect of vision in one of his eyes since his youth, which was mutilated by accident by a comrade while they were playing, and was therefore in some way deformed, it has been humbly begged of us by the said Julianus that, inasmuch as, out of devotion to holy orders, he desires to dedicate himself to divine service, we consider it worthy by apostolic generosity in this matter to provide for him and his status [...] we ask that you carefully inquire into the above-mentioned deformity and defect and the means and circumstances [of the accident] so that we may know the truth about it from your letters patent.[27]

The letter, addressed by Clement VI to the Bishop of Paris on 12 May 1346, describes the circumstances of Julianus' impairment as a central part of his supplication to enter higher orders. His mutilation, caused by a comrade while they were playing together, resulted in a 'deformity' of the eye. Games are a typical cause of impairment in children and young people in the Middle Ages.[28] Little wonder, given the fact that the most violent – and popular – medieval games involved arming children with sticks, swords, or stones.[29] Clement VI asks the episcopal addressee to demonstrate flexibility, but remain diligent in assessing the nature of Julianus' impairment and its aetiology. Whilst the reported circumstances must still be verified, the Pope seems inclined to excuse the supplicant's impairment, and not view it as an impediment to the cleric's desired promotion. Indeed, childhood accidents were considered to be extenuating circumstances in cases of clerical mutilation, since such impairments were the result of chance.[30]

27 RV 174, f. 432 V – Clement VI to the Bishop of Paris, 12 May 1346, for which I give the transcription according to the register: '*Cum sicut ex tenore oblate nobis nuper pro parte dilecti filii Juliani Boysseli clerici Cenomanensis diocesis petitionis accepimus idem Julianus patitur defectum visus in uno suo oculo quidum dudum tempore juventatis, sue oculus cum sociis ludere casualiter crepuit et ex inde aliqualiter est deformis fuit nobis pro parte dicti Juliani humiliter supplicatum ut cum ipse ex devotione in sacris ordinibus affectet se Dei servicio dedicare providere sibi et statui suo super hoc de benignitate apostolica dignaremur.* [...] *per apostolica scripta commitimus tenore presentium et mandamus quatenus de deformitate et defectu huiusmodi et eorum modo et circumstantiis cum diligentia te informans quod super hiis inveneris nobis per tuas patentes litteras*'.

28 Falls, blows, and injuries, then, can represent 20% of children's impairments, and accidents a further 9%, according to the accounts of miracles studied by Sigal, "Les Accidents de la petite enfance". Furthermore, in the English coroner sources examined by Barbara Hanawalt, falls precipitate 3.5% of miracles, and assault and battery 21%. See Hanawalt, "Childrearing among the Lower Classes", in particular pp. 11–13.

29 Consult Mehl, "Les lettres de rémission françaises".

30 On extenuating circumstances, see Chapter 1.

Julianus was therefore allowed to devote himself to divine service, despite his apparent ocular disfigurement. Notably, Clement explicitly praises Julianus' exemplary conduct in informing the Church of his impairment. By bowing to the institution as protocol demanded and following the Chancery's procedures assiduously, Julianus increased his stock at the highest levels of the Church.

Geriatric Impairments

Old age is cited as the singular cause of impairment in 12% of cases in the corpus. Yet, if we also factor in cases in which old age was a supplementary, aggravating factor in instances of mental or physical impairment, the figure rises substantially, accounting for some 35% of the corpus overall. In other words, of the total burden of impairment in the corpus, old age is a supplementary or joint factor in one thirds of cases. The prominence of age as a factor in impairment is unsurprising. Regular and secular clergy, taken as a group, had disproportionately high rates of elderly members compared with the rest of society.[31] Clerics were more insulated than the general population from the routine causes of fatality in the era – such as wars, violence, malnutrition, and epidemics – thanks to their special status, alongside the relative autonomy of their lifestyle.[32] This is particularly true at the end of the thirteenth century, which bore witness to a steady rise in the average age of clergymen.[33] Of all pontifical letters that mention 'old age' as cause of impairment, only approximately 7% disclose the writer's age: these petitioners range from 50 to 80 years old, with an average age of 68. By contrast, 21% of all petitions written by elderly petitioners provide us with their age, ranging from 45 to 80 years, with an average of 64.[34] Despite such disparities in the level of accuracy between letters and petitions, the average age of elderly supplicants remains relatively stable, between 64 and 68 years, that is, the age at which classical and medieval authors believed that the 'last period of life' began.[35] The beginning and middle of old age certainly represent the periods in which (greater) incapacity

31 See Sheehan (ed.), *Aging and the Aged*.

32 Cochelin, "*In senectute bona*", p. 126.

33 Minois, *Histoire de la vieillesse*, p. 253.

34 The petitioner's age is more frequently found in his or her petition than in the letter subsequently written by the Chancery staff, underlining that this information sometimes appears to be secondary to the institution.

35 Shahar, "Who Were Old in the Middle Ages?". On the anthropological classification of age, see Stauch, "Alt werden im frühmittelalter".

emerges, thereby preventing clerics from fulfilling their duties. However, the onset of 'old age' was tied less to a specific number than to the severity of the supplicant's impairment.[36] The corpus contains, for instance, an instance of 'age-related' impairment in a relatively youthful 45-year-old cleric. Strikingly, no documents in the corpus pertain to a supplicant over 80 years old. This appears to be the 'upper bound' for the consideration of clerical impairment.

Although its consequences were described in concrete terms in papal documents, old age was perceived in culture more generally in highly ambiguous terms.[37] This was a period of physical and moral decline, yet older people were to be valued for their wisdom and knowledge.[38] The Papal Chancery seems to equivocate similarly in its attitudes to the ravages of age and the value of the elderly. Church authorities, for example, routinely deployed negative tropes of the incompetence and immorality of old(er) men. An illustrative example is found in a letter from Alexander III, addressed to Chajalisius, Count of Pharos, and all the nobles of the island, on 1 June 1368. Alexander authorizes the electors to choose a new bishop, because the current one is far too old:

> It has come to our notice that our brother Martin, your bishop and shepherd, is no longer suitable and is causing unworthiness, at the instigation of the devil: he is said to have had an honourable youth, but at present, according to you, old age leaves him unseemly and without honour, therefore you judge that a better one should be elected to lead your church.[39]

Bishop Martin's advanced years render him unsuitable for his current episcopal position, causing indignation. Whilst the elderly bishop is not necessarily malicious in his actions, his fault lies in waiting too long to retire, after the point at which he is able to fulfil his duties satisfactorily.

36 See Stiker, "Vieillesse, pauvreté et handicap", p. 135: 'Globally, throughout history, the age of civil status is not a criterion for determining old age. It is the bodily or mental state of individuals that makes them old' (my translation).

37 Porck, *Old Age*, p. 52.

38 Le Goff and Truong, *Une histoire du corps*, p. 108.

39 Migne (ed.), *Patrologia Latina*, vol. 200, n° 574, col. 0545 D – Alexander III to Chajalisius, Count of Pharos and to all the nobles of the island, 1 June 1368: '*Insinuatum nobis esse noveritis quod erga fratrem nostrum Martinum, episcopum et pastorem vestrum, diabolo instigante, non congruam habeatis indignationem; dicitis enim eum quem in juventute honorifice habuistis, nunc senectute gravante vobis esse incongruum et inhonorum, volentes vestro arbitrio meliorem eligere, cum Dominus illum Ecclesiae vestrae diu constituit esse pastorem*'.

His continued presence in post negatively influences the management of his own, and the community's, affairs. This example demonstrates the way in which old age reorients an individual's former, youthful identity: Martin no longer embodies wisdom, and indeed is a figure of embarrassment, unworthy of holding his office.

Another, much more positive archetype of the old(er) man was also routinely used by the Church, however. In this model, old age is presented as a time of peace, prayer, and contemplation in which elderly clerics come into their own in terms of their faith practice. This is exemplified, for example, in a letter written on 28 April 1343 by Clement VI to Adus, Bishop of Winchester. The Pope authorizes the elderly bishop to install coadjutors to help him manage his diocese:

> It has been humbly requested of us that, as a reward for these efforts, and for your last days, we should provide for your tranquillity and peace, so that you may devote yourself freely to prayer and contemplation, and that you may bear with the least trouble the infirmities and oppression of old age, in which we consider it worthy to accompany you favourably.[40]

The Pope aims to support Adus in his quest for 'tranquillity and peace', despite, and in mitigation of, the otherwise 'unbearable infirmities caused by his old age'. This freedom is offered to him as a reward for the work he has done for the Church during his long life. Unlike with Bishop Martin, the Pope here actively accommodates Adus in his decline, without removing him from office.

The Church's ambivalent attitude towards old age, and indeed elderly clergymen, crystallizes in the pragmatic compassion shown by the Chancery in dealing with their affairs. Older clerics are never outright rejected or othered in the corpus, as in some literary texts.[41] Rather, the Chancery acknowledges the practical issues at hand; as in the case of Bishop Martin, age-related infirmity is a fact of life and cannot be ignored. Yet it seeks, by and large, to support elderly members of the community with respect and dignity, as long as they follow appropriate protocols and, crucially, seek

40 RV 147, f. 67 R – Clement VI on 28 April 1343 to Adus, the Bishop of Winchester, for which I give the transcription according to the register: '*Quare nobis humiliter supplicasti ut in recompensationem laborum huiusmodi et ut in extremo dierum tuorum sine per nostre operationis providentiam ea potiaris quiete et pace per quam orationibus et contemplationi te possis libere dedicare ac infirmitates et senium gravamina cum minori taedio supportare te in hac parte gratiose prosequi dignaremur*'.

41 Lalouette, "'On le voulroit veoir mourir'".

adjustments to their role before a crisis ensues. In the corpus, advanced age is determined by several operative criteria: biological age, functional age (i.e., supplicants' relative participation in society, mobility levels, and so on), and cultural age.[42] The latter depends on an individual's life circumstances (including gender, status, and occupation), and the extent to which they possessed the physical characteristics typically associated with old age (i.e., burden for Others or figure of wisdom). However, these different kinds of age are not valued equally by the Chancery. The institution privileges functionality above all in its assessment of supplications; functional age is what matters to the Chancery when determining impairments to be age-related.

Disease-related Impairment

Diseases account for up to 83% of impairment in the corpus, if we subtract conditions caused by old age alone (12%) and mutilation (5%) from the total impairment burden. The causes of diseases are sometimes provided in the documentation. In such cases, the discourse used in the letters offers invaluable insight into the conceptualization of contamination in the period. Explanations range from elaborate medical theories to divine truths, or a combination thereof, with both seeking to rationalize human suffering and give it meaning.[43] Proposed aetiologies, shared by ecclesiastical elites, vastly differ according to the principle effects of a disease (e.g., the bodily breakdown associated with leprosy vs. the sensory loss associated with ocular impairment), its presumptive longevity (if it is an acute or chronic condition, its curability, and so on), and its relative visibility.

In the medieval system of thought, good physical and mental health is rooted in the optimal balance of several factors.[44] According to the Hippocratic and Galenic traditions, the human body is composed of the four elements (fire, air, water, earth) which represent four qualities (hot, cold, wet, dry) and form four humours (yellow bile, blood, phlegm, black bile).[45] Mixed together, these criteria constitute the temperaments that characterize the 'complexion' of the patient (also called qualities). Medicine became a science in its own right in the eleventh century, developing primarily at

42 See Sprandel, "Modelle des Alterns"; Von Kondratowitz, "Alter und krankheit"; and Botelho, "Old Age and Menopause".

43 Cohen, "Towards a History of European Physical Sensibility".

44 Rose and Clark, "Psychiatric Disability", p. 67.

45 See Nutton, "Medicine in the Greek World"; or Bardinet Broso, Fantini, and Grmek, *Histoire de la pensée médicale*.

universities where Galenism and Hippocratism were taught.[46] Whilst humoral theory was predominant in the science's infancy, the theory of complexion began to emerge as a more advanced framework with which to conceptualize the balance of qualities within an organ. Indeed, it slowly took precedence over humoral theory, as medieval thinking about the human body developed.[47] In a binary framework, good and ill health are mutually exclusive states. Complexion theory, by contrast, establishes a spectrum of physical and mental experience falling between these two poles. In this way, it can account for the vast diversity, and the messy realities, of individual experiences of impairment and illness.[48] For this reason, it is a routine reference point for supplications and papal letters, especially during the fourteenth century.[49] At a basic level, petitioners were obliged to disclose their conditions in order to benefit from papal grace. But what precisely they chose to disclose and how they expressed their experiences were also crucial. At a minimum, they had to describe their ongoing suffering in a way that would both arouse the compassion of the Apostolic See and legitimize the accommodations they sought, and thus make the Pope more likely to dispense his grace.

The case of Johannes Casse, canon and chancellor of the church of Noyon, is enlightening in this context. In a letter dated 10 February 1345, Clement VI uses the medical concept of complexion to explain Johannes' illness, without doubt recapitulating information that the supplicant himself had provided on the topic. The canon wishes to return to his native land in order to regain 'the balance of qualities' that he enjoyed when he last lived there:

> Therefore, your supplications request that you, who for the care and cure of the said disease from which you have been suffering for a long time, and also moreover which is easily and conveniently aggravated, you wish to be transferred to the natural air of your homeland in order to follow medical advice, we hereby permit you to reside personally in your homeland according to the aforementioned cause, and that you may obtain the fruits, revenues and products of your office of canon and chancellor in the church of Noyon, and that for up to three years you may freely collect the daily allowances, only excepting those collected

46 Hays, *The Burdens of Disease*, p. 20.

47 Consult Jacquart, "*De crasis a complexion*".

48 On health or illness conditions, see Lugt, "Neither Ill nor Healthy".

49 On the medicalization of secular and ecclesiastical elites and for a study on their medical knowledge, see Dubourg, "*Deo iudicio percusset*".

> when you personally reside in the church or if you only intermittently visit the same church.[50]

The Hippocratic-Galenic idea that each person is formed by his or her 'natural' environment legitimizes Johannes' request and is of central interest to the Pope in his adjudication of the matter at hand.[51] Medieval thinking held that every individual possesses a complexion unique to them, albeit one that changes throughout life. According to Thomas Aquinas, abnormalities in human health are explained when the components that collectively produce the complexion (i.e., the humours) deviate from the 'normal' disposition of the human species, following some kind of balance, the one that is optimal to each individual.[52] The proper balance of their complexion was established at the moment of their birth, in accordance with the environmental conditions of their birthplace. In that context, one of the elements of an individual's complexion is a direct result of the natural environment in which they find themselves. If even a single element is out of balance, health can be lost entirely. As such, the air in a person's birth-place is the most 'healthful' for the maintenance of that proper complexion.[53] If an individual moves from this place, the mixture of qualities in their body may change detrimentally, leading to disease. Hence medical practitioners were compelled to consider the individual circumstances of the patient in order to produce treatments tailored to their situation.[54] One size would not fit all. The same is true for the papal response to Johannes' petition, and supplications more generally.

Clement VI recommends that Johannes return to his homeland, as he has not adapted to the air in Noyon. Indeed, this move had been prescribed as

50 RV 165, f. 20 R – Clement VI to Johannes Casse, canon and chancellor of the church of Noyon, 10 February 1345, for which I give the transcription according to the register: '*Tuis itaque supplicationibus inclinati tibi qui pro cura et remedio dicta infirmitas qua longo tempore te gravatum fuisse asseris et adhuc etiam aggravari facilius et commodius assequendis de consilio medicorum ad aerem naturalem tue natalis patrie desideras te transfere, auctoritate presentium indulgemus ut in dicta tua patria ex causam predictam personnaliter residendo fructus, redditus et proventus canonicatus et prebende ac cancellarie ecclesie Noviomensis quos obtines cum ea integritate, usque ad triennium libere percipere valeas cotidianis distributionibus dumtaxat exceptis cum qua illos perciperent si in ecclesia ipsa personaliter resideres et ad residendum interim in eadem ecclesia minime tenearis*'.

51 Jacquart, "The Introduction of Arabic Medicine".

52 Thomas Aquinas, *Summa Theologiae II-II*, q. 157, article 3: 'We speak of Insanity (*insania*) as the destruction of health (*sanitas*). Just as the health of the body spoils when the body deviates from the normal complexion of the human species, so we speak of madness (*insania*) when the human soul deviates from the normal disposition of the human species'.

53 Lugt, "The Learned Physician", p. 315.

54 See Riha, "Chronisch Kranke".

a form of treatment by the petitioner's medics. This reflects contemporary medical opinion: the solution to cases like Johannes' was a therapeutic return to familiar surroundings. In medieval medical discourse, the principles that make up the physiology of the human body were termed 'natural things' (*res naturales*). These 'things' comprise not just the elements, complexions, and humours, but also the body's organs and limbs, its operations, and its faculties. By influencing these six 'natural things' appropriately, individuals could re-balance their complexion and thus regain their health.[55] Interventions included the pursuit of regulation of the six 'unnatural things (*res non naturales*: air, food, exercise, sleep, starvation, and the passions of the soul), typically following specialist dietary regimens, programmes of activity in which exercise and rest, and sleep and wakefulness, were alternated, and the adjustment of one's environment in order to breathe air that was optimal for one's system. Regulation of the six 'unnatural things' became a topic of focused discussion in the first half of the fourteenth century (1300–1348) and gained significant currency in the years that followed.[56] It exerted a considerable influence on the petitions and pontifical letters.

In a conceptual sense, all illness in the Middle Ages was curable.[57] Healing was guaranteed, in theory at least, not just by advancements in medical knowledge but by God himself, thanks to divine miracles.[58] However, in petitions and papal letters, illness is presented as a condition that is destined to last, as people write to the Pope because 'cures' have failed them. So, this corpus self-selects to favour incurable illness. In the sixty cases of disease-related impairment in the corpus, two words appear again and again: *incurabilis* and *insanabilis*, and both can be translated as 'incurable'.[59] In medieval medicine, chronic conditions are considered incurable.[60] Although consideration of chronic conditions can productively illuminate episodes of temporary impairment, such conditions are rarely considered by historians of premodern disability.[61] Yet the difference between acute illnesses and chronic conditions is not always clear. The difference between acute and persistent

55 Morley, *Theories, Models, and Concepts*, p. 57.

56 Nicoud, *Les régimes de santé*, p. 4.

57 Linker, "On the Borderland of Medical and Disability History", p. 506.

58 For miracle stories, see Laes, "Disabled Children in Gregory of Tours", and Edwards Rose, "Constructions of Physical Disability".

59 These conditions are related to the third meaning of "neutral" (neither healthy nor diseased) in galenic medicine. See Lugt, "Le fœtus", p. 303.

60 Krötzl, Mustakallio and Kuuliala, "Introduction", p. 5.

61 For extensive discussion of chronic illness as impairment, with the chronically ill in the disability community, see Spencer-Hall, "Chronic Pain and Illness".

illnesses was first theorized in the fifth century by Caelius Aurelianus, a Roman physician.[62] In a pair of treatises on acute and chronic illnesses (*Acutarum or Celerum Passionum* and *Tardarum or chronicarum passionum*, respectively), Caelius proposed that chronic conditions involve episodes of severe illness followed by periods of remission.[63] In this way, chronic conditions can present, at least superficially, as a series of acute illnesses from which the patient recovers, only to fall ill once more.

Relapsing and remitting conditions are often explicitly described in the papal letters with the adjective *cronicus* (chronic). This is the case, for example, in Gregory XI's correspondence with Raphael de Luca, a professor of the order of hermits of St Augustine, Master of Theology, about Johannes Rodulphus de Luca, a professor of the same order with longstanding health issues:

> As we learn from the supplication of Johannes, who currently resides in the city of Luca, he has been suffering from a serious chronic illness (*gravi morbo cronico*) in his left leg for some time and still today, to the point that he cannot go without danger for his person to the aforementioned study in Toulouse, Johannes has humbly begged us to foresee in advance that he be absolved of this solemn promise, we consider him worthy by apostolic benevolence to be granted the badge of master.[64]

Johannes had been a brilliant student of theology in Toulouse, yet his ecclesiastic career was now in question. In his supplication, sent from his current residence in Luca, he reports suffering from a serious illness in his left leg for some time. Though he had made a solemn promise to return to Toulouse and continue his studies, such a move would now gravely endanger his health, thanks to his chronic condition. He successfully appeals to the Pope to grant a dispensation, which allowed him to renege on his vow for medical reasons and retain his title of master whilst remaining in Luca. The usage of the word

62 Riddle, *A History of the Middle Ages*, p. 58.

63 Drabkin (ed.), *On Acute Diseases and on Chronic Diseases*.

64 RA 197, f. 104 R – Gregory XI to Raphael de Luca, Franciscan professor and Master of Theology, 5 May 1375. Text analysed by Hayez, Mathieu and Yvan (eds.), *Grégoire XI*, n° 39 961, for which I give the transcription according to the register: '*Cum autem sicut eadem petitio subiungebat idem Johannes, qui in civitate Lucansi residet de presenti, adeo gravi morbo cronico in sinistro crure suo gravatus postea extiterit et existat ad presens quod absque periculo persone sue ad predictum studium Tholosanse nullatenus redire posset, pro parte ipsius Johannis fuit nobis humiliter supplicatum ut providere sibi in premissis ac ipse ab huiusmodi iuramento absolvere et huiusmodi magisterii insignia sibi concedi facere de benignitate apostolica dignaremur*'.

cronicus to describe Johannes' limb condition underscores that, whilst the affliction is permanent, its impact upon his capacity, that is, the degree of impairment it causes, varies according to the circumstances in which he finds himself.[65] Du Cange's dictionary of medieval Latin, citing the eleventh *Miracles of Saint Ruffin* as a source, states that the term *cronicus* is used to denote 'when [an] illness has been inconvenient for a long time, when there is no possible help'.[66] This definition chimes with practical sources. The term is deployed, for example, in the 1284 statutes of the Palmers' Guild in Ludlow, in which 'chronic and incurable' afflictions are recognized as conditions causing incapacity.[67]

The description of Johannes' chronic condition as an ailment that 'for some time and still today', tells us something about the ways in which medieval people conceptualized the curability of illnesses. Leprosy, for example, was considered to be a permanent condition in the Middle Ages as there was no cure. Whilst the disease certainly causes permanent disfigurement and loss of mobility, sufferers also experience periods of both of remission and relapse: their condition chronically varies.[68] Thus, leprosy is a chronic disease, that is, a long-term condition lasting for years, which is incurable but not fatal.[69] For these reasons, the chronically ill were often excluded from medieval hospitals. They could not benefit from the care provided because their condition was considered incurable.[70] Unlike acute illness, which caused only short-term, temporary impairments, chronic – permanent, sometimes varying – conditions forced supplicants to reorient their lives in order to deal with their long-term effects.[71] Johannes Rodulphus' chronic limb condition limited his ability to move from one university to another, but it did not impede his studies entirely, nor his ecclesiastical career. A dispensation of papal grace permitted him to receive his theology degree in a more suitable location. In short, the two terms chronic and incurable are used synonymously in the sources; that which cannot be cured and does not cause death inevitably returns, with some degree of frequency. The

65 For example, in the Ottoman Arab world the same word, *zamin* or *zam¯ın*, is used to refer both to people with a chronic disease or condition and to a physical disability such as a missing limb, partial paralysis or sensory impairment in relation to the ability for a man to earn a living. See Scalenghe, *Disability in the Ottoman Arab World*, p. 3.

66 Du Cange, *Glossarium*, article '*Chronicus*', vol. 2, column 321b: '*Cum vero per multum temporis morbo tam gravi laboravisset, nec ab illo, utpote jam Chronico et incurabili … auxilium invenisset.*'

67 Metzler, *A Social History of Disability*, p. 71.

68 Theilman, "Disease or Disability?", p. 198.

69 On non-fatal chronic diseases, see Wendell, "Unhealthy Disabled", p. 163. On incurable ones, see Scambler, "Long-Term Disabling Conditions and Disability Theory".

70 Kupfer, *The Art of Healing*, p. 39.

71 Falvo, *Medical and Psychosocial Aspects*, p. 2.

impairment caused by chronic conditions could vary, shifting according to the logic of the condition itself or the circumstances in which an individual found himself. Nevertheless, such conditions were permanent in terms of their continued presence, despite any periods of remission. However, the Church accepted chronically ill individuals within the ranks of the clergy.

The longevity of physical and mental conditions was thus of paramount importance in the dispensation of pontifical grace. The Chancery had to be sure that a supplicant was not merely suffering from an acute illness, after which he would regain health and full capacity, so the accommodations such clerics received were not fraudulent. Nevertheless, long-term conditions, even those with variable symptomology, were a legitimate basis for clerics' requests for accommodations to be granted. The petition process provided clerics with congenital, age-, and disease-related impairments alike the opportunity to negotiate with the Church hierarchy and secure necessary accommodations. Supplications represented a single administrative channel through which such negotiations could take place. However, the way in which clerics presented their impairment and framed the worthiness of their appeals differed substantively according to the specific cause of their impairment. In that context, the way of presenting themselves in order to appear disabled was of crucial significance.

Writing Disability

Supplicants tend to present their disability, and its cause, in vague terms. The most commonly used terminology is polysemous: *infirmitas*, *debilitas*, and *imbecilitas*. The meaning of these terms is slippery: they all denote impairment, weakness, inability to perform certain actions, and/or a disease.[72] The term *infirmitas* is commonly used to refer to all debilitating bodily conditions, whether acute or chronic.[73] On another hand, the word *debilitas* is used as a generic term for *infirmitas*, meaning illness or impairment, or sometimes more simply old age. Yet it is also used more diffusely to refer to the state of an individual's health.[74] Generally, *imbecilitas* illustrates the characteristic of something weak without any specific nuance being associated with it. Such polysemy is commonplace in the supplications and papal letters. These texts are far less concerned with establishing the biological minutiae of a

72 There are no words to encompass 'disability' in Latin, as is the case in other medieval societies. See Hsy, Pearman, and Eyler, "Introduction" and Bruce, "Unhælu".

73 On the translation of medical terms, see Barnhouse, "Languages of Experience".

74 See Goetz, "'*Debilis*'".

cleric's impairment and its aetiology than with the *consequences* of that impairment in terms of the supplicant's capabilities and his appearance.

As discussed before, the discursive material contained in papal letters is based on the information supplied in petitions. The Chancery recapitulates petitioners' own testimony in order to draft a suitable epistolary text for the official dispensation of pontifical grace.[75] This entails supplications' formal transformation, a process through which the discourse is standardized and normalized. Notwithstanding such modifications, these documents allow readers to access the authentic experiences of impaired clerics through discursive analysis. Supplicants were active participants in the petition process. They shrewdly pursued discursive strategies to present their impairments to the Chancery in the most persuasive way, and thereby maximize the chances of their success. The choice of vocabulary was of vital importance both for the petitioner and the Chancery. The former had to ensure that his condition and its effects were properly understood; the latter rendered its judgment in large part based on the avowed consequences of impairment, as disclosed by the petitioner. Ultimately, narratives legitimized the inclusion or exclusion of clerics from the ecclesial body.

Discursive Strategies

Impairment could be an asset of sorts, exploited discursively by supplicants in petitions as a means to enter negotiations with the Chancery. As long as the supplicant bore no liability for his condition, impairment provided grounds for the request of papal favours. In a letter written to Johannes, Bishop of Tusculum, Honorius IV confirms, for example, that impairment and illness are 'just causes' and legitimate impediment for the commutation of a simple vow:

> To Johannes, bishop of Tusculum and legate for the apostolic see. We hereby grant you [Johannes] the possibility of freely commuting for twenty persons the vows which they have taken and which they are unable to fulfil because of impairment (*infirmitas*), illness (*debilitas*) or any other just cause, to a different work of piety, except for the vows of continence and the visitation of the holy Jerosolomite places, God willing.[76]

75 The inclusion of the supplications content in the letters makes it possible to limit fraud, to respect increasingly precise canonical procedures, and to spread them. See Montaubin, "L'administration pontificale", p. 326.

76 RV 43, f. 206 V – Honorius IV to Johannes, Bishop of Tusculana and Legate for the Apostolic See, 31 May 1261. Text analysed by Prou (ed.), *Les registres d'Honorius IV*, n° 795, for which I give the transcription according to the register: '*Johanni, episcopo Tusculano, Apostolice Sedis legato*

The letter, dated 31 May 1261, confers only limited powers on Johannes. The Pope authorizes the bishop, as legate, to commute certain vows. He reserves for himself the ability to commute vows of continence and of pilgrimage (especially to Jerusalem), however, because of their significance.[77] It is clear, nevertheless, that impairment and illness are considered to be legitimate causes of physical or mental incapacity to the Chancery. The commutation of vows is thus justified, on the basis that such conditions prevented individuals from their fulfilment. This logic similarly governed the release of monastics from their vows monks and nuns may leave enclosure if they have a 'reasonable motive', such as illness or bodily weakness (see Chapter 5). Such scandal was a major factor in the consideration of clerical impairment because of the example they embodied for the laypeople. In theory, the presence of an impaired monastic in enclosure would generate scandal in the lay community (see Chapter 3). Yet scandal could also result from regular clerics leaving enclosure, or by their temporary presence outside of the monastery's walls – but this was not supposed to be the case for an impaired monastic (see Chapter 4). Concerning secular clerics, the Sext of Boniface VIII also recalls the precept of 'reasonable motive' in the provisions on the residence. This text stipulates that all beneficiaries must collect the income derived from their ecclesiastical office in person on a daily basis. However, all those who are physically unable to do so for 'just and rational reasons', including sickness, are excused from this obligation.[78]

Supplications should not be taken as entirely factual documents. The reality of petitioners' testimony is potentially distorted, as supplicants amplified favourable elements or omitted disadvantageous details from their narratives.[79] As Monique Maillard-Luypaert remarks, it was typical for petitioners to 'inflate their merits, feel sorry for themselves, [and] enumerate the sufferings they have endured', in attempt to garner the Pope's compassion. They might be reticent about topics that could be detrimental to their case – such as their illegitimacy, advanced age, or the number of

[...] *commutandi cum XX personis si secundum Deum videris expedire, vota eorum qui propter infirmitatem vel debilitatem aut aliam justam causam vota huiusmodi nequeunt adimplere in alia opera pietatis, votis tamen religionis continentie ac Jerosolomitano prorsus exceptis liberam tibi concedimus auctoritate praesentium facultatem*'.

77 Thomas Aquinas, *Summa Theologiae II–II*, q. 88, article 12: 'Whether the authority of a prelate is required for the commutation or the dispensation of a vow?'.

78 *Liber sextus* by Boniface VIII, edited in Friedberg (ed.), *Corpus iuris canonici,* book III, title 3, chapter 1.

79 Moyse, "Les suppliques médiévales", p. 56. To study these exaggerations, he uses the work of Baix, "De la valeur historique".

benefices that they already possessed – or even outright lie.[80] In 1924, Ursmer Berlière suspects such deception in the fourteenth-century case of Ubertino of Casale, a Franciscan friar.[81] In 1317, John XXII responded to Ubertino's petition seeking permission to join the Benedictine Order:

> Indeed, you have thought to tell us that, because of various weaknesses (*debilitas*) and impairments (*infirmitas*) of your own body, which frequently torment you, and because of other reasonable causes, you have explained to us that you wish to transfer yourself from the order of Friars Minor in which you were a teacher, to the order of St. Benedict, in order to have greater personal tranquillity and to be able to devote yourself more comfortably to the Lord.[82]

Earlier that same year, John had condemned the Fraticelli, an extremist offshoot of the Franciscan Order, as heretics. Ubertino had been accused of belonging to the heterodox sect. Berlière contends, thus, that Ubertino's avowed 'weaknesses and impairments' are feigned, serving only as a pretext for mitigating charges of heresy levied against him by transferring himself to the Benedictines. Berlière's reading of the case is supported by the opening of the letter (untranslated here), which announces that the supplicant 'argues to be ill' (*cum infirmitantibus se asserit infirmari*). Yet Berlière's suspicions do not change the fact that, despite being suspected of heresy by the Pope, Ubertino's appeal to be transferred because of his multiple impairments was successful. He was permitted to transfer to the Benedictine monastery of Gembloux on 1 October 1317, due to his ongoing ill health. Then, Ubertino could use getting accommodations for his impairments as a means to 'accommodate' (i.e., absolve) his heresy, too. It leaves room for manoeuvre by using impairment as a good excuse, even if that might not be the primary reason. But it is not for the historian to judge, since the papal institution deemed physical incapacity to be a legitimate reason for a cleric to move to another community. Then, the presence of 'authentic details' in these texts should not be dismissed or minimized.[83]

80 Maillard-Luypaert, *Papauté, clercs et laïcs*, p. 137 (my translation).

81 Berlière, *Le recrutement dans les monastères*, p. 59.

82 RV 67, f. 49 V – John XXII to Ubertino of Casale, 1 October 1317. Text analysed by Mollat (ed.), *Jean XXII*, n° 5 701, for which I give the transcription according to the register: '*Sane, nobis exponere curavisti, quod propter debilitates varias et infirmitates proprii corporis, quibus frequentibus molestaris, et propter alias etiam rationabiles causas nobis explicitas de ordine fratrum minorum, quem ab olim fuisti professus, pro maiori tuae personae quiete, et ut commodius obsequium praestare possis Altissimo, ad ordinem Sancti Benedicti desideras te transferre*'.

83 The expression 'true details' is a translation from Vallerani, "La pauvreté et la citoyenneté".

The Blurred Line between Truth and Fiction

Humanizing the supplicant was a major aim of the petition process, both for the petitioner and the Chancery. Indeed, some petitions explicitly set out the various elements that could favour the applicants' cause, including pertinent details of impairment and its consequences.[84] Petitioners sought to establish a bond of compassion and sympathy with the addressees of their supplications. The creation of such intimacy rested upon the provision of a priori truthful information, material that also made the request itself legitimate. Interacting with the ecclesiastical institution in the supplication, petitioners created a specific version of themselves and their lives. Each supplication, in a sense, invoked a temporary identity. The same petitioner might, for instance, offer a very different version of events in other supplications. This could include presenting themselves as more or less disabled, depending on the type and extent of their new request. The details of previous supplications were often included in the Chancery's forms, in order to enable the clerks to produce subsequent requests efficiently.[85] Approximately 0.3–0.5% of all letters produced by the Chancery related to clerics' disability. Even if impairment was an infrequently used criterion to ask for a pontifical grace, it was nevertheless a valid one.[86]

Petitioners disclosed their impairments in a variety of ways and for many reasons, reflecting the diverse experiences of individuals living with physical and mental conditions. Petitions were obliged to conform to rigid stylistic expectations. Nevertheless, supplicants had considerable room for manoeuvre in terms of self-expression, even after the introduction of forms, called formulary. From the start of the thirteenth century, the number of requests received by the Chancery increased sharply. This necessitated the development of forms for scribes' usage, with copyists equally provided with official forms. From the fourteenth century onwards, the Chancery circulated collections of pro forma language for applicants.[87] The Church imposed rules relating to the writing and presentation of petitions on all involved in the process – supplicants, their procurators, and internal staff – in order to streamline the petition process and increase efficiency. Such regulations were extensive, but not exhaustive: they did not correspond to

84 Kuras and Sulkowska-Kuras, "Suppliques, brouillons, lettres et registres", p. 724 (my translation).

85 Montaubin, "L'administration pontificale", p. 328.

86 The numbers are then very similar to those of Salonen, *The Penitentiary as a Well of Grace*, pp. 122–123.

87 See Auvray, "Note sur un traité".

all situations. The varied explanations used in those forms attests to the fact that petitioners could, and were incited to, offer precise descriptions of their lived experiences.

Describing experiences of impairment for maximal persuasive effect was a complex task. This is emphasized in supplications preserved in the formulary of Heinrich Bucglant. Written in the first half of the fourteenth century during the pontificate of Benedict XII (1338–1342), this collection offers examples of texts which rely only lightly on lexical convention. The vocabulary used is more varied than is typical, both when describing the impairment and its consequences. Such is the case in a petition written by a cleric known as Rokesberch, rector of the parish church of Sesterflete in the diocese of Verden (Germany). In this letter, the cleric asks to be allowed to resign from his office for a 'specific and legitimate cause': he suffers gravely from gout. The rector's condition meant that he was unable to travel to the Apostolic See to register his petition, necessitating that he sends a procurator on his behalf. Two versions of the rector's petition were presented to the Chancery and registered. Comparison of the differences between these two notionally identical texts permit to see the way petitioners could modulate their narratives, in order to most effectively describe their experiences.

Relevant sections of the documents are presented below, with text in the left-hand column from the first version of the petition, and text in the right-hand column from its second iteration:

P., known as Rokesberch, rector of the parish church of Sesterflete, in the diocese of Verden in the Holy Roman Empire, informs your Holiness that he wishes to resign freely from the office of rector in the church of Sesterflete for sound and legitimate reasons. He therefore asks that [you permit],

the Bishop of Cassino, your chamberlain	anyone you deem fit, such as cardinals,

to transmit, in person or through other letters [your decision] and that

the Bishop of Cassino	the appointed Commissioner

to legally appoints a procurator for the aforementioned P. Rokesberch because,

his gout disease (*Infirmitas podagre*)	his disease (*valetudo*)

> does not allow him to visit the Curia, and inasmuch as he has to come and collect his resignation from his parish office of Sesterflete from the Apostolic See. He therefore asked for someone to come and collect it for him, and proposed the appointment of Johannus, of the Fransoyzer, cleric of the diocese of Bremen

of good character, science and propriety	recommended for his science and letters, his morals and honest life, and other merits of multiple virtues

> to be attorney for all the proper and extensive rights of the petitioner which your authority confers and assigns, notwithstanding contradictory elements and favourable clauses.[88]

In the first version of the petition (left), the supplicant requests that Benedict XII appoints the Bishop of Cassino, his chamberlain, as a messenger to deliver his verdict to Rokesberch's procurator. In the later, updated version (right), however, the supplicant defers to the Pope in the selection of an appropriate messenger, with a mild suggestion of the use of a cardinal. Beyond this shift in logistics, the two documents present the rector's illness in connotatively different ways. Whilst the first letter explicitly identifies the petitioner's illness as gout (*podager*), the second refers only to an unspecified illness or weakness (*valetudo*) that limits the cleric's mobility. In either case, the painful consequences of the petitioner's ill health are identical. The first formulation offers a precise diagnosis. The second, by contrast, is much vaguer, evoking only the effects of the petitioner's physical impairment (i.e.,

88 Schwalm (ed.), *Das Formelbuch des Heinrich Bucglant*, nº 119, p. 68: '*Significat s. v, P. dictus Rokesberch rector parrochialis ecclesie in Sesterflete, Verd. Dyocese, quod ipse dictam (parrochialem) ecclesiam in Seterflete, quam canonice et pacifice optinet, intendit ex certis et legitimis causis libere resignare. Supplicat igitur s. v., quatinus [venerabili patri domino … episcopo Cassinensi vestre creature devote et camerario] / [alicui de reverendis patribus dominis cardinalibus vel alteri cui s. v. placuerit] vive vocis oraculo vel alias per litteras vestras committere dignemini, ut [idem espiscopus Cassinensis] / [ipse commissarius] a procuratore predicti P. Rokesberch ad hoc legitime constituto, cum predictus P. propter [infirmitatem podagre] / [valetudinem] visitare curiam s. v. non poterit, huiusmodi parrochialis ecclesie in Sesterflete resignationem apud sedem apostolicam recipiat vice vestra eaque recepta ipsam ecclesiam domino Johanni dicto Fransoyzer clerico Bremen. diocese [moribus, scientia et etate ydoneo] / [quem litterarum scientia, morum et vite honestas aliqua merita virtutum multipiciter recommendant] cum omnibus iuribus suis et pertinentiis auctoritate vestra conferat et assignet, inducentes, contradictores et cum ceteris non obstantibus et clausulis oportunis.*'

his disability). The fact that gout reduces the sufferer's mobility, or at least that this is possible, is taken as implicit in the first petition. Mention of the disease is sufficient to explain, and excuse, the petitioner's absence. The second text, however, is reticent on the subject of what, exactly, has led to the petitioner's reduced mobility.[89] Whilst illustrative, Rokesberch's case is not unique. Petitioners had no qualms in submitting multiple petitions on a single issue to the Chancery. Such redundancy indicates, above all, that petitioners adapted their testimony according to their interlocutor, and to the favour that they were requesting. It also indicates rather more practical concerns. Petitioners may need to send several letters in order to provide all the information required for the Chancery to consider their case. They had to take care, then, to describe their experiences in sufficient depth, and even from multiple angles, in their letters so that their procurator and/or the Curia's scribes could select the details, and thus the arguments, that would best support their appeal. So, the initial letter(s) had to contain enough good material that the Chancery could then use to build a solid case, which would be recapitulated in the formal papal responses.

The formalization of language thanks to the used of these formulary and petitioners' lived experiences facilitated the task of the Chancery.[90] Indeed, administrative necessity led to the extreme condensation of legal discourse and catalysed the use of stereotyped formulas.[91] In particular, it made it possible to create categories classifying supplicants according to the graces they requested in their petitions. At the same time, the standardization of descriptions of impairment allowed for the emergence of a common identity, as petitioners enunciated their unique experiences in a shared formulaic discourse. Indeed, standardized descriptors could offer individuals powerful moments of recognition, as they saw traces of their own lives captured in the administrative phraseology. Admittedly, supplications and pontifical letters tend to lack originality, to the point of arousing historians' suspicions.[92] It is essential, however, to read between the standardized lines. In fact, standard forms and vocabulary function to render the specificities of each supplicant's request that much more visible, as we discern the ways in which clerics modulated, and even diverged from, obligatory frameworks.

89 Perhaps this is a trace of the bishop's involvement in the dispensation for the rector of Sesterflete, whose incapacitating condition he knows. On the other hand, the petitioners may seek to inform the bishop. The wording of the petition to the commissioner, on the other hand, reveals a clear distancing of the rector from his interlocutor.

90 For details on the formalization of language, see Introduction.

91 Schmugge, "Female Petitioners", p. 700.

92 Verger, "Que peut-on attendre d'un traitement automatique des suppliques ?", p. 73.

Experiences of impairment, illness, and advanced age are fundamental elements in the construction of identity, both in terms of the way an individual presents – and conceptualizes – themselves, and in the way in which society categorizes them as subjects.[93] An individual's identity is thus integrally plural and constantly evolving.[94] A cleric's professional identity was anchored in his rank, for example, yet this reference point changed over the course of his career.[95] By contrast, impairment and/or disability could operate as a stable referent, one which permanently affected clerics' social identity, as demonstrated by analysis of onomastics. Clerics' physical and mental conditions were sometimes reflected in their name or nickname.[96] This is the case, for example, for Nicholas the Lame of Orgemont (*Nicolas, le boiteux d'Orgemont*). He was the son of Pierre d'Orgemont, counsellor to King Charles V of France, the first president of the Parliament of Paris, and Chancellor of France.[97] Clearly, Nicholas' mobility impairment was an important element of his identity. Strikingly, this moniker – and this impairment – did not hinder Nicholas' career.

Nicholas was the subject of three letters written by Gregory XI in the space of a few months in spring and summer 1375.[98] In these letters, we learn in great detail about Nicholas' impairment, with his lameness a result of a fistula in the tibia of his left leg. The second letter, dated 22 June, for example, explains the cleric's situation as follows:

> In this regard, you have told us that, because of the disease of fistula, which appeared by chance in the tibia of your left leg, to the point that this disease in the tibia does not allow you to move without support (*sine appodiamento*). [...] Your humble supplications asks that you will be promoted to the orders of subdeacon and deacon, and receive a cure, which nevertheless does not require the order of the priesthood, and, besides, can be received by election, and if in it there is a place in a metropolitan church or in a cathedral, you are fit to freely recover and licitly retain a benefice.[99]

93 Frohne, "Performing Dis/Ability?", p. 52.

94 See Smith, "Conflict or Compromise?".

95 Bekkum and Cobb, "Introduction", p. 4.

96 Consult Sexton, "Difference and Disability".

97 Mirot, *Les d'Orgemont*, in particular p. 93 and following.

98 Others are from RV 286, f. 60 R (RA 195, f. 353 R) – Gregory XI to Nicholas of Orgemont, 9 April 1375 and RA 197, f. 184 R – Gregory XI to Aymeric, Bishop of Paris, 24 June 1375.

99 RA 197, f. 173 V – Gregory XI to Nicholas of Orgemont, 22 June 1375. Text edited by Tihon (ed.), *Lettres de Grégoire XI*, n° 3 242, p. 114: *'Nuper siquidem pro parte tua nobis exposito quod*

Theoretically, Nicholas' mobility impairment renders him unfit to enter the orders and to receive an ecclesiastical benefice. Yet Gregory authorizes him to obtain a benefice, even one with *cura animarum*, or take up an ecclesiastical dignity in a metropolitan church or a cathedral chapter. His nickname 'the Lame' is linked to a genuine physical impairment. It is made visible due to his reliance on a cane for 'support' when walking and moving about – as the letters stated that he cannot move without support. Were it not for his usage of the assistive device, Nicholas' impairment would go unnoticed in certain circumstances, such as when he sits or stands motionless. The cane, thus, potentially stigmatizes its user. However, it is clear that Nicholas embraced his impairment as a significant part of his identity, whether as a strategy of appeasement, out of necessity, or for more affirming reasons.[100] Nicholas' situation is reported in neither vague nor elusive terms. On the contrary, Nicholas' condition and its effects are presented with clarity, precision, and empathy. Such an approach was an effective strategy to inspire papal compassion.

Strictly speaking, Nicholas should never have been granted admission to the clergy, let alone be permitted to perform the priestly office. The progression of his ecclesiastical career required successive grants of papal grace. With his decision to pursue ecclesiastical office, then, he actively placed himself outside of the norm, wilfully irregular. His supplications are entirely strategic, part of Nicholas' effort to carve out space for himself in the Church. The foregrounding of his impairment in the letter cited above, including the detail of his reliance on support when moving about, is a calculated move to achieve his aims: a grant of papal grace authorizing his receipt of a benefice, and then his use of a cane. He wishes to obtain specific favours, and consciously chooses to present himself in a way that is most likely to lead to his appeal being successful.

Documents in the corpus demonstrate that impairment was an essential part of the identity claimed by clerics making a case for the granting of grace. 'Claimed' is the operative word here, however. Such findings do not necessarily reflect the supreme importance of impairment to clerics'

propter quendam morbum fistule, quem in tibia tua sinistra casualiter incurreras, taliter in tibia ipsa debilitatus eras quod ambulare sine appodiamento non poteras [...]. *Tuis supplicationibus inclinati, tecum ut ad subdiaconatus et diaconatus ordines promoveri et dignitatem curatam, que tamen sacerdotalem ordinem non requirat, etiam si ad illam consueverit quis per electionem assumi, et in hujusmodi metropolitana aut alia cathedrali ecclesia existat, libere recipere et licite retinere valeas*'.

100 Kuuliala, *Childhood Disability*, pp. 310–315.

identity more generally. Rather, the prominence of impairment follows logically from the purpose of the texts at hand. Petitioners were compelled to craft a narrative that was both persuasive and canonically legitimate in order to stand any chance of the Pope agreeing to their request. This involved mobilizing certain elements of their identity in a strategic fashion. Nicholas of Orgemont's impairment was made obvious by his nickname, 'the Lame', a label most likely applied to him by others which he did not, or could not, cast off. Although it does not reveal Nicholas' own perceptions of his disability from day to day, the sobriquet certainly served to centre his condition as a core part of his personal identity. His impairment was unavoidable, something that he would have to take into consideration in all aspects of his life, and especially in his relationship with the Church.[101] Nicholas was clearly adept at navigating the petition process. Following Gregory XI's dispensation of grace in 1374, his ecclesiastical career went from strength to strength, bolstered no doubt by his family's prestige. He became archdeacon of Amiens, dean of Saint-Martin de Tours and canon of Péronne, and finally, at some point after 1392, a member of the chapter of Paris. Each of these promotions would require the receipt of papal grace. For Nicholas, the petition process offered the means to mitigate the impact of his impairment, as symbolized in his nickname, in the construction of his social identity. As he progressed through the Church's ranks and accrued new titles, his identity evolved.[102]

In pontifical letters, the ecclesiastical institution effectively ratified the curated identities that clerics claimed in their petitions. Indeed, it recognized the personal condition which they appropriated by allowing specific arrangements.[103] Such recognition of their disability was facilitated by the power dynamics instantiated by the supplication process. Whilst the Church held supreme authority, petitioners retained a certain agency. Petitioners chose what to disclose and how to disclose it, and the process itself could be used by clerics to achieve their own goals. Ultimately, the granting of pontifical grace allows for the recognition of the impairment as a disability.[104] Thus, it actualizes the petitioner's identity, from an institutional but probably also from a personal point of view. The Chancery classifies them as 'too disabled' to fulfil their mission properly, and as those who might be in need of accommodations.

101 See Metzler, "What's in a Name?".

102 Schmitt, "Conclusions", p. 431.

103 This topic will be discussed in depth in Chapter 4.

104 See Faure, Dab, and Tétard, *Classer les assistés*.

Conclusion

In the petitions and papal letters, the personal and the institutional are inseparable. These documents contain diverse accounts of impairment, with requests varying according to the specificities of a given cleric's circumstances. Such heterogeneity necessitated a flexible institutional response. Church authorities' treatment of impaired clerics and the irregularity generated by their conditions was a variable as the clerics' own experiences. The Chancery was far more interested in the practical consequences of impairment – petitioners' disability – than forensic examination of its physical or mental cause. The corpus indicates that, for the Church, two principal categories of impairment sufficed for administrative purposes. The first applied to clerics with facial, hand, or any bodily disfigurements who requested entrance to the major orders or other promotion. For this group, impairment was grounded in the notion of irregularity. Chronically ill and/or elderly clerics seeking accommodations fell into the second category. Petitioners of this kind requested the provision of additional assistance for their current role, or the permission to resign their office outright, all whilst retaining their benefices. Chapter 4 discusses these kinds of requests. If such clerics sought permission to leave the clergy entirely, they appealed to the Pope to continue receiving financial support, in the form of a pension. Such petitions are considered in Chapter 5. These categories highlight issues the Church considered most significant in its adjudication of impairment: clerical idoneity and the management of benefices, respectively. In this context, the aetiology of (faultless) impairment was relatively unimportant. People were grouped according to what they wanted the Church to do for them/what kind of assistance they required from the popes.

This chapter focused on the causes of clerical impairment in order to understand how narratives of aetiology affected the medieval Church's conceptualization of impairment more generally. Disability as a category includes, for example, chronically ill people, people with static physical, mental, sensory impairments. Whilst acknowledging the difference in life experiences is of course key, chronic illness was viewed as a kind of impairment, as it is today. It seems relevant, then, to include illness in the analysis of premodern disability, if only because of the ambiguity of terminology in the period. Indeed, the sources do not make a clear distinction between chronic illness and static impairment. Similarly, supplicants often offer only vague explanations of the cause of their impairment. By contrast, they were much more forthcoming about their lived experiences of disability, the ways in which their physical and/or mental condition affected their functioning in the world. Petitioners could not invent things out of whole cloth, however. Nor could they wildly exaggerate. Their accounts had to be credible, and their requests proportionate to avoid provoking the Pope's ire and the Chancery's frustration, reactions which were counter-productive to supplicants' aims. The documents in the corpus provide invaluable material for historians to analyse. With close attention to the sources, it is perhaps possible to disentangle petitioners' strategic presentation of their impairment from their authentic experiences.

Bibliography

Primary Sources

Caesar Cenci (ed.), *Supplementum ad Bullarium Franciscanum 1*, Editiones Collegii S. Bonaventurae ad Claras Aquas, 2002.

Israel Edward Drabkin (ed.), *On Acute Diseases and on Chronic Diseases*, University of Chicago Press, 1950.

Friedberg (ed.), *Corpus iuris canonici*, Akademische Druck- u. Verlagsanstalt, 1959.

Anne-Marie Hayez, Janine Mathieu and Marie-France Yvan (eds.), *Grégoire XI (1370–1378): lettres communes analysées d'après les registres dits d'Avignon et du Vatican*, École Française de Rome, 1992.

Bruno Krusch (ed.), *Gregorii Turonensis opera, pars 2*, Impensis Bibliopolii Hahniani, 1885.

Giulio Silano (ed.), *The Sentences*, Pontifical Institute of Mediaeval Studies, 2007–2010.

Jacques Paul Migne (ed.), *Patrologiae Cursus Completus, Series Latina*, Migne, 1844–1855.

Guillaume Mollat (ed.), *Jean XXII (1316–1334): lettres communes analysées d'après les registres dits d'Avignon et du Vatican*, Albert Fontemoing, 1923.

Germain Morin (ed.), *Sancti Caesarii Arelatensis Sermones*, Brepols, 1953.

Maurice Prou (ed.), *Les registres d'Honorius IV (1285–1287)*, E. Thorin, 1888.

Andrea Sartori, *Archivio Sartori, documenti di storia e arte francescana II/1: La provincia del santo dei fratri minori conventuali*, Padova, Giovanni Luisetto, 1986.

Jakob Schwalm (ed.), *Das Formelbuch des Heinrich Bucglant: an die päpstliche Kurie in Avignon gerichtete Suppliken aus der ersten Hälfte des 14. Jahrhunderts*, Gräfe, 1910.

Thomas Aquinas, Summa Theologiae II–II, ed. By The Aquinas Institute and transl. by Fr. Laurence Shapcote, URL consulted on 31 July 2021: https://aquinas.cc/.

Camille Tihon (ed.), *Lettres de Grégoire XI, 1371–1378: textes et analyses*, Tome III, Institut belge de Rome, 1958.

Secondary Sources

Lucien AUVRAY, "Note sur un traité des requêtes en cour de Rome du XIIe siècle", *Mélanges d'archéologie et d'histoire*, 10.1 (1890), pp. 112–117.

Carole AVIGNON, "Les mariages clandestins: impasse disciplinaire, scandale ou moteur de la réflexion doctrinale?", *Médiévales*, 71 (2016), https://doi.org/10.4000/medievales.7911.

François BAIX, "De la valeur historique des actes pontificaux de collation des bénéfices", *in Hommage Ursmer Berlière*, H. Lamertin, 1931, pp. 57–66.

Maria Laura BARDINET BROSO, Bernardino FANTINI and Mirko Drazen GRMEK, *Histoire de la pensée médicale en occident 1, Antiquité et Moyen Âge*, Seuil, 1995.

Lucy BARNHOUSE, "Languages of Experience: Translating Medicine in MS Laud Misc 237", *in* Stefanie KÜNZEL and Erin CONNELLY (eds.), *New Approaches to Disease, Disability, and Medicine in Medieval Europe*, Archaeopress, 2018, pp. 94–108.

Wout Jac van BEKKUM and Paul M. COBB, "Introduction: Strategies of Medieval Communal Identity", *in* BEKKUM and COBB (eds.), *Strategies of medieval communal identity: Judaism, Christianity and Islam*, Peeters, 2004, pp. 1–10.

Ursmer BERLIÈRE, *Le recrutement dans les monastères bénédictins aux XIIIe et XIVe siècles*, M. Lamertin, 1924.

John BOSWELL, *The Kindness of Strangers: The Abandonment of Children in Western Europe from Late Antiquity to the Renaissance*, Pantheon Books, 1988.

Lynn BOTELHO, "Old Age and Menopause in Rural Women in Early Modern Suffolk", *in* Lynn BOTELHO and Pat THANE (eds.), *Women and Aging in British Society since 1500*, Harlowe, 2000, pp. 43–65.

Karen Anne BRUCE, "Unhælu: Anglo-Saxon Conceptions of Impairment and Disability", thesis in philosophy from the Ohio State University, 2014.

Isabelle COCHELIN, "*In senectute bona*: pour une typologie de la vieillesse dans l'hagiographie monastique des XIIe et XIIIe siècles", *in* Henri DUBOIS and Michel ZINK (eds.), *Les âges de la vie au Moyen Âge*, Presses de l'Université de Paris-Sorbonne, 1992, pp. 119–138.

Esther COHEN, "Towards a History of European Physical Sensibility: Pain in the Later Middle Ages", *Science in Context*, 8.1 (1995), pp. 47–74.

Carole M. CUSACK, "*Graciosi*: Medieval Christian Attitudes to Disability", *Disability and Rehabilitation*, 19.10 (1997), pp. 414–419.

Ninon DUBOURG, "*Deo iudicio percusset* – l'idée de contamination d'après les suppliques et les lettres pontificales", *in* Sylvia CARARO (ed.), *Alter-habilitas. Perception of Disability Among People, Towards the Creation of an International Network of studies*, Alteritas, 2018, pp. 89–114.

Charles Du Fresne DU CANGE, *Glossarium mediae et infimae latinitatis*, Akademische Druck-U. Verlagsanstalt, 1954.

Martha L. EDWARDS ROSE, "Constructions of Physical Disability in the Ancient Greek World: The Community Concept", *in* David T. MITCHELL and Sharon L. SNYDER (eds.), *The Body and Physical Difference: Discourses of Disability*, University of Michigan Press, 1997, pp. 35–50.

Donna R. FALVO, *Medical and Psychosocial Aspects of Chronic Illness and Disability*, Jones and Bartlett Publishers, 2005.

Olivier FAURE, Sandra DAB and Françoise TÉTARD, *Classer les assistés (1880–1914), Les cahiers de la recherche sur le travail social*, 19 (1990), pp. 46–47.

Bianca FROHNE and Klaus Peter HORN, "On the Fluidity of "Disability" in Medieval and Early Modern Societies", *in* Sebastian BARSCH, Anne KLEIN and Pieter VERSTRAETE (eds.), *The Imperfect Historian: Disability Histories in Europe*, Peter Lang, 2013, pp. 17–40.

Bianca FROHNE, "Performing Dis/Ability? Constructions of "*Infirmity*" in Late Medieval and Early Modern Life Writing", *in* Christian KRÖTZL, Katariina MUSTAKALLIO and Jenni KUULIALA (eds.), *Infirmity in Antiquity and the Middle Ages: Social and Cultural Approaches to Health, Weakness and Care*, Ashgate, 2015, pp. 51–65.

Jennifer Mary GIANFALLA, "'Ther is moore mysshapen amonges thise beggeres': Discourses of Disability in Piers Plowman", *in* Joshua EYLER (ed.), *Disability in the Middle Ages: Reconsiderations and Reverberations*, Ashgate, 2010, pp. 119–134.

Hans-Werner GOETZ, "'*Debilis*'. Vorstellungen von menschlicher Gebrechlichkeit im frühen Mittelalter", *in* Cordula NOLTE (ed.), *Homo debilis. Behinderte-Kranke-Versehrte in der Gesellschaft des Mittelalters*, Didymos-Verlag, 2009, pp. 21–56.

Barbara A. HANAWALT, "Childrearing among the Lower Classes of Late Medieval England", *The Journal of Interdisciplinary History*, 8.1 (1977), pp. 1–22.

J. N. HAYS, *The Burdens of Disease: Epidemics and Human Response in Western History*, 2e ed., Rutgers University Press, 2009.

Jonathan HSY, Tory V. PEARMAN and Joshua R. EYLER, "Introduction: Disabilities in Motion", in HSY, PEARMAN, and EYLER, *A Cultural History of Disability in the Middle Ages*, Bloomsbury, 2020, pp. 1–18.

Sarah IRWIN, "Repositioning Disability and the Life Course: A Social Claiming Perspective", *in* Mark PRIESTLEY (ed.), *Disability and the Life Course*, Cambridge University Press, 2009, pp. 15–25.

Danielle JACQUART, "*De crasis a complexio*: note sur le vocabulaire du tempérament en latin médiéval", *in* Guy SABBAH (ed.), *Mémoires du centre Jean Palerme, volume V, textes médicaux latin antiques*, Publications de l'Université de Saint-Étienne, 1984, pp. 71–76.

Danielle JACQUART, "The Introduction of Arabic Medicine into the West. The Question of Etiology", *in* Sheila D. CAMPBELL (ed.), *Health, Disease and Healing in Medieval Culture*, Palgrave MacMillan, 1997, pp. 186–195.

Ladislav KLICMAN, *Monumenta vaticana res gestas Bohemicas illustrantia T. 1-Acta Clementi VI*, Typis Gregerianis, 1903.

Kristjana KRISTIANSEN, Simo VEHMAS and Tom SHAKESPEARE, *Arguing about Disability: Philosophical Perspectives*, Routledge, 2009.

Christian KRÖTZL, Katariina MUSTAKALLIO and Jenni KUULIALA, "Introduction: *Infirmitas* in Antiquity and the Middle Ages", *in* KRÖTZL, MUSTAKALLIO, and KUULIALA (eds.), *Infirmity in Antiquity and the Middle Ages: Social and Cultural Approaches to Health, Weakness and Care*, Ashgate, 2015, pp. 1–11.

Marcia A. KUPFER, *The Art of Healing: Painting for the Sick and the Sinner in a Medieval Town*, Pennsylvania State University Press, 2003.

Stanislaw KURAS and Irena SULKOWSKA-KURAS, "Suppliques, brouillons, lettres et registres de la Chancellerie apostolique relatifs à la Pologne à l'époque d'Avignon (1305–1378)", *Mélanges de l'École française de Rome*, 96.2 (1984), pp. 719–725.

Jenni KUULIALA, *Childhood Disability and Social Integration in the Middle Ages: Constructions of Impairments in Thirteenth and Fourteenth-Century Canonization Processes*, Brepols, 2016.

Christian LAES, "Disabled Children in Gregory of Tours", *in* Katariina MUSTAKALLIO and Christian LAES (ed.), *The Dark Side of Childhood in Late Antiquity and the Middle Ages: Unwanted, Disabled and Lost*, Oxbow Books, 2011, pp. 39–62.

Anne-Laure LALOUETTE, "'On le voulroit veoir mourir'. Vieillesse et exclusion au miroir des sources du Moyen Âge central", in Nicole Gonthier (ed.), *L'exclusion au Moyen Âge*, Université Jean Moulin-Lyon III, 2006, pp. 107–125.

Jacques LE GOFF and Nicolas TRUONG, *Une histoire du corps au Moyen Âge*, Seuil, 2003.

Didier LETT, *L'enfant des miracles: enfance et société au Moyen Âge (XIIe–XIIIe siècle)*, Aubier, 1997.

Didier LETT, "Les lieux périlleux de l'enfance d'après quelques récits de miracles des XIIe–XIIIe siècles", *Médiévales. Langues, Textes, Histoire*, 17.34 (1998), pp. 113–125.

Beth LINKER, "On the Borderland of Medical and Disability History: A Survey of the Fields", *Bulletin of the History of Medicine*, 87.4 (2013), pp. 499–535.

Maaike van der LUGT and Charles de MIRAMON (eds.), *L'hérédité entre Moyen Âge et époque moderne: perspectives historiques*, Edizioni del Galluzzo per la Fondazione Ezio Franceschini, 2008.

Maaike Van Der LUGT, "Neither Ill nor Healthy: The Intermediate State between Health and Disease in Medieval Medicine", *Quaderni Storici*, 136 (2011), pp. 13–46.

Maaike van der LUGT, "The Learned Physician as a Charismatic Healer: Urso of Salerno (Flourished End of Twelfth Century) on Incantations in Medicine, Magic, and Religion", *Bulletin of the History of Medicine*, 87.3 (2013), pp. 307–346.

Maaike van der LUGT, "Le fœtus entre science, théologie et droit (XIIe–XVe siècle)", Unpublished HDR thesis, Université d'Orléans, 2016.

Monique MAILLARD-LUYPAERT, *Papauté, clercs et laïcs: le diocèse de Cambrai à l'épreuve du grand schisme d'occident (1378–1417)*, Publications des Facultés universitaires Saint-Louis, 2001.

Jean-Michel MEHL, "Les lettres de rémission françaises: une source pour l'histoire des jeux médiévaux", *in* María BARCELÓ CRESPÍ and Bernat SUREDA (eds.), *Espai i temps d'oci a la història*, Institut d'Estudis Baleàrics, 1993, pp. 33–45.

Irina METZLER, *Disability in Medieval Europe: Thinking about Physical Impairment during the High Middle Ages, c. 1100–1400*, Routledge, 2006.

Irina METZLER, "What's in a Name? Considering the Onomastics of Disability in the Middle Ages", *in* Wendy J. TURNER and Tory Vandeventer PEARMAN (eds.), *The Treatment of Disabled Persons in Medieval Europe*, Edwin Mellen Press, 2010, pp. 15–50.

Irina METZLER, *A Social History of Disability in the Middle Ages: Cultural Considerations of Physical Impairment*, Routledge, 2013.

Irina METZLER, "Disabled Children: Birth Defects, Causality and Guilt", *in* Naoë Kukita YOSHIKAWA (ed.), *Medicine, Religion and Gender in Medieval Culture*, D.S. Brewer, 2015, pp. 161–180.

Georges MINOIS, *Histoire de la vieillesse en Occident: de l'Antiquité à la Renaissance*, Fayard, 1987.

Léon MIROT, *Les d'Orgemont: une grande famille parlementaire aux XIVe et XVe siècles*, Champion, 1913.

Pascal MONTAUBIN, "L'administration pontificale de la grâce au XIIIe siècle, l'exemple de la politique bénéficiale", *in* Hélène MILLET (ed.), *Suppliques et requêtes: le gouvernement par la grâce en Occident, XIIe–XVe siècle*, École française de Rome, 2003, pp. 321–342.

Neville MORLEY, *Theories, Models, and Concepts in Ancient History*, Routledge, 2004.

Gérard MOYSE, "Les suppliques médiévales: documents lacunaires, documents répétitifs?", *Publications de l'École française de Rome*, 31.1 (1977), pp. 55–72.

Marilyn NICOUD, *Les régimes de santé au Moyen Âge: naissance et diffusion d'une écriture médicale, XIIIe–XVe siècle*, École française de Rome, 2007.

Vivian NUTTON, "Medicine in the Greek World, 800–50 BC", *in* Lawrence I. CONRAD, Michael NEVE, Vivian NUTTON, Roy PORTER and Andrew WEAR (eds.), *The Western Medical Tradition: 800 BC to AD 1800*, Cambridge University Press, 2011, pp. 11–38.

Tory Vandeventer PEARMAN, "'O Sweete Venym Queynte!': Pregnancy and the Disabled Female Body in the Merchant's Tale", *in* Joshua EYLER (ed.), *Disability in the Middle Ages: Reconsiderations and Reverberations*, Ashgate, 2010, pp. 25–38.

Thijs PORCK, *Old Age in Early Medieval England: A Cultural History*, Boydell, 2019.

Carole RAWCLIFFE, "Sickness and Health", *in* Richard G. WILSON and Carole RAWCLIFFE (eds.), *Medieval Norwich*, Hambledon and London, 2004, pp. 301–324.

John M. RIDDLE, *A History of the Middle Ages, 300–1500*, Rowman & Littlefield, 2016.

Ortrun RIHA, "Chronisch Kranke in der medizinischen Fachliteratur des Mittelalters. Eine Suche nach der Patientenperspektive", *in* Cordula NOLTE (ed.), *Homo debilis: Behinderte, Kranke, Versehrte in der Gesellschaft des Mittelalters*, Didymos-Verlag, 2009, pp. 99–120.

Martha L. ROSE and Patricia A. CLARK, "Psychiatric Disability and the Galenic Medical Matrix", *in* Christian LAES, Chris F. GOODEY and Martha L. ROSE (eds.), *Disabilities in Roman Antiquity: Disparate Bodies, a Capite ad Calcem*, Brill, 2013, pp. 45–72.

Kirsi SALONEN, *The Penitentiary as a Well of Grace in the Late Middle Ages: The Example of the Province of Uppsala 1448–1527*, Academia Scientarum Fennica, 2001.

Marilyn SANDIDGE, "Changing Contexts of Infanticide", *in* Albrecht CLASSEN (ed.), *Childhood in the Middle Ages and the Renaissance: The Results of a Paradigm Shift in the History of Mentality*, Walter de Gruyter, 2005, pp. 291–306.

Sara SCALENGHE, *Disability in the Ottoman Arab World, 1500–1800*, Cambridge University Press, 2014.

Sasha Jane SCAMBLER, "Long-term Disabling Conditions and Disability Theory", *in* Nick WATSON, Alan ROULSTONE and Carol THOMAS (eds.), *Routledge Handbook of Disability Studies*, Routledge, 2012, pp. 136–150.

Connie L. SCARBOROUGH, *Viewing Disability in Medieval Spanish Texts: Disgraced or Graced*, Amsterdam University Press, 2018.

Jean-Claude SCHMITT, "Conclusions", *in* Peter von MOOS (ed.), *Unverwechselbarkeit: persönliche Identität und Identifikation in der vormodernen Gesellschaft*, Koln, Böhlau, 2004, pp. 429–438.

Ludwig SCHMUGGE, "Female Petitioners in the Papal Penitentiary", *Gender & History*, 12.3 (2000), pp. 685–703.

John E. SEXTON, "Difference and Disability: On the Logic of Naming in the Icelandic Sagas", *in* Joshua EYLER (ed.), *Disability in the Middle Ages. Reconsiderations and reverberations*, Ashgate, 2010, pp. 149–166.

Shulamith SHAHAR, "Who were Old in the Middle Ages?", *Social History of Medicine*, 6.3 (1993), pp. 313–341.

Michael M. SHEEHAN (ed.), *Aging and the Aged in Medieval Europe*, Pontifical Institute of Mediaeval Studies, 1990.

Tobin SIEBERS, "Disability in Theory: From Social Constructionism to the New Realism of the Body", *American Literary History*, 13.4 (2001), pp. 737–754.

Pierre-André SIGAL, "Les Accidents de la petite enfance à la fin du Moyen Âge d'après les récits de miracles", *in* Robert FOSSIER (ed.), *La petite enfance dans l'Europe médiévale et moderne*, Presses Universitaires du Mirail, 1997, pp. 59–76.

Caroline SMITH, "Conflict or Compromise? Identity and the Cathedral Chapter of Girona in the Fourteenth Century", *in* Laura DELBRUGGE (ed.), *Self-Fashioning and Assumptions of Identity in Medieval and Early Modern Iberia*, Brill, 2015, pp. 277–297.

Alicia SPENCER-HALL, "Chronic Pain and Illness Reinstating Chronic-Crip Histories to Forge Affirmative Disability Futures" in Jonathan HSY, Tory V. PEARMAN and Joshua R. EYLER, *A Cultural History of Disability in the Middle Ages*, Bloomsbury, 2020, pp. 51–66.

Rolf SPRANDEL, "Modelle des Alterns in der europäischen Tradition", in Michael ERBE and Hans SÜSSMUTH (eds.), *Historische Anthropologie: der Mensch in der Geschichte*, Vandenhoeck & Ruprecht, 1984, pp. 110–122.

Carmen STANGE, "*Oculi cordis*: Verstümmelung, Wahrnehmung und Erkenntnis in Herrands von Wildonie Die treue Gattin" *in* Gabriela ANTUNES and Björn REICH (eds.), *(De)formierte Körper 2 die Wahrnehmung und das Andere im Mittelalter*, Universitätsverlag Göttingen, 2014, pp. 83–102.

Eva STAUCH, "Alt werden im frühmittelalter", *in* Brigitte RÖDER, Willemijn de JONG and Kurt W. ALT (eds.), *Alter(n) anders denken: kulturelle und biologische Perspektiven*, Böhlau, 2012, pp. 133–162.

Sylvie STEINBERG, *Une tache au front: La bâtardise aux XVIe et XVIIe siècles*, Albin Michel, 2016.

Henri-Jacques STIKER, "Pour une nouvelle théorie du handicap. La liminalité comme double", *Champ Psychosomatique*, 45.3 (2007), pp. 7–23.

Henri-Jacques STIKER, "Vieillesse, pauvreté et handicap dans l'histoire", *Revue d'histoire de la protection sociale*, 8, 2015, pp. 132–144.

John THEILMAN, "Disease or Disability? The Conceptual Relationship in Medieval and Early Modern England", *in* Wendy J. TURNER and Tory Vandeventer PEARMAN (eds.), *The Treatment of Disabled Persons in Medieval Europe: Examining Disability in the Historical, Legal, Literary, Medical, and Religious Discourses of the Middle Ages*, Edwin Mellen Press, 2010, pp. 197–229.

Claude THOMASSET, "La représentation de la sexualité et de la génération dans la pensée scientifique médiévale", *in* Willy VAN HOECKE and Andries WELKENHUYSEN (eds.), *Love and Marriage in the Twelfth Century*, Presses Universitaires de Louvain, 1981, pp. 1–17.

Massimo VALLERANI, "La pauvreté et la citoyenneté dans les suppliques du XIVe siècle", *L'Atelier du Centre de recherches historiques. Revue électronique du CRH*, 13, https://doi.org/10.4000/acrh.6547.

Jacques VERGER, "Que peut-on attendre d'un traitement automatique des suppliques?", *Publications de l'École française de Rome*, 31.1 (1977), pp. 73–78.

Hans-Joachim VON KONDRATOWITZ, "Alter und krankheit. Die dynamik der diskurse und der wandel ihrer historischen aushandlungsformen", *in* Joseph EHMER and Peter GUTSCHNER (eds.), *Das alter im spiel def generationen*, Böhlau, 2000, pp. 109–155.

Susan WENDELL, "Unhealthy Disabled: Treating Chronic Illnesses as Disabilities", *in* Lennard J. DAVIS (ed.), *The Disability Studies Reader*, Routledge, 2013, pp. 161–173.

3 Joining the Clergy

Abstract
This chapter interrogates the tests used by the Church to determine disability. These were required at several stages of the clerical profession: canon law stipulates that all candidates applying for admission to the secular and regular orders, and all clerics wishing to receive a promotion, must be examined before their appointment. Supposedly a 'quality-control' measure to guarantee the uniformity of the clerical condition at all levels, this evaluation was required from a cleric's first tonsure to their entrance into the priesthood, up until his election as bishop or abbot, when the Pope himself, in theory at least, conducted the examination.

Keywords: Examination; Promotion; Election; Education; Black Death

The Papal Chancery routinely blocked the entry of disabled clerics into minor and major orders, alongside preventing their receipt of a benefice attached to the care of souls (*cura animarum*). Restrictions of grace of this kind were more prevalent in the thirteenth century, when the number of such promotions granted to disabled churchmen remained low.[1] Analysis of the relevant petitions addressed to the Papal Chancery by the disabled clerics and papal letters sent in response suggests, however, an openness to the inclusion of disabled clerics within major orders in the following century. While the thirteenth century saw a large proportion of resignations by disabled secular clerics (51% of letters, compared to 15% in the fourteenth century, see Chapter 5) the pontifical institution received significantly more requests for secular promotions during the fourteenth century, with the topic figuring in 33% of letters (94) and 26% of petitions (22) in the latter period, compared to just 17% of thirteenth-century letters (32) (see Figure 3.1).

1 It is impossible, however, to compare the number of refused requests, since they are not registered by the Papal Chancery. We have access only to the records pertaining to restrictions of grace, which sometimes include partial or even total rejections.

Dubourg, N., *Disabled Clerics in the Late Middle Ages. Un/suitable for Divine Service?*
Taylor & Francis Group, 2023
DOI: 10.5117/9789463721561_CH03

Figure 3.1 Promotions granted for major and minor orders, with or without cura

	Letters from 13th c.	Letters from 14th c.	Petitions from 1342-1366	Total
With cura	9	34	7	50
Without cura	20	19	11	50
Major Orders	3	41	4	48
Minor orders	8	12	6	26
Total promotions	32	94	22	148

These numbers show that the pontifical institution granted graces to receive a benefice with the care of souls and/or a promotion to the major orders to disabled clerics more willingly during the fourteenth century. Indeed, the Papal Chancery authorized the request of 64% of petitioners seeking to accede to a pastoral role, that is, benefices *cum cura* (vs. 31% in the thirteenth century), and 77% of those wishing to join major orders (vs. 27% in the previous century). The results for petitions to join the minor orders are in line with letters of the thirteenth century, with most petitioners prohibited from joining major orders (four out of six cases), alongside fewer spontaneous requests to enter minor orders (two cases out of six). However, if we read the content of the petitions and papal letters carefully, we can understand how the dispensation process worked and we can see how disabled clerics could be integrated within the clergy following an examination.

One hundred and twenty letters in the corpus explicitly mention the examination of the disabled clerics at the time of their entry or their promotion in the orders. Thirty of these grant dispensations enabled disabled men to join the clergy, by accessing minor order and/or without a cure of souls, whilst ninety authorized the entrance of disabled clerics to major orders and/or with a cure of souls. This disproportion in the number of cases between the access of the minor/major orders and/or the reception of a benefice with/out a cure of souls illustrates the strong pontifical control regarding who is supposedly suitable to enter into divine service, depending on whether they will have a more or less active role in it. The substantial shift evident between the thirteenth- and fourteenth-century data – from a significant proportion of resignations to an overt increase in promotions – illustrates the evolution of curial interest over the period as well as the emergence of favourable conditions.

Ultimately, it appears that the focus switched to the physical and/or mental, practical, and social capacities of active clergy members that were needed to perform their duties, with less emphasis on those who wished, or were forced by their circumstances, to leave the clerical state. Secular clerics no longer wrote to resign due to difficulties engendered by their impairment, but rather sought accommodations: the receipt of a curial benefice or entrance into major orders.

Examination of Future Clerics

Canon law stipulates that all candidates applying to enter the secular and regular orders, and all clerics wishing to receive a promotion, must be examined before their appointment. The recommendation for the time of ordination and the expected qualities of the applicant are found in the provisions of Lateran IV, taken up in Gregory IX's *Decretals*:

> The person responsible for confirming the appointment must first carefully examine the form, qualities, morals, science and age of the person elected.[2]

Supposedly a 'quality-control' measure to guarantee the homogeneity of the clerical condition at all levels, this evaluation was required from a cleric's first tonsure to their entrance into the priesthood, up until his election as bishop or abbot, when the Pope himself, in theory at least, conducted the examination. Any free boy over seven years of age and of legitimate birth could receive the tonsure by the bishop, if he attested the requisite minimal knowledge and was accompanied by two witnesses.[3] The examination to enter orders took place at the diocesan level for all clerics. Although there are few pontifical letters about disability dealing with clerical entry, the examples we do have shed light on the conditions levied against people with so-called 'defects' of body and/or mind concerning their access to minor benefices and regular orders, through the grant of 'irregular' nominations.[4]

Access to Benefices

The Church has seven levels, or degrees, of holy orders. These seven degrees are defined by the precepts of the *Liber officialis*, written by Amalarius in 832.

2 *Decretals of Gregory IX*, book I, title 11: *'de temporibus ordinatiunum et qualitate ordinandorum'* (on the time of ordination and the qualities of the ordinate).

3 Tabbagh, "Effectifs et recrutement du clergé", p. 182.

4 There are many more letters regarding the age (5%) or illegitimacy (14%) of the future clerics or clerics wishing to be promoted, whereas letters concerning the defects of body and/or mind represent between 0.3% and 0.5% of those between 1455 and 1492. See Salonen and Schmugge, *A Sip from the "Well of Grace"*, p. 19.

Doormen, readers, exorcists, and acolytes form the minor orders; subdeacons, deacons, and priests compose the major orders. The bishop inhabits the highest rank, above these seven degrees entirely.[5] Notwithstanding this hierarchy, allocation of an individual's benefice is arguably more enlightening than their further access to minor orders in terms of developing our understanding of how disability impacted entrance into the clergy. Indeed, little is known of this crucial initiatory step: there are only few traces left in the source, no doubt illustrating the fact that the Roman Curia assigned it little importance. For example, the ministry of acolyte (the highest of the minor orders) could either be received at the same time as the tonsure, or on the same day that the supplicant entered the major orders as a subdeacon. In total, the corpus contains seventeen letters regarding the examination for entering the clergy and obtaining a simple benefice (with an active role in the Mass, but no care of souls), alongside documents recording twenty grants of a sinecure (benefice without care of souls).

All clerics had to undergo a diocesan examination conducted by the bishop at the time their benefice was assigned. The process was fixed, unfurling according to a defined set of steps. First, a survey was launched among the relatives of the future ordained to gather information about him before his meeting with the bishop.[6] During this encounter, the candidate had to give the bishop several letters of recommendation, called *litterae dimissoriales*, written by other ecclesiastical authorities. These referees indicated that they supported the candidacy, and that they found the would-be cleric worthy of receiving orders.[7] However, these letters were not sufficient in and of themselves to verify the applicant's eligibility, according to canon law. Indeed, the supplicant then had to undergo the bishop's thorough inspection few days before the ordination ceremony, which was organized by the head of the diocese.[8] In this, the candidate's character, qualifications, and knowledge were subject to scrutiny.[9] In non-contentious cases, the candidate was then granted a benefice.

The process was significantly less smooth for disabled clerics, who faced dismissal during the first diocesan examination because of their physical and/or mental impairments. This was the case for Johannes Fernandus of Ruppefideli, a poor cleric of the diocese of Palencia, who had to appeal to the

5 Barrow, *The Clergy in the Medieval World*, p. 38.

6 Burger, *Bishops, Clerks, and Diocesan Governance*, p. 36.

7 Dohar, "*Sufficienter literatus*", p. 307.

8 Dohar, "Medieval Ordination Lists", p. 21.

9 Testimonies and examinations were also used to judge the fitness of a person with dementia under curatorship in the Paris Parliament. See Ternon, *Juger les fous*, p. 56.

Papal Chancery. Johannes probably passed the initial exam and advanced to the next stage of the process. Yet the over-zealous bishop refused to grant him a benefice, because of his congenital impairment: Johannes was born without his left fist. By consequence, he needed pontifical grace to enter into orders and receive a benefice. In a petition addressed to Urban V registered on 25 October 1363, Johannes asked to be able to hold a sinecure, despite the bishop's opposition:

> Blessed Father, it is with great devotion that your Johannes Fernandus of Ruppefideli, a poor cleric of the diocese of Palencia in the province of Toledo in Spain, was examined *in forma communi pauperum* for an ecclesiastical benefice, that was given to him *in forma communi* by the examiners that your holiness deputized, and was recognized as suitable and sufficient to receive the titles, since he obtained the grade of '*bene*' in all the examinations but had been refused [by the diocesan examination] since he was born missing his left fist. That is why it is asked to your holiness that the same Johannes, through your compassionate paternal affection, may dedicate all his days to study and work for science, and, if he studies skilful and docilely, and if he does not soil the clerical honour by being forced to beg, that he may receive a benefice notwithstanding the above-mentioned defect, and be considered worthy to receive the benefices already requested above *in forma pauperum*, and that he can been dispensed *in forma dispensamus* for the grace of receiving a benefice without *cura*.
> [In the margin] Add on the original letter. B. It is pleasing to admit the grace of a sinecure, B. May 10, 1364.[10]

10 RS 40 f. 209 V – Johannes Fernandus of Ruppefideli, poor cleric of the diocese of Palencia, province of Toledo to Urban V, 25 October 1363. Text analysed by Hayez, Mathieu, and Yvan (eds.), *Urbain V*, n° 1 647, for which I give the transcription according to the register: '*Beatissime pater cum nuper devotus vester Johannes Fernandi de Ruppefideli, pauper clericus Palentinensis diocesis, provincie Toletanensis, in Ispania, fuerit examinatus in forma communi pauperum ad beneficium ecclesiasticum in forma communi obtinendum per examinatores per s. v. deputatos et repertus fuerit idoneus sufficientesque titulos habuit quia videlicet "bene" per omnia verum ab assignatione collationis eidem, fiente dictus Johanni fuit repulsus ex eo quod pugno manus sinistre caret a nativitate, unde supplicat e. v. s. quatenus eidem Johanne paterno compatientes affectu cum desideret pro scientia laborare diesque suos in studio consumere sitque habilis et docibilis ad illa et ne in cleri opprobrium mendicare cogatur ut beneficium sine cura obtinere valeat predicto defectu non obstante secum dignemini seu ad assignationem collationis in predicta forma pauperum mandare admitti, cum eodem nunc dispensatur et alia in forma dispensamus ut admittatur ad gracia ad beneficium sine cura.* [*Additis in originali. B. Placet quod admittatur ad gratiam ad beneficium sine cura, B. Datum Avinione sexto id. maii anno secundo.*]'.

The interest of this case lies in the existence of a *second* examination conducted by several examiners at the Pope's request, offering additional testing before Johannes was permitted to collect his benefice. This verification was *in forma communi pauperum*, because the petitioner was a poor clerk without income. A candidate's success in terms of overturning the earlier ruling *in forma pauperum* depended entirely on his moral and intellectual qualities.[11] The applicant had to pass examinations in reading and singing, unless he was a graduate of a university, in which case the knowledge test was deemed unnecessary and thus waived. The candidate had to therefore pass an oral and a written examination in front of adjudicators appointed by the Holy See. There are few sources that directly report on this secondary evaluation, however.[12] Theoretically, judges limited themselves to checking the applicant's fluency in Latin and his ability to sing choral music, essential skills for a serving priest, but even cases to determine sinecure benefices entailed rigorous interrogation.[13] The petition reports that, during the evaluation carried out by the papal investigators, Johannes was considered suitable to receive the tonsure, as well as a benefice without the care of souls. He was deemed to possess sufficient knowledge as he received the best rating (*bene*) in all subjects.[14] Subsequently, Johannes obtained a *cedula super hujusmodi examines cum secreto examinatorum* (statement about the private review by examiners), as did all clerics who passed the evaluation with flying colours. He was then authorized to receive a simple benefice from Urban V, as indicated by the marginal notion added by the Papal Chancery, confirming that the appeal request had been granted. Johannes was personally informed of this decision in a letter dated 25 October 1363.[15]

The core purpose of clerics, secular and regular alike, was to enable lay people to save their souls.[16] This function was advantageous, placing clerics in the highest ranks of medieval society, but also required them to fulfil certain responsibilities and duties.[17] Clerical obligations were more or less burdensome, dependent on two key criteria: if the cleric was a member

11 Montaubin, "L'administration pontificale de la grâce", p. 339.

12 Dohar, "*Sufficienter litteratus*", p. 306.

13 Telliez, *Les institutions de la France*, p. 207.

14 Berlière, "Épaves d'archives pontificales", p. 46. The scores given by the examiners for each subject are, from the best to the worst grade: *bene*, *competenter*, and *male*.

15 RV 252, f. 157 V (RA 154, f. 644 V) – Urbain V to Johannus Fernandus of Ruppefideli, poor cleric of the diocese of Palencia, province of Toledo in Spain, on 25 October 1363. Text analysed by Avril, Botineau, Gaborit, Gaborit-Chopin, Hayez, Hayez, and Laurent (eds.), *Urbain V*, n° 5738.

16 Bishops and priests could also provide manual work, as recommended by numerous councils, especially that of Orléans in 511. See Le Goff, "Travail, techniques et artisans".

17 Lis and Soly, *Worthy Efforts*, p. 127.

of major orders (subdeacons, deacons, priests), and if he held a benefice with care of souls (*cum cura*). Clerics in other roles were less constrained by strictures relating to physical and/or mental perfection, though they remained subject to the same rules concerning access to the clergy, under the pretext that all orders can, in theory, lead to the priesthood and then to a benefice with cure of souls.[18] Thus, disabled men granted a benefice without care of souls (sinecures) were required to obtain a pontifical dispensation, even though their impairment may not be directly relevant in terms of their capacity to undertake the desired role. This was the case, for instance, with Petrus Blasii of Boemia, a student of the diocese of Prague, whose right ear had been amputated by an angry nobleman. A letter from Nicholas IV (1227–1292), sent by the Papal Chancery on 13 June 1291, attests:

> The wise petition you sent us reports that, while you were passing time with fellow schoolchildren who were fishing while you were staying by the water's edge, you saw a horse ridden by a nobleman approaching, and [the animal] became scared, and, though you did not do anything to provoke him, he ran away. However, this noble, thinking that you had annoyed his horse, cruelly amputated your right ear, even though you had not committed any fault. That is why you humbly ask us to be able to receive the minor orders that are a prerequisite to join the military orders as is your wish. Thus, your supplications incline us to dispense you, by apostolic authority, notwithstanding the above-mentioned defect of your ear, so that you may be promoted to minor orders and obtain an ecclesiastical benefice, provided that it is not with care of souls.[19]

18 Guaydier, *Les irrégularités*, p. 89. Other rules fluctuated depending on whether the cleric was a member of minor or major orders. For example, at this time, celibacy was only imposed from the subdiaconate degree onwards.

19 RV 46, f. 58 R – Nicolas IV to Petrus Blasii of Boemia, student of the Diocese of Prague, 13 June 1291. Text analysed by Langlois (ed.), *Les registres de Nicolas IV*, n° 5 389, for which I give the transcription according to the register: '*Sane petitio tua nobis exhibita continebat, quod cum tu olim cum quibusdam scolaribus sociis tuis spatiatum ivisses, tandem eisdem sociis in quadam aqua piscantibus, tu existens in litore dicte aque, et aspiciens quendam nobilem versus te venientem in equo propter timorem eius licet eum nullatenus offendisses fugam arripere procurasti. Sed idem nobilis te cum eodem equo insequens importune tibi quem violenter cepit dextram auriculam sine aliqua culpa tua inhumaniter amputavit. Quare nobis humiliter supplicasti, ut cum tu sicut asseris ascribi desideres militie clericali et ex hoc minus habilis habearis, providere tibi super hoc paterna diligentia curaremus. Nos itaque tibi supplicationibus inclinati, quod defectu auricule huiusmodi non obstante possis libere ad minores dumataxat ordines promoveri, et ecclesiasticum beneficium obtinere cui cura non imineat animarum, tecum auctoritate apostolica dispensamus*'. This letter is also sent to the Bishop of Prague, according to op. cit., n° 7 584 (in the appendix of the Nicolas IV's register, unknown folio).

This is an elucidating example of the pontifical institution's handling of the requests of disabled men: joining the clergy was permissible, though the cleric should preferably join minor orders, and avoid pastoral and sacramental duties entirely. Indeed, when the Chancery refused such requests, it centred the need, above all, to prevent disabled clerics from accessing the altar, performing rites. The integral sacredness, or perfection, of the clergy could not be called into question by any cleric's putative moral weakness, or his obvious physical 'defect'.

The case of Johannes of Sancto Quintino is particularly revealing. The cleric wrote to Pope Clement VI on 21 May 1349, folding his request into the *rotulus* (a gathering of several papal requests collated by an institution) sent by the University of Medicine in Paris.

> Idem, the Master Johannes of Sancto Quintino, from the diocese of Tournai, master of arts and medicine, having obtained no ecclesiastical benefice, because of his birth defect, from which he suffers to have only one eye, because of which he has been previously granted by your holiness the right to be promoted to the orders of sub-deacon and deacon and to obtain a benefice without *cura* [following a letter dated 20 June 1342]. He now asks to be recognized as capable and worthy of being promoted to the priesthood and to be able to obtain an ecclesiastical office or benefice *cum cura*, or to entrust to him a canon's office that would be exempted that the bishop or the chapter of the church of Thérouanne could entrust to him; notwithstanding that the St. Donatian of Bruges' canon obtains his expected prebend. We cannot dispense in this way, but he can have the prebend of provost of the Church of Beata Maria in Bruges, diocese of Tournai, in order to dedicate himself to a benefice without care of souls.[20]

20 RS 19, f. 123 V – Johannes of Sancto Quintino of Bruges, cleric of Tournai, master of arts and medicine to Clement VI, 21 May 1349. Text edited by Berlière (ed.), *Suppliques de Clément VI*, n° 1588, p. 428: '*Item, magistro Johanni de Sancto Quintino, Tornacensis diocesis, in artibus et medicina magistro, nullum beneficium ecclesiasticum assecuto, super defectu natalium quem patitur unicum oculum a nativitate sua habenti, super quo* [*ut*] *ad subdiaconatus et diaconatus ordines promoveri possit et beneficio sine cura obtinere alias dispensavit, ut ad presbiteratus ordinem promoveri valeat et dignitas personatum vel officium aut beneficium ecclesie cum cura, si sibi canonice conferatur, obtinere, dignemini dispensare ac de beneficio ad collatio episcopi et capituli ecclesie Morinensis providere; non obstantibus quod canonicus ecclesie Sancto Donatiani Brugensis, dicte diocese, obtineat sub expectatione prebenda. Non possumus ita dispensare, sed habeat ad collatio prepositi Beata Maria in Brugis, Tornacensis diocesis, ad beneficia que habet conferre sine cura*'. Johannes refers to his earlier petition: RV 151, f. 229 R (RA 61, f. 267) – Clement VI to *Johannes of Sancto Quintino* of Bruges, 20 June 1342. Text analysed by Berlière and Van Isacker (eds.), *Lettres de Clément VI*, n° 166.

Whilst acknowledging Johannes' situation, Clement VI closed his letter by refusing to grant him any dispensation; Johannes had to be satisfied with a sinecure. The Pope issued a counter-offer: the position of Provost Marshal at the Church of St. Mary in Bruges, in the same diocese. The invocation of his new diploma and the support of his university, which interceded on his behalf, were not enough for Johannes to obtain a benefice *cum cura*. Active participation in worship was, indeed, a crucial issue for the ecclesiastical institution. Theoretically, the papacy strongly preferred to prohibit disabled clerics from celebrating Masses and performing other tasks comprising the *cura animarum*. After all, there was a lot at stake: the holy purity of the altar, the sacraments' honour, and even the reputation of the Church itself.[21]

Nevertheless, Johannes de Sancto Quintino tried assiduously to negotiate with the Church, petitioning to receive pontifical grace by acceding to a canon's office. Canonical prebends were generally an appropriate solution for disabled clerics: they were attractive benefices, especially because not all canons participated in worship. This is further evidenced by a petition sent by Petrus Karaszim, rector of the Church of St. John the Baptist in Jászberény, in the diocese of Veszprém (Hungary) to Urban V, on 2 July 1363.

> Your holiness is informed by your devoted Petrus Karaszim, rector of the church of St. John the Baptist in Jászberény, diocese of Veszprém, that, as he was walking towards his parish with another priest from the city of Segesd, he found himself facing bandits who, incited by the devil, shouted enormous insults at them, stole all their property and then, drawing their sword, deprived him of two fingers of his right hand, before letting him flee, striking him down with final blows and insults, half dead, afflicted by many evils and in shock. Then, it is true, Holy Father, that he continued to celebrate the divine services in his church with his two missing fingers when he was no longer suitable. The said Petrus begs your holiness to receive a special grace to be judged worthy to receive a canonical prebend from St. Peter's church in Old Buda, diocese of Veszprém, vacant or soon to be vacant, notwithstanding that said parish church of St. John is abandoned at the time of writing this letter.[22]

21 Montford, "Fit to Preach and Pray", p. 99.

22 RS 39, f. 161 R – Petrus Karaszim, rector of the Church of St. John the Baptist of Jászberény, in the diocese of Veszprém to Urban V, on 2 July 1363. Text analysed by Hayez, Mathieu, and Yvan (eds.), *Grégoire XI*, n° 1 530, for which I give the transcription according to the register: '*Significat s. v. devotus vester Petrus Karaszim, presbiter rector parrochialis ecclesie Sancti Johannis Baptiste de Berensis, Vesprimiensis diocesis, quod cum olim ipse cum alio presbitero de Villa Segusdiensi ad parrochiam propriam pergeret, accedit quod quidam latrones eumdem obviantes,*

No longer able to fulfil this clerical duty because of this tragic accident, Petrus had to resign or, alternatively, find another more suitable position in the Church. It is for this reason, then, that Petrus, fully aware of his recent rule-breaking, asked for a canonical prebend without *cura* at St. Peter's Church in Old Buda, Hungary. The objective was certainly to increase his quality of life: a canon's benefice was more profitable than the type of sinecure that he would have likely received because of his disability – if only in terms of the income from Masses and alms that he would have lost from his original position.[23]

Then, it appears that the pontifical institution used the minor orders and benefices *sine cura* to authorize otherwise unsuitable people to join the Church's ranks, without risking the salvation of Christians. The Apostolic See sought to strictly control the care of souls, an issue which caused great apprehension. Similarly, the inclusion of disabled churchmen in monasteries was a topic of much concern for the papacy.

Access to Regular Orders

The social role of regular clerics was close to that of secular clerics: both embodied a model of Christianity.[24] Whilst secular clerics remained in the world, however, monks left their earthly families to join a spiritual community when they entered a monastery as novices and ultimately made their vows.[25] They abandoned, in theory, their lay identity in order to adopt monastic garb and comply with monastic rules.[26] Although the status of monks diverged according to certain characteristics – for example, if they were juvenile or late converts to religious life – all inhabitants of a monastery nevertheless were united according to a common set of criteria. Entering the community was an essential step, setting male and female monastics

diabolo instigante, multis verbis enormibus ipsum vituperaverunt et omnia bona sua abstulerunt, tandem, gladio evaginato, duobus digitis manus sue dextre privaverunt et, ultimis plagis et verberibus eumdem affligendo, semivivum dimittentes, abierunt, vero sanctissime pater, cum pro digitorum suorum perditione dictam suam ecclesiam deserviendo divina officia celebrare super quo meretur non valet. Supplicat e. v. s. idem Petrus quatenus sibi graciam facientes specialem de canonicatu sub expectatione prebende ecclesie Sancti Petri de Veteribuda, Vesprimiensis diocesis, vacante vel vacaturo eidem dignemini nunc providere, cum acceptus etc, non obstante dicta parrochiali ecclesia Sancti Johannis quam presenti supplicatione signata paratus est dimittere'.

23 The income from Masses and alms can be an important complementary income. For Franciscans see, for example, the study of Lenoble, *L'exercice de la pauvreté*, pp. 226–238.

24 Swanson, "Angel Incarnate", p. 160.

25 Trexler, "Introduction", p. 11.

26 Murray, "Masculinizing Religious Life", p. 29.

clearly apart from the wider lay community, since both monks and nuns renounced the expected roles of husband and wife, father and mother.[27] The process comprised a conversion ritual, entailing scrupulous preparations, ceremonies, and so on, which allowed the future monk to prepare adequately and thoughtfully for their newly sworn religious way of life. The reception of an oblate (a person given to the monastery during his or her childhood) similarly functioned as a rite of passage, an initiation following symbolic steps for an individual's entrance into their new community.[28]

Following such ritualized initiation processes, people who joined orders adopted a particular mode of identity and behaviour. Shared values held by all monks contributed to the formation of a unifying social identity grounded upon imitation of a worthy model.[29] Indeed, monastic rules encouraged brothers to imitate the life of Christ in prayer, preaching and penance, alongside adopting an ascetic way of life.[30] Uniformity was key: each member of the community must acquire, or attempt to acquire, the same exemplary spiritual, moral, and social qualities.[31] This posed a significant challenge for disabled clerics, whose group identity was called into question by the 'difference' of their impairment. In such cases, according to the pontifical letters, some clerics could no longer follow the rules to which they were subject, nor work for the monastery as they were supposed to do.[32] For example, ordinances regarding the observance of canonical hours and the ban on eating meat were commonly followed by all regular clerics – derogating from them was thus tantamount to abandoning a part of one's monastic identity.[33]

The petitions and pontifical letters additionally testify to the supreme importance of suitability (whether an individual conforms to set criteria as established by an order, a community, even an individual monastery) when accepting monastics into an order. This imperative was found in the rules of community life and in the various prescriptions followed by each order, even by each monastery; and this was the case for male and female

27 Thibodeaux, "Introduction", p. 5.

28 The comparison between the rite of conversion and the rite of passage is done by Miramon, *Les "donnés" au Moyen Âge*, p. 24, quoting Turner, *The Ritual Process*.

29 Buser, *L'inconscient aux mille visages*, p. 182.

30 Coon, *Dark Age Bodies*, p. 89.

31 Pansters, "Norm and Form", p. 100.

32 The debate between monks and canons on the superiority of the active or the contemplative life became heated at the beginning of the twelfth century. See Le Goff, "Métier et profession", p. 50.

33 On disability and monastic identity, see Chapter 4.

entrants alike. The Papal Chancery was certainly aware of the constitutions, customs, and statutes specific to individual religious houses. Yet the popes rarely took them into account when granting grace. Indeed, the popes relied above all on canon law, and the rule followed by the given order, to adjudicate the matters at hand. The omission of hyper-local specificities allowed the popes to unify the clergy through common rules, imposing a general definition of suitability on regular entrants, both men and women.

Historians have long been interested in the entry of young disabled people into the orders through the mechanism of oblation.[34] From as early as the twelfth century, this practice was viewed negatively by legislators, whose views were exemplified by Peter the Venerable in his *Statuta* around 1122. Peter proclaims that one must 'abhor and fear deformity' when recruiting future monks, especially during childhood, if one did not want to hire 'lame, contracted, one-eyed, squinting, blind or maimed' people.[35] In reality, however, many children with disabilities were given to monasteries. Nevertheless, oblation was definitively prohibited in canon law by an undated papal bull written by Alexander III (1159–1181), setting the age of entry of boys at fourteen years or over, and by another act of Clement III (1187–1191), proscribing the donation of girls under twelve years old to convents.[36] Various religious orders adopted age-based restrictions. The Cistercians, for example, fixed the lower-bound for entering convents at fifteen years old in 1134, rising to eighteen years old in 1157.[37]. The Abbot of Cluny, acknowledging that some monasteries accepted the 'infirm and the useless', ordered in his *Statutes* that such controls must be strengthened so that only individuals deemed 'useful' for community life were accepted.[38] However, the practice of oblation of disabled persons persisted. In his reports of pastoral visits dated 1248–1269, Bishop Eudes Rigaud, for instance, noted the existence of two nuns with mental deficiencies (*fatue*) in the Cistercian

34 On oblation, see Lemesle, *La société aristocratique*, p. 92 on familial strategy.

35 Constable (ed.), "Statuta Petri Venerabilis", chapter 35, p. 70. Quoted in Lynch, *Simoniacal Entry*, pp. 44–45: '*abhorruit et expavit deformitatem gregis. Quidam enim claudi, quidam contracti, quidam monoculi, quidam strabones, quidam ceci, quidam vero manci inter eo apparebant*' (my translation).

36 *Decretales Gregory IX*, edited in Friedberg (ed.), *Corpus iuris canonici*, book III, title 31, chapters 11 and 12. Some have traced this condemnation back to the *Decretum Gratiani*, quoting its more liberal attitude towards oblation. See Metz, "L'entrée des mineurs", p. 200.

37 See Peters, "Offering Sons to God".

38 Charvin (ed.), *Statuts, chapitres généraux*, p. 42: '*et quoniam ex susceptione debilium et inutilium personarum, ista precipue pestis irrepsit, precipimus, ut nonnisi tales recipiantur in monachos qui apti sint servitio Dei et non onerosi fratribus, et utiles monasterio*', quoted in Peters, *A Companion to Priesthood*, p. 281.

monastery of Bondeville, alongside three disabled monks at the Benedictine abbey of St. Marie of Valmont.[39] Oblation was in decline from the eleventh century onwards, and more or less disappeared during the twelfth century. Yet the practice did not die out entirely, with instances recorded in the fourteenth century, and recurring in following centuries.[40]

The corpus of petitions and pontifical letters contains the cases of fifteen disabled people who asked to enter a monastery. Of these, five wished to join an institution without having previously belonged to the secular clergy; ten others made their request after resigning from their secular office. Possession of a papal letter of authorization was theoretically mandatory for disabled applicants attempting to enter a monastery. The priest Ulricus, canon of the old chapel of Regensburg and chaplain of the Archbishop of Mainz, explained to the Pope that, since he currently 'suffered from illness until he despaired of life', he promised to enter the Order of Preachers, if they accepted him:

> The dear son priest Ulricus canon of the old chapel of Regensburg, chaplain of the Archbishop of Mainz, explained to us that, since he has been suffering from a serious infirmity, and, because he was desperate for life, he promised that he would enter the order of friars preachers at the suggestion of one of them. However, the prior and brothers of this order deny being able to receive him while he is still sick, swearing that they cannot receive him until he is in good health according to the rules of their order. They say that if he enters before he is healthy, he will not be able to observe the rules. That is why he humbly begs us to provide on this subject so that we can force his detractors with paternal foresight. Thus, according to the circumstances of which we have become aware, we mandate that, after having initiated an investigation to establish the truth, and if things turn out to be so, Ulricus should not force himself to obey the monastic rules.[41]

39 Peters, *A Companion to Priesthood*, p. 283.

40 Berend, "La subversion invisible", p. 125.

41 RV 22, f. 41 R – Innocent IV to Hermannus, Bishop of Wurtzbourg, 9 February 1251. Text edited by Berger (ed.), *Les registres d'Innocent IV*, n° 5033: '*Dilectus filius Ulricus presbyter, canonicus Veteris Capelle Ratisponensis, capellanus bone memorie ... archiepiscopi Maguntini, nobis exposuit quod ipse olim, gravi infirmitate detentus, cum de vita desperaretur ipsius, ad suggestionem quorumdam fratrum de ordine Predicatorum promisit quod ordinem eorum intraret, sed ... prior et fratres ipsius ordinis ei adhuc in infirmitate posito dare habitum ejusdem ordinis denegarunt, asserentes quod ipsi aliquem nisi sit in sanitate positus non possunt recipere secundum ipsius ordinis instituta. Cum autem idem canonicus esset sanitati pristine restitutus, ipse affectum non applicavit observantie regulari. Quare nobis humiliter supplicavit ut providere sibi super hoc, ne [quid] quis emulus in ipsum detractionis impingat, paterna providentia curaremus. Quia vero de*

However, the prior and brothers of the order refused to let him join their ranks, because they were unable to receive a sick person. They decided that he would be welcomed only when he was deemed to be entirely healthy again. So Ulricus was writing to get a papal letter to force the Order to let him join in his current state of sickness and exempt him from following the rules – which he got. Disability could indeed constitute an obstacle to acceding to the monastic state, even in cases of late or *ad succurendum* vows.[42] The Council of Trent (1545–1563) strictly regulated admission to convents with its decree 'on regulars and nuns'. Even before this edict, though, entrance to orders was already subject to canon law, and the specific rules of the various religious orders, in the thirteenth and fourteenth centuries.[43] Access to mendicant orders followed the same rules as for traditional orders, perhaps even more strictly because of their rigorous lifestyle. Entry into monastic or mendicant orders was subject to several precepts, defined at various levels, from local conventions to the higher-level regulations of the Church.

In the letter addressed to Ulricus, the Pope asked that an investigation be carried out to determine if the applicant had regained his health or not, and if so, if he might thus be able to follow the monastic rules. For this type of evaluation, the brothers gathered in committee to rigorously examine the candidate's fitness for monastic life. Directly after his tonsure, the future ascetic entered his novitiate, a probationary period. This step allowed time for supervisors to assess the apprentice's physical fitness for work and his adaptation to community life.[44] If successful, the applicant was authorized to progress, taking their vows to join the order formally. However, because it was a papal grace, if the examiners were to find that Ulricus could not obey the rules, he would be accepted into the order anyway.

The various religious orders of the thirteenth century used the novitiate system in order to identify, and ultimately incorporate, future brothers and sisters who were 'capable and useful' to the monastic community. As the Master General of the Order of Preachers, Humbert of Romans, explained in his *Work of Regular Life*, brothers must possess great physical strength to carry out the work for which they were responsible.[45] These responsibilities

facto et facti circumstantiis habere poteris notitiam pleniorem, mandamus quatinus, inquisita super hiis diligentius veritate, si rem inveneris ita esse, denunties eundem canonicum propter hoc ad regularem observantiam non teneri'.

42 On *ad succurendum* vows, see Chapter 5.

43 Waterworth (transl.), "The Council of Trent", "On regulars and nuns", p. 236.

44 Rost, Inauen, Osterloh, and Frey, "The Corporate Governance", p. 94.

45 Montford, "Fit to Preach and Pray", p. 96, quoting Berthier (ed.), *Opera de vita regularis*, volume 2, p. 407: *'expedit eum habere vires corporales, ut possit vigilas in studendo, clamorem in*

were determined by the separate provisions for each house, adapted to a given institution's way of life. Rules were set down in customary laws which were fixed and normalized in the twelfth and thirteenth centuries, or in institutional statutes adopting specific provisions.[46] In an article on the reception of friars, the *Constitutions of the Friars Preachers* (valid from 1256 to 1375) required that three suitable Dominicans be elected from the chapter to examine those who wished to commit themselves to the order.[47] This restricted council, composed of 'mature and wise men', evaluated the morals and knowledge of the applicant. Examiners had to verify, additionally, that the candidate was not hiding any infirmity or illness that would prevent him from wearing the monastic habit.[48] Following this high-level interrogation, brothers at the local level took care of the applicant's recruitment, in order to integrate people who were beneficial to their community, able to follow the novitiate and conform to their way of life.[49]

Whilst monks were subject to the assessment of an individual house and to other ecclesiastical regulations specific to the order they wished to join, their highest authority remained the Pope. Letters written by Innocent IV between 1245 and 1254 and by Alexander IV in 1261 testify to the crucial role that popes played in such entrance examinations. The two popes addressed the Abbot of Cîteaux, the head of the Cistercian order, and his co-abbots, as well as all Cistercian convents. They were obliged to act, as it was well known that some Benedictine monks had been ordained without first passing any tests as to their suitability:

> Thus, as your petition read out to all states, the monks of your order are promoted to the institution without recommendation of ecclesiastical

praedicando, labores in discurrendo, penuriam in indigentiis et huiusmodi multa sustinere sicut fecerunt Apostoli'.

46 Vauchez and Caby, *L'histoire des moines*, pp. 75–76. See, for Clunisian order: Charvin, *Statuts, chapitres généraux et visites*, volumes I to IV, or Canivez (ed.), *Statuta capitulorum generalium*, volumes 9, 10, and 11.

47 These provisions are preceded by an amendment promulgated in 1239, according to Montford, "Fit to Preach and Pray", p. 103, quoting Cenci (ed.), "De Fratrum", p. 76: '*si infirmitate aliquem habeat vel praevamcorporis qualitatem propter quam foret postea onerosus si membrum aliquod mutilatum habeat vel inefficax quoquomodo*'.

48 Istituto storico domenicano S. Sabina (eds.), *Constitutiones et acta*, chapter 13: '*In quolibet conventu tres ydonei fratres eligantur de comuni consilio capituli qui recipiendos in moribus et sciencia diligenter examinent, et examinacionem priori et capitulo referant, eorum iudicio an recepi debeant relinquentes.* [...] *Lectio. Nullus recipiatur nisi requisitus an sit coniugatus an servus an raciociniis obligatus an alterius professionis vel occultam habeat infirmitatem*'.

49 For a full presentation of the formation of Dominican novices, see Mulchahey, "*First the Bow is Bent in Study...*", chapter 2.

> prelates and without having undergone any examination, we ask you on this subject, since some monks of this order who should be excluded from it are vitiated by notorious crimes or vitiated bodies, and we decree by our apostolic authority that they be systematically examined by a prelate.[50]

Those two popes used their letters to point out the intolerable consequences of the lack of supervision in the recruitment of future monks, and to remind all Cistercians of the rules. It was the Church's duty to ensure that criteria regarding physical perfection were respected, even in monasteries and convents.[51] The petitions and papal letters evidence the multiple mechanisms of control at play, from examinations by local commissions to delegations appointed by the Apostolic See, in the verification of an individual's suitability for entrance into an order. What becomes clear, as with Innocent IV and Alexander IV's interventions, is that the papacy exerted a strong influence in defining the suitability of monks and nuns, and the processes by which institutional 'fit' was determined.

The popes had the authority to adapt the rules of each house by means of letters of grace, in particular by mediating between the various local authorities. Thus, Clement VI wrote on 5 October 1344 to the abbots of the monasteries of Saint-Thibéry (diocese of Agde), Florac (Orléans), and Bonne-Aigue (Limoges) to intercede in the case of Heliades, daughter of the noble Geraldus Dalvernh ('of Auvergne') of the diocese of Tulle who wished to join the Benedictine convent of Brageac (Clermont-Ferrand) as a nun, despite the 'stains' (*macula*) on her eyes:

50 Innocent IV, 2 May 1245, L 244, n° 73 (olim n° 72), RV 21, f. 180, for which I give the transcription according to the original letter: '*Cum itaque sicut lecta coram nobis universitatis vestre petitio continebat monachi ordinis vestri ab institutione ipsius soliti sint a prelatis ecclesiarum sine aliqua examinatione ad ordines promoveri, nos devotionis vestre precibus inclinati ut hoc ipsum cura monachos eiusdem ordinis eis dumtaxat exceptis in quibus fuerit notorium crimen vel enorme corporis vitium a prelatis eisdem perpetuis temporibus observetur, auctoritate presentium duximus statuendum*'. Text also analysed by Berger, *Les registres d'Innocent IV*, n° 1223, p. 189. See also Innocent IV, 12 October 1245, L 245, n° 100 (olim n° 99) (text analysed by Barbiche, *Les actes pontificaux*, n° 552, p. 212); Innocent IV, 19 March 1254, L 248, n° 245 (text analysed in op. cit. n° 736, p. 280); Alexander IV, 28 March 1261, L 966, n° 49 (olim L 1146 (9)) (text analysed in op. cit. n° 1080, p. 416)

51 Bishops and archbishops were also taking up the issue, as Dominicans were often called to order by provincial chapters. They seemed not to respect the rules and admitted into the clergy people who were too young, uneducated, or afflicted with physical 'defects'. See Mulchahey, "*First the Bow is Bent in Study...*", p. 84. For examples, prioresses who thus received unsuitable candidates were deprived of the right to admit new candidates into the order.

> The dear daughter Heliades, born of the noble Geraldus Dalvernh, a literate girl from the diocese of Tulle, wishes to join the ranks of the abbess and daughters of the convent of the monastery of Brageac, of the order of St. Benedict in the diocese of Clermont and live under the habit and in the service of God in this same place, which is what we accept to comfort the praiseworthy wishes of this young girl. That is why we ask that you or two of you or someone else, check that, as it is said, this young girl has a stain in one of her eyes and see if she is suitable, and if there is no canon against it, that she be received into the monastery, provided that it has room for her.[52]

The Pope tasked the abbots to determine whether Heliades could be received in the monastery – a proposition he broadly supported – despite her visible disability. Admission would be permissible if there were room available in the convent for her, and if the committee of appointed experts decided that it was appropriate. If so, Heliades could become a nun at Brageac, regardless of her ocular impairment and of Brageac's specific statutes and customs, or those of the Benedictine order itself.[53] According to canon law, physical 'defects' – encompassing illness, old age, and even more diffuse bodily 'weakness' – constituted 'impediments', in a legal sense, to joining orders. Papal letters were necessary in order to authorize any contravention of such legislation. A pontifical favour was therefore needed to allow Heliades to enter the monastery despite her disability. The name of the applicant's father, Geraldus Dalvernh, was given in the letter, certainly as a guarantee of the quality of her lineage and her upbringing, given the fact the was a nobleman from the Tulle area. He sought to admit his daughter to the convent by using his *patria potestas* (paternal authority), probably with the help of a substantial dowry.[54]

52 RV 138, f. 98 V – Clement VI to the abbots of the monasteries of Saint-Thibéry (diocese of Agde), Florac (Orléans) and Bonne-Aigue (Limoges), 5 October 1344. Text edited by Déprez, Glénisson and Mollat (eds.), *Clément VI*, n° 1 150: '*Cum itaque dilecta in Christo filia Heliadis, nata dilecti filii nobilis viri Geraldi Dalvernh puella litterata, Tutellensis diocesis, cupiat, sicut accepimus, una cum dilectis in Christo filiabus... abbatissa et conventu monasterii de Bragiaco, ordinis Sancti Benedicti, Claromontensis diocesis, in eodem monasterio sub regulari habitu virtutum domino famulari, nos volentes eandem puellam in hujusmodi suo laudabili proposito confovere, mandamus quatenus vos vel duo aut unus vestrum per vos vel alium seu alios, si predicta puella que, sicut asseritur, habet in altero suorum occulorum maculam, alias sit ydonea, et aliud canonicum non obsistat, in dicto monasterio, si in eo certus monialium numerus non habetur recepi faciatis*'.

53 Cygler, "“unité des cœurs”", pp. 174–175.

54 Neiske, "Les enfants dans les monastères", p. 231.

It is likely that Heliades' impairment represented a decisive factor in her family's, and her own, resolve for her to enter a convent: she did not correspond to the perfect physical image prized by the noble elite.[55] This 'solution' could be part of a family strategy, more or less agreed upon by the applicant, facilitated by a financial transaction with a convent, one that was less expensive than marriage.[56] A father might, for example, prefer to entrust his daughter to God's care rather than to see her fail at her socially defined function of finding a husband and having children. The Dalvernh family seem to be part of the (probably lesser) nobility, and obviously have enough resources to pay for Heliades to join a monastic community, and thus overcome her disability to some degree. Moreover, it remains quite possible that the literate Heliades spearheaded her entrance into Brageac, preferring to dedicate herself to intellectual work than the marriage market.[57] As a nun, she would obtain more independence than in an earthly marriage.[58] She might also be motivated to become a nun to withdraw from the earthly world and thereby to avoid (further) social ostracism rooted in the putative shame her impairment caused her family, and herself.[59] In any case, the result of the abbots' review remains unknown: no petition subsequently mentions it. What is clear, nevertheless, is that the pontifical institution established and managed a stringent framework through which to measure the physical and moral perfection of those wishing to enter religious orders, in order to include only men and women deemed worthy of belonging to the superior monastics.

Once authorized to settle in a diocese or religious house (whether by usual examination or dispensation), newly tonsured clerics were placed on an ordination list. Other additional information was recorded, such as the date and place of their enthronement ceremony, the identity of the bishop who presided at it, their regular (order and house) or secular (diocese of origin) status, and the title for which they were ordained.[60] Such details

55 The noble elite celebrated beauty and physical perfection, but, nonetheless, other qualities can be proven equally important, such as education or value in combat. See Kuuliala, "Nobility, Community and Physical Impairment".

56 On family strategies, see Kuuliala, "Infirmitas in Monastic Rules".

57 On nuns' choices to leave a freer life, away from the gendered violence of earthly life, see Von Tippelskirch, "Spiritualités en captivité".

58 Donahue, *Law, Marriage, and Society*, p. 86.

59 Metzler, *A Social History of Disability*, p. 31. The author recounts, for example, the case of Anna, from the diocese of Basel. In 1455, she refused to remain cloistered after being locked away by her parents because she was missing a hand, a fact they wished to hide. The difficulty in getting married when disabled is also addressed by Von Tippelskirch, "Spiritualités en captivité".

60 Dohar, "Medieval Ordination Lists", p. 18.

became useful if any irregularities were found following an individual's admission. If a case of fraud was proven, for example, it was possible to take action against overly lax examiners. Indeed, canon law, including the Fourth Lateran Council (1215, canon 27), ruled that bishops who committed such fraudulent acts would lose the authorization to confer orders, and would have to leave their own office:

> If in the future they presume to ordain ignorant and unformed men (a defect that can easily be discovered), we decree that both those ordaining and those ordained be subject to severe punishment. In the ordination of priests especially, it is better to have a few good ministers than many who are no good, for if the blind lead the blind both will fall into the pit (Matt. 15:14).[61]

Notwithstanding such strict regulations, the improper receipt of benefices without *cura* or admission to regular orders were not the Curia's foremost concern in terms of controlling the clergy. 'Unsuitable' individuals' elevation to major orders, as we shall see, aroused extensive attention from all quarters, local superiors and popes alike.

Promotions and Elections

The promotions of secular (and, on occasion, regular) clerics to major orders and benefices with *cura* represent 13% of the cases found in the thirteenth- and fourteenth-century letters, and 10.5% of the petitions sent to the Pontifical Curia between 1342 and 1366. Of the 90 clerics for whom the question of access to major orders arose, eighteen were authorized to say Mass (receiving a simple benefice) while fifty were permitted to join the full major orders (receiving a cure of souls) despite their disability; however, fourteen disabled clerics were barred from sacramental worship, and a further eight were blocked from joining major orders entirely. Promotion to the priesthood was a crucial issue for the pontifical institution. The Church sought to drastically restrict elections, as evidenced, in particular, by the Investiture Controversy, during which the papacy reasserted its right to install senior church officials by undercutting secular (mainly imperial) powers. Eventually, the Church succeeded in imposing pontifical theocracy as a mode of governance: the popes functioned as monarchs ruling over

61 *The Canons of the Fourth Lateran Council, 1215*, canon 27.

the territory of all Christianity. From the twelfth century onwards, the papacy – and not secular elites – exerted its power by appointing members of the high clergy and influencing the recruitment policies of major clergy at the diocesan level.

Access to Major Orders

Bishops and archbishops were theoretically authorized to grant petitioners grace in terms of contravening institutions' admission policy, as they were delegates of the Pope's ordinary power over the relevant jurisdiction. However, their power was largely circumscribed in practice: they could only overturn a ruling they themselves (or their predecessors) have made previously, or those promulgated in a diocesan council in their own territories. They were thus only empowered to offer pardons (exemptions) in minor cases within their own diocese. The clarification, and strengthening, of pontifical prerogatives first begun in the twelfth century led steadily to a reduction of the archbishops' and bishops' powers. They could no longer go against canon law. Towards the end of the thirteenth century and during the fourteenth century, the popes assumed control over several prerogatives that had, until that point, been the exclusive purview of regional ecclesiastical prelates. Gradually, then, local and institutionally specific hierarchies were being weakened, and ultimately displaced, by pontifical authority.

In contrast to the limited powers of bishops and archbishops, the Pope had the full range of ecclesiastical laws at his disposal, whether universal – regional and ecumenical councils – or particular (i.e., local statutes and institutional conventions), due to his supreme authority. Indeed, Christ conferred on the apostle Peter, and thus on all popes, the power to exempt individuals from canon law.[62] Owing to the primacy of his dominion, the Pope functionally concentrated jurisdictional power: he was the repository for all Christian law, following the model of a bishop in charge of his diocese.[63] The Apostolic See therefore reserved for itself the most complex questions of canon law, in particular cases pertaining to clerical exemptions from altar service.[64] This is evidenced in the eleventh-century *Dictatus Papae*, written (but never published) by Gregory VII, which established the Pope as the sole authority governing all churches in Christendom, to whom

62 Besson, "Dispensation".

63 Benson, *Bishop-Elect*, p. 173.

64 Parlopiano, "*Propter Deformitatem*", p. 94.

all important cases (*major causae*) should be referred, thereby centralizing ecclesiastical powers (chapter 21).[65]

The popes' expanding role in the management of the clergy after the Gregorian Reform prevented bishops from governing their own dioceses as they saw fit, which put a stop to bishops ignoring the prerogatives of canon law. As the papacy tightened its grip, becoming more present in regional administration, the authority of the head over its members became ever stronger. In this way, St. Peter's successors claimed the full extent of the papacy's power, to the detriment of local ecclesiastical elites. This is amply illustrated by the case of Master Guillelmus of Sayssac, whose promotion was refused by the canons of the cathedral of Puy-en-Velay following false accusations that he had only one disabled hand, whose circumstances were considered by Boniface VIII on 18 June 1302:

> We have supported your candidacy because you are worthy of it, a scholar of letters, honest morals, commendable conversation and life among other virtues, and we therefore wish to freely give you a special grace. You recently personally disclosed to us that, in the past, when you were examined in civil law, you were recognized as suitable and you could receive an ecclesiastical benefice [...] since then, some people continue to say, sowing wrongly and mistakenly, that you are suffering from a vice of the body, that you have only one hand and that you therefore cannot conveniently or properly celebrate the divine offices, and that in addition, you suffer from an incurable and deforming disease in your other hand at that moment which has since passed, and for which you have been helped, in the same way as it would have been decreed for a one-eyed person (*luscus*), but those people have called several times to the Apostolic See so that you cannot celebrate the divine services.[66]

65 On the rights reserved to the Pope resulting from the *plenitudo potestatis*, see Herghelegiu, *Reservatio Papalis*, p. 27.

66 RV 50, f. 218 V – Boniface VIII to Guillelmus of Sayssac, Canon of Le Puy-En-Velay, 18 June 1302. Text edited by Digard, Fawtier, Faucon, and Thomas (eds.), *Les registres de Boniface VIII*, n° 4770: '*Quia igitur litterarum scientiam, honestatem morum, conversationem vite laudabilis et aliarum virtutum merita tibi accepimus suffragari, personam tuam libenter prosequimur favore gratie specialis. Nuper siquidem in nostra proposuisti presentia constitutus, quod nos olim pro te, quem in jure civili examinari fecimus quique per examinationem hujusmodi fuisti repertus ydoneus ad ecclesiasticum beneficium obtinendum* [...] *dicitur postmodum adhesisse, falso ac mendaciter asserentes te fore in proprio corpore vitiatum, quod unicam tantum manum habebas, cum qua comode ac congrue posses divina officia celebrare, pro eo quod in altera manu morbum incurabilem et deformitatem patiebaris tunc, et passus fueras ante, nec te juvare poteras de eadem, ac ex eo*

The letter informs us that Guillelmus was first recognized as suitable for the clergy during his civil law examination. The evaluation, which he passed with top marks, was a precursor to obtaining a benefice with care of souls, because membership of major orders carried with it the possibility of celebrating Mass. As with any ecclesiastical promotion, the entrance exam for major orders was carried out by the bishop, or his delegate. However, examiners in these cases had to be even more rigorous when it came to the ordination of a person in receipt of a benefice *cum cura*.[67]

Entering major orders symbolized a point of rupture between simple clerics (relegated to minor orders), and those who fulfilled a higher mission of preaching and giving the sacraments. This line of demarcation had been constituted long before the medieval era and formed the rationale for ecclesiastical examinations. In his book *Laws* (written between 358 and 356 BC), the ancient Greek philosopher Plato maintains that all would-be priests must be subject to an assessment of their physical and mental capacities, in order to exclude the disabled from the ranks of the clergy. Regulations regarding the purchase of priestly roles in Cos, moreover, stated that Greek priests must be both healthy (*hugies*) and 'unmutilated' (*holokanos*) to be able to lead worship.[68] Ecclesiastical legislation prohibited disabled and/or ill people from acceding to the priesthood or taking on core priestly duties, with the aim of preserving the purity of ministerial functions, not to mention of the ministry itself.[69] The conditions for access to major orders are much more stringent than those pertaining to minor orders for this reason. This fear crystallized in particular around the sacrament of the Eucharist.[70] To reinforce the solemnity of the entry in major orders, it was only possible for a bishop to give the permission to celebrate Mass to one of his cleric four times a year.[71] It was mandatory for the head of the diocese to refuse this promotion to a disabled cleric in order to receive only suitable priests, and then bring the case before the Pope to obtain a pontifical grace.

Following his first examination in civil law, Guillelmus was authorized by his superiors – thanks to his education and moral virtues – to receive a canonical benefice in the cathedral of Le Puy-en-Velay or in another

etiam quod luscus fueras et eras taliter, quod discernere, ut decebat, divina officia non valebas, ad Sedem Apostolicam semel et iterum appellaverunt'.

67 Hanska and Salonen, *Entering a Clerical Career*, p. 14.

68 Wilgaux, "'Υγιὴς καὶ ὁλόκλαρος", pp. 232–233, quoting Plato, *Laws*, tome VI, 759 b–c.

69 Thomas Aquinas, *Summa contra gentiles*, q. 39, q. 82; *Decretum Gratiani*, edited in Friedberg (ed.), *Corpus iuris canonici,* distinctio 55; *Decretals of Gregory IX*, op. cit., book I, title 20, chapter 3.

70 Dubourg, "*Deformitas* et célébration de l'eucharistie".

71 Tabbagh, "Effectifs et recrutement du clergé", p. 183.

collegiate church. After securing this permission, he sought the prebend of the late Dalmatius of Gorsia, Canon of Le Puy-en-Velay. The other canons, however, refused to let Guillelmus enter the cathedral chapter, because of his supposed physical impairment: he had only one hand, which, according to his detractors, did not allow him to properly perform divine services, especially since it was wracked by an incurable and deforming disease. Guillelmus was therefore considered insufficiently pure to touch the objects used during worship. Whilst minor and major orders shared the same conditions for entry in theory, suitability was more fraught for clerics with *cura animarum*, who must be exemplary and above reproach.

Faced with the canons' resistance, Guillelmus appealed to Boniface VIII, making a case for a papal grant of grace. Guillelmus' rejection, he testified, was orchestrated by Bertrandus of Sereis and three other canons, one of whom was Bertrandus' brother, and further supported by the Bishop of Le Puy-en-Velay, who refused to allow his promotion to canon for the same reason. In Guillelmus' appeal, his reputation, tainted by these slanderers, is foregrounded as the reason why the decision should be overruled. No clarification is given regarding his physical state, whether he actually was disabled and/or ill or not. Nevertheless, the Pope confirmed Guillelmus' appointment. According to canon law, 'infirmity' does not prevent promotion to the sacred orders: limb loss, ocular conditions, congenital impairment, emasculation, and missing nails are all conditions that were eligible for papal graces allowing a supplicant to enter major orders, as set out in Gregory IX's *Decretals* – a precedent to which the Papal Chancery alludes in its response, with a reference to the figure of the one-eyed cleric.[72]

Whilst the Papal Chancery could look favourably on disabled supplicants, it was essential that they were informed of the situation at hand, including the specificities of an individual's impairment, a responsibility borne by the disabled clerics themselves. In Guillelmus' case, as in most cases, it is impossible to know if he did, in fact, live with a disease ravaging his remaining hand: the Pope did not request a full examination, even if the cleric requested one in order to clear himself of all accusations once and for all. To clear his name, the Pope addressed his letter – which basically stood as an equivalent to a successful examination – to the Bishop of Le Puy-en-Velay, the abbot of the monastery of Saint-Chaffrey and the Master Uguitonus of Vercellis, chaplain of the Pope, canon of the dioceses of Bruges, Le Puy-en-Velay, and Tournai. These individuals may well have subsequently

72 *Decretals of Gregory IX*, book I, title 20: '*De corpore vitiatis ordinandis vel non*' (On the bodily defects that make it possible to be ordained or not).

initiated an investigation into Guillelmus' impairment. Unfortunately, we will never know. Nevertheless, the rumoured condition of his remaining, 'diseased' hand, did not prevent Guillelmus from becoming a canon, an outcome entirely dependent on his receipt of a papal dispensation.

Subdeacons, deacons, and priests all participated in the celebration of Mass; as members of major orders, they were authorized to touch holy objects during worship. Within the remit of a benefice with care of souls, priests could also administer the sacraments and issue penance. This obligatory roster of duties allowed the pontifical institution to limit access to major orders, especially in the case of clerics with physical and/or mental disabilities. The petitions and pontifical letters demonstrate that restrictions from those clerical duties were commonly levied in the thirteenth century, but became rarer during the fourteenth century, though this latter period may well have witnessed more rejections that were simply not recorded. In any case, the granting of a papal exemption remained subject to the two criteria enshrined in canon law in determining the suitability of disabled individuals: their physical capacity and their unimpeachable image on the flock (see Chapter 1). Suitability was formally assessed when promotion took place. However, the suitability of a priest with *cura animarum* was, practically speaking, tested every day in terms of his ability to celebrate worship.

A letter from Pope Alexander III, dated 1168–1169, addressed to Desiderius, provost of Lille, regarding a seriously ill priest from the same city, reveals how the pontifical institution handled situations in which priests could not say Mass daily:

> We have been informed that a priest voluntarily dedicates himself to a prebend in your communal church, in such a way that he is supposed to celebrate the Mass of Saint Mary daily despite the fact that his body is weighed down by illness. Your church is not only common but also provostal, i.e., the consensus of the chapter can resign or assign the prebend each year. In this practice that we have confirmed so far, the priest who previously held the prebend, prevented by the illness of his body, could not perform his divine service diligently, even if, when he was sometimes able to do so in cases of solemn Masses, he celebrated them honestly and devoutly. Because this is forbidden, he has to be transferred to another church or he has to retire for a good cause. By ordering accordingly, we ensure that no man can violate or go against our confirmation in any way.[73]

73 Archive of Lille, Saint Pierre's cartulary, 89, D.3. 11 f. 40 and Library of Lille, collegiate church of Saint Pierre's cartulary, D.3. 8, f. 12 – Alexander III to Desiderius, provost and canon of Lille,

Whilst the unnamed cleric was unable to lead worship regularly due to his ill health, he was nonetheless able to offer solemn Masses on occasion, and with exemplary conduct. Yet this fluctuating capacity was not sufficient in terms of allowing the priest to keep his office without accommodation. In the end, the Pope reconsidered the consensual election by the chapter, because a priest must be able to give mass every day. He then authorized the cleric's transfer to another church, likely removing the care of souls from his responsibilities, or even withdrawing him permanently from divine service. Since the initiating petition wrote by unnamed priest has not been preserved, we cannot know whether this decision came from the Pope directly, or whether the matter was submitted for his sign-off by Desiderius (acting in his role of the priest's superior), or if the unknown priest himself lodged the case. In any case, the letter indicates that clerics must be able to celebrate Mass daily, for a lengthy period of time, as part of their duties. Clerics were allowed no 'half measures' – for instance, leading worship occasionally – in terms of accommodating their disability within the remit of the *cura animarum*.

Logically, for a cleric to be suitable for his role, he must be able to fulfil his duties, however the ecclesiastical powers define them. A letter written by Nicholas IV on 1 August 1290 to Hugonus (surnamed Galant), rector of the church of Loberge in the diocese of Thérouanne, highlights the issue of priests' representation in worship rites. According to the summary contained in the first lines of the Pope's letter, Hugonus was authorized to join the orders of subdeacon and deacon by the Bishop of Thérouanne, despite a 'defect' in his left eye. The Bishop of Arras later sanctioned his promotion to the priesthood, a decision to which the Bishop of Thérouanne now objected. According to the latter, Hugonus was obliged to secure a pontifical dispensation in order to celebrate the Divine Office. Even if he retained some vision, his impairment was nevertheless an issue to be adjudicated

13 January 1168–1169. Text edited by Von Pflugk-Harttung (ed.), *Acta pontificum Romanorum*, n° 261, p. 241: '*Significatum est nobis, quod cuidam sacerdoti prebendam unam in ecclesia vestra communi voluntate dedistis, ita quidem, ut missam de sancta Maria, nisi corporis sit infirmitate gravatus, debeat cotidie celebrare. Qui ecclesiam vestram non nisi communi tam prepositi, quam capituli consensu potest dimittere, nec cuiquam prebende illius anniversarium delegare. Quam siquidem institutionem eatenus confirmamus, ut predictus sacerdos ecclesie memorate, nisi infirmitate corporis fuerit impeditus, assidue debeat obsequium suum impendere, et quanto frequentius potest, salva honestate sua et debita devotione, missarum sollempnia celebrare. Nec liceat sibi, hoc illi se ad aliam ecclesiam transferendo, aut voluptatis causa subtrahere. Decernimus ergo, ut nulli omnino hominum liceat, hanc paginam nostre confirmationis infringere vel ei aliquatenus contraire*'.

by the pontifical institution. Thus, the future priest appealed to Nicholas IV to receive his grace. The Pope responded:

> It is true that you have stated before the Bishop of Thérouanne about your deformity – that you have a slight stain of your left eye, present since your youth, even if it does not completely deprive it of light – and you have asked to be dispensed by the Apostolic See to serve in the [major] orders: what you humbly ask for has been provided by the grace of the Apostolic See. Yet we will ensure about it, provided that the deformity does not cause scandal, and because a reliable and esteemed witness has testified to your good morals and honest life, and we respond favorably to your requests by the use of special grace, so that you may be promoted to the priesthood despite the deformity or defect from which you suffer: we consent by the authority of this letter that you may join the divine service freely and lawfully.[74]

The Pope's grace is conditional: it holds only if Hugonus' ocular impairment does not cause scandal among the people. Hugonus is only partially blind, and thus able to read, fulfilling an essential task of the priesthood and rendering him suitable for the role from this perspective. The question of capacity is linked here to that of social representation: is the disability hidden enough to permit Hugonus to become a priest?[75] The problem for the Papal Chancery laid mainly in the way in which the supplicant may damage the clergy's public image. Initially, although in a situation of irregularity, Hugonus was authorized to serve and listen to the confessions of the faithful as deacon, subdeacon, or minor cleric by the authority of his superior, the Bishop of Thérouanne. In this period, his partial blindness and the visible stain on his eye were not an issue. A priest with *cura*, however, must be physically capable of essential clerical work: reading, consecrating the

74 RV 45, f. 64 R – Nicolas IV to Hugonus said *Galant*, rector of the church of Loberge (Thérouanne), on 1 August 1290. Text analysed by Langlois (ed.), *Les registres de Nicolas IV*, n° 3 031, for which I give the transcription according to the register: '*Verum dictus episcopus Morinensis pretendens tecum non esse super deformitate quadam quam tenuis macula inducta a tui pueritia in sinistro oculo quamquam non existas illius totali lumine destitutus, per Sedem apostolicam dispensatum te non patitur in susceptis ordinibus ministrare: super quo suppliciter petiisti tibi per ipsius Sedis graciam provideri. Nos igitur attendentes quod huiusmodi deformitas scandalum non inducit, ac volentes tibi cui de bonis moribus et honesta vita a fidedignis laudabile testimonium prohibetur, graciam facere specialem tuis supplicationibus inclinati, ut deformitate seu defectu huiusmodi quod te talem fecisti taliter in presbiterum promoveri, nequaquam obstante possis in susceptis ordinibus libere ac licite ministrare devotioni tue auctoritate presentium indulgemus*'.

75 See Dubourg, "Un/Acceptable Disability?"

host, and so on. His impairment must be minimal enough, functionally invisible or thereabouts, not to be noticed by congregants, so that he may freely perform divine services without sullying the reputation of the clergy. Thus, it is implied that Hugonus' infirmity must remain hidden from the flock – or at least, non-scandalous – in order for the grace licensing his priesthood to remain valid.

Pontifical letters could erase the apparent irregularity of a priest, in terms of their access to ecclesiastical benefices. In Hugonus' case, the Bishop of Thérouanne was circumspect: he did not wish to bear the responsibility for a potentially contested decision – and even accusations of fraud associated with the promotion. He chose instead to oppose another prelate, and thereby leave the last word to the Pope. The Pope granted the favour, we learn, because of the positive testimony he had received (perhaps from one of the two bishops) regarding Hugonus' honest morals and lifestyle. In theory, the Papal Chancery could not afford to grant undeserved favours. The words of supplicants, their superiors, and any supporters had to be verified. The version of accounts offered by interested parties to the Pope might not be objective, or could be false, exaggerated. For this reason, the Papal Chancery often added to letters an injunctive clause ordering one or more ecclesiastical officers to ensure that the measures being sanctioned were justified. Letter writers similarly inserted hedging asides such as *si est ita* ('if this is how it is'), *si verum esset* ('if this is true'), or *si preces veritate nitantur* ('if your pleas are well-founded'), which make it clear that all exemptions are voided if the supplicant has lied.[76] The objective here was to prevent any grace being issued as a result of fraudulent appeals, but such phrases also functioned as control mechanisms more generally: to specify restrictions to, or issue conditions upon, pontifical sentences.[77]

The extreme control exercised by the papacy was not limited to the Church's lower ranks, but rather intensified for appointments to higher orders which could be subject to pontifical examinations, though they were not always mandatory. The rationale for such supplementary assessment is found in canon law, notably in Gregory IX's *Decretals*. This text observes that an exemption to the assessment criteria might be ratified by a bishop following the receipt of a pontifical letter, so that a solicitor could join the orders and become a minister of God without having to undergo any examination. Taken from a letter written by Alexander III to the Archbishop

76 Zutshi, "Petitioners, Popes, Proctors", p. 286.

77 Hayez, "La personnalité d'Urbain V", p. 8. For example, Urban V restricted its grace by this process in more than a quarter of cases.

of Salerno, the following passage from the *Decretals* ensured that the bishops played a key role in granting exemptions even if this is the popes that makes the final decision:

> About the priest of Campania, who spontaneously and consciously participated in a battle during which he loses a part of his finger, we reply that if this is the true then and now, as we see it now, he has not lost so much of his finger that he can celebrate solemn Masses without scandal, not enough so that he cannot, after having done penance by acting mercifully, serve in his order despite the existing unhealthy excess.[78]

This exchange between the bishop (the superior of the priest in question) and the Pope aimed to determine whether a cleric's visible bodily difference could be the source of scandal – and thus disqualify an individual from the priestly role – according to the prominence of any deformity and its impact upon an individual's capacity to fulfil essential clerical tasks. To gauge such effects, the Apostolic See typically referred the case to third parties, called *commissarii*, who were then responsible for certifying the veracity of the supplicant's statement on occasions in which an evaluation could not be carried out in person at the Curia. In the case under discussion here, we cannot be sure whether the priest came to the Pope to undergo the examination or if the Pope saying that he saw the mutilation is only a discursive stylistic. Indeed, the inclusion of the phrase *si est ita* in papal documents did not necessarily suggest that the supplicant appeared at the Apostolic See to undergo the examination. Probably, in most cases, the *commissarius* certified the claim's veracity to the Pope, who then wrote to the disabled cleric and his superior. Moreover, the executors of pontifical grace appointed by the Pope were generally the supplicant's bishop or one of his officials, facilitating the conduct of the examination.[79] Yet there were no specific legal considerations governing the choice of such executors, and a decision regarding suitable examiners was effectively made on a case-by-case basis. Typically, the (successful) proceedings ran as follows: the bishop applied the sentence set out in the papal bull – for example, examining the supplicant – and if he passed successfully, conferred the ecclesiastical office to the supplicant (*collaudatio*), and received him in his

78 *Decretals of Gregory IX*, book I, title 20: '*De corpore vitiatis ordinandis vel non*' (On the bodily defects that make it possible to be ordained or not), chapter 1.

79 Clarke and Zutshi, *Supplications from England and Wales*, p. xvi.

church.[80] The letters from Gregory IX's *Decretals* discussing the unnamed priest in Campania indicate that both the bishop and the Pope acknowledged the supplicant's partial limb loss. Nevertheless, they both testified as to the priest's suitability for Divine Offices despite his condition, not least because his limb loss occurred on the battlefield, through no 'fault' of his own. As such, he could receive papal grace via the bishop.

The phrase *si est ita* thus constituted an effective diplomatic guarantee in the Curia's administrative and governmental system.[81] It signified the imposition of additional checks and balances upon petitioners: supplementary assessment of supplicants' physical and/or mental capacity, carried out by the Apostolic See or its official deputies, depending upon the circumstances of the specific case. Unfortunately, historians only have access to part of the overarching audit structure in which such examinations were embedded. We do not know, for example, the selection criteria for papal executors nor the identity of the person appointing them.[82] Nevertheless, without the approval of the addressee (i.e., the deputized executor), the pontifical authority contained in the document became null and void. The executor might refuse to follow through with the papal exemption, if he considered an impairment to be too severe, for instance, or if the applicant proved to be unworthy in other respects. In this case, the petitioner was authorized to call upon the Pope and request another *comissarius* to conduct the investigation, alleging bias or excessive severity on the part of his first evaluator.[83] The *si est ita* clause reveals that, in certain situations, clerics at the local level were invested by the Apostolic See with real decision-making power, in terms of appointing appropriate individuals to benefices for which the local cleric was responsible.[84] Nonetheless, bishops and their officials tended to accept the initial ruling on a case from the Papal Chancery and perform examination only under pressure, with the aim of maintaining a good relationship with the Apostolic See.[85]

In the most complex cases, the Papal Chancery used a 'double-dispatch' system to have their orders executed by third parties. This process allowed the papal authorities to verify that the local hierarchy complied with their requests.[86] Several letters were thus sent: one gracious missive

80 De Collenberg, "Le choix des exécuteurs", p. 394.
81 Smith, "Papal Executors and the Veracity of Petitions", p. 682.
82 Hitzbleck, *Exekutoren*, p. 553.
83 Clarke and Zutshi, *Supplications from England and Wales*, pp. xvi–xvii.
84 Smith, "Papal Executors and the Veracity of Petitions", p. 675.
85 Morris, *The Papal Monarchy*, p. 549.
86 De Collenberg, "Le choix des exécuteurs", p. 395.

to the supplicant or a third-party addressee, and another communiqué containing the mandate to apply the exemption, sent to executors.[87] Letters sent by the Chancery could thus have many interlocutors in the form of named executors to whom the relevant additional letter was sent. The two documents have strictly the same content; the only variance comprises an additional execution order appended to the letters to executors.[88] Papal registers record this method of dispatch with the following notation: the letters are followed by as many *in eodem modo* ('in the same way') entries as necessary, according to the number of executory recipients.[89] As Figures 3.2 and 3.3 show, 57% of the letters dating to the thirteenth century (8 out of 14) and 81% of fourteenth-century examples (62 out of 76) containing an *in eodem modo* clause ('in. e. m.' letters) were sent at first to the supplicants.[90] De facto, there were many more executors than supplicants, at a rate of almost three to one; 'in. e. m.' letters were sent, on average, to 2.8 and 2.9 recipients in the thirteenth and fourteenth centuries, respectively.[91]

Recipients of 'in. e. m.' letters were, by and large, powerful people, whether active in the lay or ecclesiastical community. They were responsible for enforcing the pontifical sentence themselves, or for delegating its enforcement to one or more agents.[92] They formed a committee established to adjudicate matters of benefices under discussion. This typically comprised a senior member of the secular clergy (generally from the province in which the petitioner resided, but from a different bishopric) or an abbot from a different diocese, a representative of the Pontifical Curia, and a person chosen by the petitioner.[93] In both the thirteenth and fourteenth centuries,

87 Maillard-Luypaert and Cauchies, *Papauté, clercs et laïcs*, p. 192.

88 The pontifical letters containing the 'in.e.m.' clause represent only 5% of the total corpus of documents discussing physical and mental disability in the thirteenth century (14 out of 276), and 12% of those in the fourteenth century (76 out of 624). All of them contain an additional execution order.

89 Gasnault, "L'élaboration des lettres secretes", p. 212: this formula opens with a shorter copy of the letter, usually the first three words, until the duties of these recipients appear.

90 These figures contain the cross-referenced data from supplicants (lines) and executors in the 'in e. m.' letters (INEM, rows) in the thirteenth century (Figure 3.2) and the fourteenth century (Figure 3.3). They group the supplicants according to their ecclesiastical statutes and put them in contact with the executors' statutes.

91 The total of executors is 40 for 14 supplicants in the thirteenth century (or 2.8 per supplicant), and 220 for 76 applicants in the fourteenth century (or 2.9 per supplicant). There is only one case in which the letter 'in e. m.' was send to the supplicant himself (not explicit here).

92 Giry, *Manuel de diplomatique*, p. 688: This obligation is signified in the deeds by the formula '*quocirca mandamus, quatenus vos vel duo aut unus vestrum per vos vel alium seu alios*'. The final protocol is also summarized in the registers, since it is similar to the body of the letter.

93 De Collenberg, "Le choix des exécuteurs", pp. 397–398.

Figure 3.2 Cross-referenced data from supplicants and executors 'in e. m.' in the thirteenth century

			Lay people (6)		Secular orders (20)			Monastic orders (14)		
	Supplicants	INEM	Individuals	Groups	Major orders	Minor orders	Groups	Individual s	Groups	Total INEM
Lay people	Individuals	0								0
	Groups	0								0
Secular orders (12)	Major orders	9	1	4	6		5	8	2	26
	Minor orders	3			4	3		2		9
	Groups	0								0
Monastic orders (2)	Individuals	2		1	2			1	1	5
	Groups	0								0
	Total	14	1	5	12	3	5	11	3	40

Figure 3.3 Cross-referenced data from supplicants and executors 'in e. m' in the fourteenth century

			Lay people (9)		Secular orders (147)			Monastic orders (64)		
	Supplicants	INEM	Individuals	Groups	Major orders	Minor orders	Groups	Individuals	Groups	Total INEM
Lay people (2)	Individuals	2			1	3		2		6
	Groups	0								0
Secular orders (53)	Major orders	28	1	2	29	21	3	18	1	75
	Minor orders	25			32	26		21		79
	Groups	0								0
Monastic orders (21)	Individuals	21	1	5	25	7		15	7	60
	Total	76	2	7	87	57	3	56	8	220

the composition of the committee varied according to the ecclesiastical rank of the petitioner. Secular clerics from the major or minor orders and regular clerics played an almost equal role in the granting of pontifical grace (see Figures 3.2 and 3.3). Nevertheless, the controls put in place to examine the validity of papal grants of grace were intrinsically hierarchical. Indeed, for a bishop or an archbishop, the initial executors were often abbots, priors, and/or archbishops or bishops. The canons of the relevant diocese also took part in the process, probably for informative or even coercive purposes. For a monk or abbot, the executory committee was usually composed of another abbot and/or a bishop, along with representatives of the institutional community to which the supplicant belonged. The makeup of the committee was not left to chance. Indeed, it was precisely strategic for all involved. On the one hand, the supplicant was permitted to engage his supporters in order to sway things in his favour. At the same time, the Apostolic See stacked the committee with intermediaries in order to control the process. The corpus reveals that the committees were compiled on a case-by-case basis to optimize supervision. Whilst the Pope delegated certain powers to the recipients *in eodem modo*, they were not independent actors, but rather, traditional relays of pontifical authority. Deputized by the papacy, these executors, in fact, ensured that edicts issued at the top of the ecclesiastical hierarchy flowed down to, and were respected at, the local level.

Whilst it was true that supplicants who wanted to join major orders could bypass local authorities, ultimately, they had to respect the theoretical standards of suitability – physical and/or mental ability and unimpeachable image – found in canon law and adjudicated by the papacy. Indeed, permission to bend regulations as to physical and/or mental 'defects' was the sole purview of the Pope. Disabled clerics who wanted to enter major orders, or their superiors, had to contact the Papal Chancery. The election of a disabled subdiaconate, diaconate, priest, or canon was under strict papal control. And the process became even more stringent when ascending the ecclesiastical hierarchy, when disabled clerics petitioned to become bishops or abbots.

Access to the Bishopric and the Abbacy

The election of a bishop or an abbot entailed a rigorous adjudication process. The manner in which the election procedure was conducted could be subject to assessment, as could the individual standing for election himself. Once more, an applicant's superiors judged his physical and/or mental capacities, despite any previous examinations in this vein. Access to the priesthood already represented a key stage in the ecclesiastical career, but in the case of bishops or abbots – directly under the authority of the Holy See, and thus with a hotline to power themselves – the need to strictly control membership became even more urgent. Promotion to the higher echelons of the Church required applicants to journey to the Roman or Avignonese Curia and pay tribute to the Pope, alongside undergoing another assessment of their skills and physical suitability to their new role, one which came with substantially increased visibility and responsibility. With these measures, the pontifical institution sought to guarantee the suitability of clergy at the highest level of the organization's hierarchy, with the aim of admitting only those who could best fulfil the diverse requirements of the office.

Clerics with disabilities were not barred from seeking promotion to the bishopric or abbacy. Nevertheless, if they pursued such a promotion, they were required to request a pontifical dispensation for their eventual election to be authorized. Whilst a successful appeal to the Pope was mandatory, making such a request was only permissible, however, after the recognition of their promotion at the local level. This is the case, for example, with the cleric Nicolaus. After his promotion to the bishopric by the superintendent, deacon, and chapter of the cathedral of Verdun, Nicolaus was obliged to submit himself to an examination of conformity, because, according to the relevant papal source, it was well known that he suffered from a 'stain' (*macula*) on his eye. In his letter dated 27 August 1310, Pope Clement V (1264–1314) summarized the various stages in the recognition of Nicolaus' election:

> The petition you bring to our attention contends that, because Thomas, the former Bishop of Verdun had just died, the Superintendent, the Deacon and the chapter of that church – following the custom of choosing the future suitable pastor all together – unanimously elected you as Bishop of Verdun. Then, the prosecutors of the said superintendent, deacon and chapter met with your metropolitan, Ditherius of good memory, Archbishop of Trier, to inform him of this election, which he immediately confirmed. The same Archbishop has proposed in his general letters that a proclamation be issued in your church in Verdun so that, if some people wish to oppose your election, they can appear before the Archbishop in a given time. However, no one appeared during the delay to complain about your election. The same Archbishop has carefully examined your merits and dedication in a diligent investigation of your person and the form of your election. He recognizes by his learned opinion that you are an appropriate person, able to celebrate according to the precepts of the Church notwithstanding the stain from which you suffered and from which you still suffer now in your eye with which you were able to see and you are still able to see. Then, this metropolitan authority confirms that you may serve as bishop and consecrates you according to your election by the Superintendent, Deacon and chapter mentioned above, confirming and consecrating the above election by the letters of the said Archbishop, bearing seals called 'complete'. Consequently, we respond favourably to your requests, confirming and consecrating your election, notwithstanding the stain above-mentioned.[94]

94 RV 57, f. 142 R – Clement V to Nicolaus, Bishop of Verdun, 27 August 1310. Text analysed by Benedictine monks (eds.), *Registres de Clément V*, n° 5670, for which I give the transcription according to the register: '*Sane petitio tua nobis exhibita continebat quod dudum ecclesia tua Virdunensi per obitum bone memorie Thomae Virdunensis episcopi predicti tui pastoris regimine destituta dilectus filius … primicerius … decanus et capitulum eiusdem pro futuri substitutione pastoris, ut moris est, convenientes in unum, te in Virdudensis episcopum concorditer elegerunt. Demum vero procuratoribus eorumdem primicerii, decani et capituli ad hoc specialiter constitutis*

Nicolaus' case is emblematic of the stringent regulations to which elections to the bishopric were subject, grounded in canon law with examinations *in forma electionis*. Gregory IX's *Decretals* observed, for example, that a bishop must be questioned in depth before being confirmed.[95] In Nicolaus' case, the investigation, conducted *in forma electionis* by the archbishop, established that the would-be bishop was an appropriate individual, despite the stain on his eye, especially because his disability did not affect his vision.

Clement's letter details the examination of Nicolaus' moral and intellectual qualities in its latter portion. Its opening section sheds further light, however, on the way in which the relative visibility of an individual's disability impacted their supposed suitability for serving in the clergy. It chronicles a rather extraordinary decision undertaken, it seems, due to the fact that Nicolaus' impairment was so well known. Ditherius, the archbishop responsible for the investigation, issued a decree in the church of Verdun, allowing those opposed to Nicolaus' appointment to make themselves, and their objections, known. This was certainly not a standard part of the promotion process, even for disabled clerics, because there is no other letter that mentions it. Ditherius' invitation to the faithful, the *populo* (the people), to weigh in on the election – itself a means of 'warning' them of Nicolaus' potential installation as bishop – proves that a senior cleric's reputation and decency, including their 'reputation' for disability (i.e., the visibility thereof), was of fundamental importance for the ecclesiastical institution.

The local ecclesiastical hierarchy to which Nicolaus reported presumably already knew about his disability. He had, after all, undergone several compulsory examinations, administered by local authorities, to progress

ad bone memorie Ditherii archiepiscopi Treverensis, metropolitani tui, tunc viventis presenciam accedentibus et dictam electionem petentibus ab eo cum instantia confirmari. Idem archiepiscopus in dicta tua ecclesia Virdunensi per suas litteras generale citationis proponi fecit edictum, ut si qui huiusmodi electioni se vellent opponere, coram eodem archiepiscopo certo peremptorio ad hoc in eisdem litteris termino constituto legitime comparerent. Et quia nullus adhoc comparuit coram ipso in termino supradicto. Idem archiepiscopus de tuis meritis et eligentium studiis ac electionis forma diligentius inquisita ac persona tua et forma electionis ipsius examinatis sollicite electionem ipsam, quia illam de te persona iidonea invenit canonice celebratam de consilio sapientum non obstante macula, quam tunc patiebaris sicut adhuc pateris, in altero oculorum, de quo tunc videbas et etiam adhuc vides auctoritate metropolitica confirmavit tibique postmodum servatis in hoc statutis a iure temporibus propriis manibus munus consecrationis impendit, prout de electione huiusmodi per decretum super hoc confectum primicerii, decani et capituli predictorum et confirmatione ac consecratione predictis per litteras eiusdem archiepiscopi sigillo munitas plenius dicitur apparere. Nos igitur tuis supplicationibus inclinati, electionem, confirmationem, et consecrationem huiusmodi, non obstante macula supradicta'.

95 *Decretals of Gregory IX*, edited in Friedberg (ed.), *Corpus iuris canonici*, book I, title 12: '*De scrutinio in ordine faciendo*'.

in the seven degrees of minor and major orders, necessary steps to becoming a bishop.[96] We can also assume that parishioners were informed of his disability, since they were called upon to give their opinion on his election to the bishopric. In any case, it is clear that the archbishop was especially concerned about congregants' reaction to Nicolaus' election, evidenced by his decision to draw attention to this issue in his response to the Apostolic See. Through his rhetoric, Ditherius thus presents himself in an almost hagiographical light: he preferred to seek the opinion of the common laity before settling on his own decision, in order to satisfy his own political (and pontifical) ambitions, and protect himself against any potential objection to Nicolaus' appointment on the basis of his putative lack of decency. Nicolaus' election was, in fact, uncontested; he was eventually confirmed as bishop by Ditherius himself, as no *scandalum* arose following the election. Canon law, it seems, considered suitability as one of the principal conditions that had to be satisfied in the appointment of a bishop. Ocular stains or limb loss did not always constitute prohibitive impediments to acceding to the bishopric, as long as such impairments did not impact clerics' decency and did not induce *scandalum*.[97]

Awareness of the potential rejection of disabled clerics by lay worshippers prompted the Papal Chancery to compel all high-ranking clergy, such as archbishops, bishops, or abbots, to visit the Apostolic See for confirmation of their appointment. The Pope, their ultimate hierarchical superior, must meet newly elected members in person in order to enthrone them, but also – and more importantly – to personally verify their moral and intellectual qualities. This rule is found in particular in canon 26 of Lateran IV issued in 1215:

> Those who are immediately subject to the Roman pontiff, must appear personally before him for confirmation if this can be done conveniently, otherwise they may send suitable persons from whom may be ascertained the necessary information regarding the process of the election and the person of the one elected; so that only after a thorough investigation by the Pope will those elected obtain the plenitude of their office, provided, of course, there be no canonical obstruction. Those who live at a great

96 Barrow, *The Clergy in the Medieval World*, p. 38.

97 *Decretus Gratiani*, edited in Friedberg (ed.), *Corpus iuris canonici*, distinctio 55, canon 8: '*Licite ordinetur episcopus, qui per hominum insidias eunnchizatur*': '*Eunuchus, si per insidias* (=*ex insultus et iniuria*) *hominum factus est, uel si in persecutione eius sunt amputata uirilia, uel si ita natus est, et est dignus, fiat episcopus*'; *Decretales Gregory IX*, op. cit., book I, title 20, chapter 3: '*quod eunuchus, si per insidias hominum factus, vel ita natus sit, aut etiam in persecutione sint ei amputata virilia, et dignus est, possit in episcopum promoveri*', quoting the canon of the apostles.

> distance, that is outside of Italy, if they have been elected unanimously, may in the meantime and by way of exception (dispensative), on account of the needs of the churches, administer the respective offices in matters spiritual and temporal, so, however that they alienate absolutely nothing belonging to the churches. The consecration or benediction let them receive as has so far been the custom.[98]

Despite Ditherius' anxiety surrounding congregants' potentially negative reaction to Nicolaus, the requirement for an audience with the Pope was waived for the new bishop, as he was elected unanimously and resided far from the Curia. In other words: clerics' disability did not automatically compel greater face-to-face interaction with, and surveillance by, the papacy.

Notwithstanding Nicolaus' situation, meeting the Pope in person was not simply a bureaucratic 'box-ticking' exercise for disabled clerics. Indeed, decisions made by local authorities in clerics' favour could be overturned, and disabilities that were deemed prohibitive for clerics acceding to more senior roles within the ecclesiastical hierarchy could be 'discovered' during this supplementary assessment stage. A letter from John XXII, concerning Galterus of Fournis, monk of the Benedictine Abbey of La Trinità della Cava in the diocese of Salerno, allows us to address this question:

> Since the Benedictine monastery of St. Nicholas and St. Cataldo in Lecce no longer has a pastoral guide because of the abbot Petrus's recent death, the dear brothers of the convent of this monastery called all those who wanted, should and could easily be present to discuss the future election of the abbot, to set a suitable day for all. During this assembly, Galterus of Fournis, monk of the Benedictine Abbey of La Trinità della Cava in the diocese of Salerno was elected abbot of this monastery thanks to a compromise, despite the defect and deformity he notably had to his right hand. The so-called elected monk, as a result of this consensus, out of habit of respecting the law, personally came to the Apostolic See to confirm his election – as requested by the law promulgated at the time of our predecessor Nicholas III – placing his trust in our judgment and that of our brothers present to whom he explained the situation. We have asked our venerable brother Berengarius, Bishop of Portus, our dear sons Gaucelmus, priest of Saint Marcelin and Saint Peter, and Raymundus, deacon of Santa Maria Novella, to form a commission to examine this case. But, since the monk Galterus had exposed his deformity to us [the Pope and a bishop],

98 *The Canons of the Fourth Lateran Council, 1215*, canon 26.

> and his deformity being such enormous in his right hand, and the monk himself having acknowledged that his deformity cannot in any way be tolerated for an abbot, the said monk does not wish to undergo further examinations at the Roman Curia by the above-mentioned bishops and cardinal since he cannot receive a licence from us on this subject.[99]

Galterus had been elected abbot of the monastery of St. Nicholas and St. Cataldo in Lecce, after the death of his abbatial predecessor, Petrus. Galterus' election was a 'compromise', as his impairment meant that he was not an ideal candidate. Unlike Nicolaus, he was not elected unanimously but by consensus. For this reason, and following an earlier decree made by Nicholas III, Galterus was obliged to visit the Apostolic See to have his appointment ratified. This case demonstrates the logistical minutiae of the episcopal appointment procedure, including conventional standards and exemptions therefrom. As a general rule, monks gathered in chapter to choose their next abbot. Then, in cases where the abbot was subject to diocesan authority, the appointment had to be ratified by the bishop. The latter blessed the newly elected official in a ceremony, during which he verified that the monastic community had taken part in the election.[100] In the event of a dispute, however, the Pope or archbishop might consecrate

99 RV 74, f. 50 V (RA 18, f. 58 V) – John XXII to Christophorus, provost of the Benedictine monastery of San Angelo de Valleregia (Diocese of Valva), 6 October 1322. Text analysed by Mollat (ed.), *Jean XXII*, n° 16 393, for which I give the transcription according to the register: '*Dudum siquidem monasterio sanctorum Nicolai et Cataldi Liciensis ad dictam Romanam ecclesiam nullo medio pertinente ordinis sancti Benedicti per obitum quondam Petri, abbatis ipsi pastoris regimine destituto dilecti filii conventus eiusdem monasterio vocatis omnibus qui voluerunt, debuerunt et potuerunt comode interesse ad tractandum de futuri substitutione abbatis die ad hoc prefixa convenientes in unum, Galterum de Fournis, monachum monasterio Cavensis dicti ordinis, Salernitanae diocesis, quamvis in dextera manu deformitatis defectum notabiliter pateretur, per viam compromissi in abbatem elegerunt dicti monasterii Liciensis. Cumque idem monachus post consensum electioni huiusmodi per eum sui superioris habita super hoc licentia prestitum ad Sedem apostolicam pro confirmatione electionis huiusmodi personaliter accessisset, seque etiam niteretur in nostra et fratrum nostrorum constitutus presentia excusare quod in veniendo ad dictam Sedem iuxta formam constitutionis felicis recordationis Nicolai pape III predecessoris nostri super hoc edite tempora non servarat, nos huiusmodi negotium venerabili fratri nostro Berengario episcopo Portuensis, et dilectis filiis nostris Gaucelmo, titulo sanctorum Marcellini et Petri, presbitero, ac Raimundo sancte Marie Nove diacono, cardinalibus examminandum commissimus et nobis postmodum referendum et cum idem episcopus cui idem Galterius dictam deformitatem ostendit nobis exposuisset quod ipse sic enormem deformitatem in dicta manu dextera monachi eiusdem conspexerat quod huiusmodi deformitas non erat in abbate aliquatenus toleranda, idem monachus nolens eiusdem episcopi et dictorum cardinalium ulterius examen subire de Romanam curia sine licentia nostra huiusmodi negotio sic pendente, recessit*'.
100 Gaudemet, *Les élections dans l'Église latine*, p. 236.

the abbot in the bishop's stead. Abbots were, at times, impelled to pledge their obedience to the Pope alone, especially if they were appointed to head a house otherwise exempted from episcopal authority. Visiting the Roman or the Avignonese Curia was thus an essential step to confirm their appointment and receive pontifical blessing.

In Galterus' case, the Pope was called upon to resolve the conflict at hand. Following convention, the pontiff called upon to resolve the conflict launched an investigation to determine whether the election had been conducted properly, and whether the would-be abbot was even suitable for promotion in the first place.[101] The examination commission organized by the Holy See in this matter for Galterus was composed of a trio of illustrious clerics: Berengarius, Bishop of Portus; Gaucelmus, priest of Saint Marcelin and Saint Peter; and Raymundus, deacon of Santa Maria Novella. These investigators were tasked to determine, as papal agents, whether Galterus' deformity was 'enormous', and thus intolerable. The use of the adjective 'enormous' (*ex normis*) here, a term which literally means 'outside the norms', reveals that certain disabilities were potentially impossible to 'forgive' because of their potential incompatibility with the highest clerical offices, which is further confirmed by the use of the formula *aliquatenus toleranda* ('tolerable to a certain extent').[102] Galterus, however, decided not to wait for the commission to even be formally convened, perhaps on the understanding that their judgment was a foregone conclusion, and not in his favour. The Pope had already considered that his deformity was to be incompatible with the abbot's office, and it was his decision that held the most weight. As Galterus did not contest the sanction, he was no longer obliged to present himself before the committee, and the process of electing an alternative abbot began. Indeed, the Pope asked the college of voters to appoint another abbot, and wrote directly to Christophorus (addressee of this letter and intendant of the Benedictine monastery of St. Angela de Valleregia in the diocese of Valva), to take over the management of the community of St. Nicholas and St. Cataldo in Lecce in the interim.

Petitions and papal letters were written for clear-sighted reasons: to enable disabled clerics to contravene canon law and/or specific clerical or monastic rules concerning the entry in the minor or major orders, alongside those governing the benefices with or without cure. Exemptions were given according to the severity of the disability, judged not only in terms of an individual's physical and/or mental capacity but also of his public image.

101 Berlière, *Les élections abbatiales*, p. 11.

102 On 'enormity', see Théry, "*Atrocitas/enormitas*".

But the flexibility facilitated by grants of pontifical grace could also be increased following certain favourable conditions, either in terms of the supplicant's desirable qualities at the time the request was made or to the ongoing needs of an institution.

Favourable Circumstances

The dialogue between the disabled applicant and the pontifical institution was a negotiation. Whilst the former presented his specific capabilities, the latter set the bar in terms of which role (and concomitant duties) they would allow the would-be entrant to fulfil. For disabled applicants, two major factors increased their bargaining power: their own educational prowess, and any exigent circumstances affecting the institution, or indeed the Church as a whole. Firstly, it was hard to find well-educated clerics. As such, applicants with a strong educational background potentially had an advantage over their able-bodied, less-educated peers. Secondly, moments of crisis, notably epidemics of disease, presented opportunities for irregular candidates to enter orders as suitability criteria were relaxed. The Black Death pandemic in the second half of the fourteenth century, for example, led to a shortfall in the number of clerics. The Church's emergency recruitment drive opened the door for disabled clerics. In this context, then, it becomes clear that the rules governing clerical bodies were more malleable than one might first expect. They could be selectively softened by the papal institution, if the needs were pressing enough.

Educational Attainment

The letters issued by the Papal Chancery show that disabled clerics were not dismissed out of hand by the pontifical institution. Indeed, such clerics could be extremely useful, and they often possessed rare and sought-after capacities.[103] In their rhetoric, disabled supplicants sought to market themselves in terms of their aptitudes according to the Curia's ongoing needs and expectations. Despite their disability, they offered solutions to some of the Church's unmet needs. The ecclesiastical profession required a bedrock of education, with future clerics achieving certain qualifications that were understood as essential to becoming an effective member of the clergy. Yet not all applicants had the same skills; the quality of education varied, often

103 Abberley, "The Limits of Classical Social Theory", p. 37.

as a result of students' social background.[104] Educational excellence was thus a highly desirable recruitment criterion in the eyes of the ecclesiastical institution – hence the rigorous entrance examinations to ensure that only the most competent individuals were hired. As discussed above, the Pontifical Institution proposed a definition of capacity in which 'being suitable' for the clergy was no longer entirely synonymous with 'being able'. Clerics might have the requisite knowledge base, yet lack the physical and/or mental capacity to progress projects or works further, in practical terms. This was not a deal-breaker for the Curia, however. In the cases we have been able to study, the Papal Chancery invariably prioritized, and promoted, clerical education, rather than being swayed by concerns regarding clerical disability.[105] A high degree of education could functionally neutralize the 'problem' of a cleric's disability. Popes managed this trade-off by, at times, limiting the expectations levied on disabled clerics in order to integrate them more easily into the fabric of the Church. This is the logic, for instance, underpinning the grant of benefices without *cura* to disabled clerics.

Lack of education amongst the clergy posed a significant challenge to the Church. Popes were frequently forced to give advice to their subordinates on how to deal with poorly educated clergymen. Such clerics put the Church and its message at an even greater risk than the potential damage wrought by their disabled counterparts. Ill-educated clergy could unwittingly spread misinformation and heretical ideas to their flock, since they were responsible for the laity's religious instruction.[106] To remediate this risk, the pontifical institution made instruction at the local level mandatory for all clerics, with the explicit aim of protecting the Christian message from distortion, as set out in canon 27 of Lateran IV, issued in 1215.[107] Synods, organized for this purpose, provided a framework for the continued professional development of ecclesiastics, through the verification of their knowledge and use of Latin. Records of such meetings offer us a portrait of a typical parish priest in the

104 Lis and Soly, *Worthy Efforts*, p. 114. These authors point out that more and more priests and clerics came from the poorest classes during the medieval period.

105 A parallel can be drawn here with the medieval urban economy: the working population was highly knowledgeable, even if such knowledge was not always put into practice. See Chevalier, "Corporations, conflits politiques et paix sociale".

106 The contemporary study of the clergy in Castile at the end of the medieval period, carried out thanks to a pastoral visit of the Archdiaconate of Madrid dated to 1427, reveals the extent to which the Church wished to offer clergy a minimal education. See Rucquoi, "La formation culturelle du clergé". The author relies on the number of books (especially liturgical books), their language (not necessarily in Latin), and the university education of clerics to highlight the difficulty of judging their cultural level.

107 The role of the popes in local education is studied by Boyle, *Pastoral Care*.

thirteenth century, as well as illustrating the anguish of the Church caused by its poorly educated workforce.[108] Canon law was a prominent subject on the synodal curriculum, as it was difficult for village priests to understand and, in any case, its dissemination to the Church's rank and file remained relatively narrow.[109] Synodal statutes, moreover, aimed to strengthen the spiritual and intellectual education of clerics, thereby highlighting the evident shortcomings of the appointment system.[110]

Education, then, was a solid factor in gaining access to a grace. The training of clerics who wished to access major liturgical functions was becoming a priority for the Church. This is demonstrated, for example, in the case of Rigaldus of Komeffe, who lost the vision in his left eye as a result of a 'fortuitous' blow when he was a child:

> Your petition brought to our attention mentions that, when you were a child, playing with a friend, you take a blow to the left eye, without any fault of your own and by accident, but this blow caused you to lose the vision in the left eye, even though you say you are able to read and sing and that you were received as suitable without fraud in the church of Liège. That is why you humbly ask us to do what is necessary so that, notwithstanding this defect, you can be promoted in all orders. We hereby dispense with special grace that you may assume the minor orders and the position of sub-deacon notwithstanding this defect.[111]

The letter notes that Rigaldus himself initiated the request, highlighting in the appeal his skills as a reader and singer. These two talents attested to his ability to pass the examinations necessary to be appointed as a cleric and thereby gain entrance to major orders. Crucially, as the letter underscores, Rigaldus proved himself without committing any fraud. For this reason,

108 Rapp, "Les synodes diocésains", p. 27.

109 Belin, "Les statuts synodaux", p. 29.

110 Consult Pontal, "Le rôle du synode diocésain".

111 RV 44, f. 143 R – Nicholas IV at Rigaldus de Komeffe, canon of Liege, on 20 April 1289. Text edited by Langlois (ed.), *Les registres de Nicolas IV*, n° 862: '*Exhibita siquidem nobis tua petitio continebat quod olim, in etate puerili existens, cum tuis ludendo coetaneis, ab uno ipsorum percussionem, sine culpa tua, in oculo sinistro, casu fortuito, recepisti, cujus percussionis occasione visum ejusdem oculi perdidisti, sed ad legendum et cantandum adeo habilis esse diceris quod Leodiensis ecclesia in te debitis obsequiis non fraudatur. Quare nobis humiliter supplicasti ut tecum quod, hujusmodi non obstante defectu, possis ad omnes ordines promoveri, dispensare misericorditer curaremus. Nos igitur* [...] *ut minores et subdiaconatus ordines assumere valeas, hujusmodi non obstante defectu, tecum auctoritate presentium de speciali gratia dispensamus*'.

he was authorized for promotion to minor orders and the subdiaconate.[112] Rigaldus' thirteenth-century case is indicative of the increasing importance attached to education in ecclesiastical recruitment as well as the care given to the applications during the ordination exams. This trend, beginning at the end of the eleventh century, perhaps reflects the Church's desire to recruit more mature and capable servants, reorienting the clerical career.[113] Clerical candidates were instructed through the observation and imitation of their betters, confirmed clerics who acted as teachers and mentors, even before this practice was mandated at the Council of Trent on 22 May 1542.[114] Such pedagogical relationships were sometimes formalized with an apprenticeship contract that specified the reciprocal obligations of teacher and student, an arrangement similar to that of many other professions.[115]

Well-educated ecclesiastics could be something of a rarity in the clergy, which explains why impairments were sometimes minimized. This provided useful leverage for disabled clerics. At the same time, the papacy could also exploit the situation to their advantage: the granting of a papal exemption was sometimes subject to the disabled supplicant obtaining certain qualifications or developing their knowledge in key areas. This is evidenced by a letter written by Boniface VIII on 22 April 1295 to the cleric Jacobus:

> Your petition brought to our attention mentions that, during the time of our predecessor Pope Nicholas IV, you were exempted by apostolic

112 See also another letter RA 169, f. 524 R – Urban V to Martinus Roderici, canon of the Church of Toledo and Didacus Fernandi, treasurer of the same church, on 9 July 1369. It addresses the case of Alfonsus Lupi, cleric of Cordoba. The latter can neither sing, nor read, nor even speak intelligently (i.e., construct a sentence). However, Alfonsus asks to be appointed Canon of Toledo, even as if he is described by the Pope as 'almost totally mentally deficient'. Urban V announces that the grace will only be valid if Alfonsus can perform at least two of the three expected performances (singing, reading, or speaking). The pontiff therefore reduces the expectations of the canon's role so that this supplicant may one day be suitable for the position. Text analysed by Avril, Botineau, Gaborit, Gaborit-Chopin, Hayez, Hayez, and Laurent (eds.), *Urbain V*, n° 24 707, for which I give the transcription according to the register: '*Dictus Alfonsus legere et construere et cantare nesciebat, imo erat quasi penitus idiota, attendentes quod in statutis ipsius ecclesie aliquibus non conferantur nisi scientibus bene legere et construere ac cantare vel saltem duo ex ipsis*'.

113 Barrow, *The Clergy in the Medieval World*, p. 70.

114 Council of Trent, Session 23, chapter 7: 'The examination that the bishop must make of those who present themselves to the Orders', quoted in Dohar, "*Sufficienter litteratus*", p. 317.

115 Bornstein, "How to Behave in Church". The author studies an apprenticeship contract signed in 1340 in Treviso between the cleric Giovanni di Nascimbene of Monselice and the priest Pietro, rector of San Lorenzo, to allow Giovanni to stay for five years with the priest in order to learn the clerical art and function (*ars et officum clericatus*).

> authority from the defect from which you suffer, that is, you were born without a right hand, as it pleased God that you were born, but that you nevertheless devoted yourself to the study of literature and it is said that you are making notable progress, notwithstanding this defect and after having received this exemption, you were able to serve as a cleric and receive the clerical tonsure. Following this, we accept that, after having studied civil law for five years with insistence, having obtained commendable results, we improve this grace, notwithstanding your defect and we dispense you by apostolic grace so that you can be promoted to minor orders and receive a benefice without cure of souls.[116]

The missive begins with the Pontiff pointedly reminding all parties that Jacobus was authorized by Nicholas IV, his papal predecessor, to receive the tonsure despite being born without a right hand, because of his exemplary dedication to developing his knowledge of literature and grammar. Five years later, Boniface increased the remit of his predecessor's grace, now authorizing Jacobus, who had already received the clerical tonsure thanks to Nicholas' dispensation, to be promoted to minor orders. This is a direct result of Jacobus' admirable studiousness, having diligently studied civil law for the past five years alongside achieving excellent results during his apprenticeship. Regardless of his praise, the Pope reiterated, albeit implicitly, the potential threat posed by Jacobus' impairment to the care of souls: the cleric is still prohibited from accessing major orders. Nevertheless, the fact that Jacobus secured a benefice, even one without *cura animarum*, highlights the ways in which spiritual and intellectual qualities could compensate for clerics' bodily 'defects'. Indeed, education appears to have been a valuable commodity for disabled men wishing to join divine orders, even if an individual's disability was highly visible and prevented him from

116 RV 47, f. 35 R – Boniface VIII to Jacobus, cleric born of the noble Johannes Judicis de Clausura, a Roman citizen, on 22 April 1295. Text analysed by Digard, Fawtier, Faucon, and Thomas (eds.), *Les registres de Boniface VIII*, n° 130, for which I give the transcription according to the register: '*Petitio tua nobis exhibita continebat quod olim felicis recordationis Nicolaus Pape IIII predecessoris nostri tecum super defectu quem pateris ex eo quod sine manu dextera sicut Domino placuit ortus fuisti quoque diu insistens studio litterarum in grammaticalibus profecisse commendabiliter dicebaris, auctoritate apostolica dispensavit ut huiusmodi non obstante defectu posses clericalem tonsuram tamen recipere, et cum clericis Domino deservire tuque post dispensationem huiusmodi prefatam clericalem tonsuram te asseris recepisse. Cum autem, sicut accepimus, postmodum iuris civilis per quinquennium insistens studio, in eo laudabiliter profecisse noscaris, nos volentes tibi graciam facere ampliorem ut defectu predicto nequaquam obstante possis ad omnes minores ordines promoveri et ecclesiasticum beneficium cui animarum cura non immineat obtinere auctoritate apostolica dispensamus*'.

performing Mass or administering the sacraments. Flexibility of this kind allowed the Papal Chancery to recruit high-calibre clerics. At the same time, it enabled the Church to recruit much-needed clerics when they were in otherwise short supply, educated or otherwise, as became apparent during the Black Death plague pandemic.

The Black Death and Its Aftermath

Public-health crises initially led to a reduction in the number of papal dispensations granted. This decline was due to the difficulties inherent in travel, identified, for example, during the 1347–1352 outbreak of plague – the Black Death – and its many resurgences, when plague became a somewhat routine part of late fourteenth-century life. The pandemic caused mortality rates to skyrocket, thereby causing a substantial reduction in the number of clerics who were available and suitable for parish leadership. In consequence, there was an uptick in petitions and papal letters regarding many different ecclesiastical matters, among which were irregular nominations. With a catastrophe on its hands, the Curia relaxed criteria for the receipt of papal dispensations, with the aim of recruiting and installing much-needed clergymen as soon as possible.

The Black Death, a contagious disease that swept across Europe between 1347 and 1352, arrived in Avignon in 1348 under the reign of Clement VI, later returning to the region in 1361 at the end of the reign of Innocent VI. The end of each epidemic episode marked the beginning of an increase in the number of petitions received and letters sent. Applicants took advantage of the severe shortage of clerics caused by the disease's high mortality rate: the plague killed about a third of the continent's population.[117] This sharp demographic decline forced ecclesiastical evaluators to become less picky, alongside the adoption of non-standard protocols. As such, a letter written on 15 December 1349 by Clement VI authorized the Bishop of Uzès to accept entrants into the sacred orders during epidemic episodes, in contravention of the usual regulations:

> We have heard from you that, because of the epidemic and the deadly disease, there are only a few people left capable in a little time in your city and diocese of Uzès, you are facing a shortage of priests since many died during the plague or the deadly disease, none or very few are among the surviving priests to ordain and celebrate divine services to the point

117 Gottfried, *The Black Death*, pp. 43–55.

> that there is almost no divine worship and the devotion of the Christian people is neglected. Therefore, you beg us to allow you, for the reasons mentioned above, the right to give both minor and sacred orders in your city and diocese of Uzès, at times that are not ordinary and outside the times established by the apostolic constitutions, provincial customs and synods. For these reasons we grant by this apostolic authority and by special grace that you may lawfully and according to the rites celebrate the orders at the above-mentioned additional times and notwithstanding all the objections mentioned.[118]

The Pope acknowledged the bishop's testimony as truthful: the Uzès diocese simply did not have enough priests to perform services and serve the local community. High mortality rates among priests impacted directly upon religious practice, threatening the souls of the laity and the Church itself. The situation needed to improve, urgently. It is for this reason, then, that Clement backed emergency measures – like this exceptional procedure – to make it easier and faster to ordain clerics. During the Black Death, finding enough applicants to guarantee continuous spiritual provision to the laity became especially challenging. Indeed, the number of petitions and letters authorizing clerical examinations to be held according to irregular schedules, and supporting the ordination of unqualified individuals, sharply increased.

Checks on the suitability of clerics necessarily became less rigorous at certain times, not just during plague epidemics but in the aftermath. Even after the Black Death abated, the remaining priests were not numerous enough to provide divine services adequately, nor were they necessarily suitable for undertaking the task properly. Disabled clerics or 'bastards' (i.e., individuals of illegitimate birth or the children of priests) could thus take advantage of the relaxed entrance requirements, rooted in the shortage of

118 RV 187, f. 315 R – Clement VI to the Bishop of Uzès, 15 December 1348, for which I give the transcription according to the register: '*Cum itaque sicut ex parte tua accepimus tam propter epidemiam et mortalitatem plurimum personae que per non modicum tempus in tuis civitate et diocesi Uticensis viguit quam etiam propter presbiterorum carentiam qui tempore pestis seu mortalitatis huiusmodi in illis partibus obierunt nulli vel paucissimi inibi reperiuntur presbiteri qui divinis velint aut possint officia celebrari propter quod divinus cultus minuitur et devoto remittitur populi christiani nos tuis supplicationibus inclinati ut temporibus quibuscumque etiam non consuetis et extra tempora a iure constituta, omnes tam minores quam sacros ordines in tuis civitate et diocesi Uticensis supradictis quibuscumque constitutionibus apostolicis ac statutis et consuetudinibus provincialibus et synodalibus licet tu nuper ex parte dictis causis excessione per nos specialiter tibi facta ordines celebraveris extra tempora supradicta ac aliis contariis nequaquam obstantibus semel dumtaxat alias tamen rite licite valeas celebrare tibi de speciali gracia auctoritate apostolica tenore presentium indulgemus*'.

priests, to join sacred orders from which they would previously have been rejected. A letter from Gregory XI, sent on 3 December 1371 to the Archbishop of Nidaros (now Trondheim) in Norway, describes the severe impact of the Black Death on the clergy as follows:

> Your petition mentions that in the city and diocese of Nidaros, there are generally about 300 priests, but because of the plague that has ravaged this region, there are only 80 priests left, almost all of them old and decrepit, so that everywhere divine worship is reduced and in the province of Nidaros little or no legitimate person wants or is suitable to be promoted to the priesthood. [...] According to your supplications we dispense by our authority that 20 persons of illegitimate birth and 10 other persons born of priests and single parents, from the aforementioned city, diocese and provinces but worthy of being clerics, may be elected notwithstanding this birth defect.[119]

Trondheim was affected by the Black Death later than Central Europe, with plague first erupting around 1349.[120] The epidemic arrived in several successive waves, at an interval of approximately ten years between resurgences. The third outbreak reached Trondheim with full force in 1370.[121] The archdiocese was home to some 300 priests before this episode; as of 1371, only about 80 remained. The surviving clerics, as observed in the letter, were all 'old and decrepit': the clergy of Trondheim was on the verge of extinction. The Pope thus authorized the archbishop to recruit a total of 30 men who would previously have been deemed unfit for clerical office. Despite their less-than-ideal parentage, these 'bastards' could now be promoted to sacred orders and receive a benefice *cum cura*. However, Gregory XI underscores the fact that these irregular new recruits must be

119 RV 282, f. 92 V (RA 174, f. 380 V) – Gregory XI to the Archbishop of Nidaros (Trondheim, Norway), December 3, 1371. Text analysed by Hayez, Mathieu, and Yvan (eds.), *Grégoire XI*, n° 11 032, for which I give the transcription according to the register: '*Tua petitio continebat quod in tuis civitate et diocesi Nidrosiensi, in quibus consueverunt esse trecenti presbiteri vel circiter, propter mortalitatum pestes que in illis partibus viguerunt non sunt nunc ultra quadraginta presbiteri, qui quasi omnes antiqui et decrepiti existunt, propter quod cultus divinus est inibi non modicum diminutus et in provincia Nidrosiensi pauci vel nulli legitime nati existunt qui velint et valeant ad sacerdotium promoveri.* [...] *Huiusmodi supplicationibus inclinati hac vice auctoritate nostra cum viginti de solutis et decem aliis personis civitatis et diocesis ac provincie predictarum de presbiteris et solutis parentibus genitis, clericali caractere insignitis, quas duxeris eligendas ut huiusmodi natalium defectum nequaquam obstante*'.

120 Biraben, "Les maladies en Europe", p. 309.

121 Benedictow, *The Black Death*, pp. 199–201 for the years 1371 to 1373.

fundamentally worthy of entering into God's service, suitable on all other levels. They must have good intentions, for instance, with a virtuous lifestyle and moral behaviour. It stands to reason that pious clerics with physical and/or mental disabilities could equally have benefited from a relaxation of the rules, although the letter does not mention this explicitly. The exigent circumstances of plague epidemics, and the concomitant needs of the Papal Chancery, justified the softening of canon law. Other demographic shifts, such as population growth in the laity, similarly compelled a relaxation of standards in clerical recruitment, due to the urgency of installing enough priests to serve communities adequately.[122]

Conclusion

In theory, 'defects' of body and/or mind rendered individuals unfit for clerical office. Yet the corpus of petitions and letters demonstrate that the Curia could, and did, circumvent such regulations when it was in its best interest. The cases discussed above, representative of the general terrain, testify as to the value that the papal institution placed on ecclesiastical education, but above all they demonstrate a staunch commitment to offering high-quality guidance to the faithful. The Black Death, and its cascading effects, created the conditions in which the Papal Chancery could reasonably and legitimately bypass canon law, making it easier for non-standard applicants including (we may presume) disabled men, to access divine offices. Nevertheless, it seems that disabled supplicants were more readily attributed minor benefices without *cura*; the major orders remained that much more difficult to access for disabled churchmen than for their able-bodied peers. Such difficulties notwithstanding, however, the letters show a great degree of flexibility at play regarding the entrance of disabled clerics into major orders and their access to *cura animarum*, especially during the fourteenth century.

The petition and papal letters equally highlight how the popes asserted their *plenitudo potestatis* (full power) over local clerical hierarchies. Documents sent by the Papal Chancery functioned to affirm the Curia's authority over all Christendom, including the most senior members of the clergy.[123] The Chancery also strengthened its control over regional churches by tasking local bishops with verifying if papal grants of grace were justified, forcing

122 Peters, *A Companion to Priesthood*, p. 18.

123 Montaubin, "L'opposition des clercs", p. 229.

such deputies to accept favours – even if the institutional response to the requests for exemption did not match the first appeals of the petitioners, without, however, refusing them altogether. The archival evolution of the Papal Chancery is the result of the consolidation of the pontifical theocracy through *plenitudo potestatis*, a mechanism which endowed popes with the power to interfere in numerous aspects of medieval society. The pontifical institution could intervene in any and all clerical affairs, even minor issues at the local level. Consequently, petitions substantively increased access to minor and regular orders for 'unsuitable' disabled clerics, who could appeal to the pontiff and thereby bypass local ecclesiastical elites. This process further entrenched the Church's control over all aspects of clerical life, but especially entrance in major orders and attribution of benefices with cure of souls. The sources show that the supplication system did not operate on a 'one-size-fits-all' mandate. Rather, the individual specificities of the case at hand were taken into account; the Papal Chancery drew up categories for each type of supplicant, according to the subject of their request. And in this process, physical and/or mental disability constituted a valid criterion for requesting a papal dispensation.

Nonetheless, responsibility for the distribution of exemptions (i.e., whether granting dispensations was the purview of the Pope alone, and/or under control of regional powers) had not yet been finalized by the end of the medieval period. Indeed, this distribution of authority was still being resolved during the fourteenth century.[124] The exclusive papal right of derogation, dating back to the Gregorian Reform, was not fully applied from the twelfth to the fourteenth century. In fact, bishops continued to grant graces to the clergy in their diocese. Supplicants thus appealed to the Apostolic See in two cases: either when the bishop opted to defer the decision entirely to the Pope; or when the supplicant wished to protect themselves from episcopal bias by obtaining an unquestionable grace. Episodes in which the Papal Chancery assessed petitioners' disability echoed similar examinations conducted at the local level by representatives of the regional ecclesiastical hierarchy. The Pope was only invited to intervene following a ruling made by the diocesan and/or archdiocesan authorities, when the supplicant needed to be granted a papal grace. Appealing to the pontiff made it possible to bypass canonical legislation in order to integrate disabled clerics into secular or regular, minor or major orders, or to grant them benefices without care of souls. The Apostolic See might follow the recommendations of clerics' superiors and endorse the requests contained

124 See also Stöhr, *Körpermakel – Arbeits(un)fähigkeit – Kirchenrecht*.

in the petition. Alternatively, it could delegate its observer function to others less directly involved in the case than the superiors, or individuals judged to be more honest. It is likely that many entrants were able to conceal their physical and/or mental disability altogether, either acting alone or with the assistance of their investigation committee. Such cases are not, of course, captured in the Chancery's records. However, in cases that do figure in the Pontifical Registers, we gain insight into the experiences of disabled clerics: they describe their impairments, explain the consequences of their conditions in terms of their capacity to carry out clerical rights and duties, and convey their desire to receive papal grace and dedicate their life to divine service.

Papal power, initially purely consultative, gradually became coercive, as demonstrated in the examples presented in this chapter. The Chancery had the power to endorse or reject decisions taken at the local level. Rejection of this kind amounted to the Chancery overruling regional authorities, who were then tasked with enforcing the popes' decision. It is for this reason, then, that we find more and more pontifical letters in this context, testifying to the institution's keen attention to issues of clerics' capacity and *claritas* during the thirteenth century, an interest that grew even stronger in the fourteenth century. This explains, then, why fewer secular clerics wrote to resign their role – and why more clerics asked to receive benefices with *cura animarum*, or to join major orders – during the fourteenth century. The Papal Chancery could, at times, be a powerful ally for disabled would-be clerics, and their counterparts in post.

Bibliography

Primary Sources

François AVRIL, Pierre BOTINEAU, Jean-René GABORIT, Danielle GABORIT-CHOPIN, Michel HAYEZ, Anne-Marie HAYEZ and Marie-Hyacinthe LAURENT (eds.), *Urbain V (1362–1370): lettres communes analysées d'après les registres dits d'Avignon et du Vatican*, Bibliothèque des Écoles françaises de Rome et d'Athènes, 1954.

Bernard BARBICHE, *Les actes pontificaux originaux des archives nationales de Paris 1, 1198–1261*, Vatican, Biblioteca Apostolica Vaticana, 1975.

BENEDICTINE MONKS (eds.), *Registres de Clément V*, E. de Boccard, 1948.

Élie BERGER (ed.), *Les registres d'Innocent IV (1243–1248)*, E. Thorin, 1884.

Ursmer BERLIÈRE (ed.), *Suppliques de Clément VI (1342–1352)*, Institut historique belge, 1906.

Ursmer Berlière and Philippe Van Isacker (eds.), *Lettres de Clément VI (1342–1352): Tome I (1342–1346)*, Institut historique belge, 1924.

Joachim-Joseph Berthier (ed.), *Opera de vita regularis*, Marietti, 1956.

Joseph Marie Canivez (ed.), *Statuta capitulorum generalium Ordinis Cisterciensis*, Bureaux de la Revue, 1933.

Cesare Cenci (ed.), "De Fratrum Minorum Constitutionibus Praenarbonensibus", *Archivum franciscanum historicum*, 83 (1990), pp. 50–95.

Gaston Charvin (ed.), *Statuts, chapitres généraux et visites de l'ordre de Cluny, tome 1, 1030–1289*, Boccard, 1965.

Eugène Déprez, Jean Glénisson and Guillaume Mollat (eds.), *Clément VI (1342–1352): lettres closes, patentes et curiales se rapportant à la France*, Boccard, 1961.

Robert Digard, Antoine Fawtier, Maurice Faucon and Antoine Thomas (eds.), *Les registres de Boniface VIII: recueil des bulles de ce Pape publiées ou analysées d'après les manuscrits originaux des Archives du Vatican*, Bibliothèque des Écoles françaises d'Athènes et de Rome, 1884.

Friedberg (ed.), *Corpus iuris canonici*, Akademische Druck- u. Verlagsanstalt, 1959.

Anne-Marie Hayez, Janine Mathieu and Marie-France Yvan (eds.), *Urbain V: suppliques de 1362 à 1365 (années I à IV)*, [electronic version: *Ut per litteras apostolicas*], Brepols, 1978.

Anne-Marie Hayez, Janine Mathieu and Marie-France Yvan (eds.), *Grégoire XI (1370–1378): lettres communes analysées d'après les registres dits d'Avignon et du Vatican*, École française de Rome, 1992.

Istituto storico domenicano S. Sabina (eds.), *Constitutiones et acta capitulorum generalium ordinis fratrum praedicatorum, 1232–2001*, Directmedia, 2002.

Ernest Langlois (ed.), *Les registres de Nicolas IV: recueil des bulles de ce pape publiées ou analysées d'après les manuscrits originaux des Archives du Vatican*, E. Thorin, 1886.

Guillaume Mollat (ed.), *Jean XXII (1316–1334): Lettres communes analysées d'après les registres dits d'Avignon et du Vatican*, Albert Fontemoing, 1923.

Giles Constable (ed.), "Statuta Petri Venerabilis abbatis cluniacensis IX (1146/7)", in, *Consuetudines benedictinae variae (saec. XI–saec. XIV)*, Corpus consuetudinum monasticarum vol. 6, F. Schmitt, 1975, pp. 37–106.

The Canons of the Fourth Lateran Council, 1215, transl. from the *Internet Medieval Sourcebook*, URL consulted on 31 July 2021: https://sourcebooks.fordham.edu/basis/lateran4.asp.

Thomas Aquinas, *Summa contra gentiles*, transl. Laurence Shapcote, edited and revised by The Aquinas Institute, URL consulted on 31 July 2021: https://aquinas.cc.

Julius VON PFLUGK-HARTTUNG (ed.), *Acta pontificum Romanorum inedita 1 (748–1198)*, Akad. Dr.- u. Verl.-Anst., 1958.

James WATERWORTH (transl.), "The Council of Trent", in *The canons and decrees of the sacred and oecumenical Council of Trent*, Dolman, 1848.

Secondary Sources

Paul ABBERLEY, "The Limits of Classical Social Theory in the Analysis and Transformation of Disablement", *in* Len BARTON and Michael OLIVER (eds.), *Disability Studies: Past, Present and Future*, Disability Press, 1997, pp. 25–44.

Julia BARROW, *The Clergy in the Medieval World: Secular Clerics, Their Families and Careers in North-Western Europe, c. 800–c. 1200*, Cambridge University Press, 2015.

Morgane BELIN, "Les statuts synodaux: un outil au cœur de la transmission de la loi de l'Église aux pasteurs et à leurs fidèles", *Kritische Zeitschrift für Überkonfessionelles Kirchenrecht/Revista crítica de Derecho Canónico Pluriconfesional*, 1 (2014), pp. 27–58.

Ole Jørgen BENEDICTOW, *The Black Death and Later Plague Epidemics in the Nordic Countries: Perspectives and Controversies*, Walter de Gruyter GmbH & Co KG, 2015.

Robert Louis BENSON, *Bishop-Elect: A Study in Medieval Ecclesiastical Office*, Princeton University Press, 2015.

Nora BEREND, "La subversion invisible: la disparition de l'oblation irrévocable des enfants dans le droit canon", *Médiévales. Langues, Textes, Histoire*, 13.26 (1994), pp. 123–136.

Ursmer BERLIÈRE, "Épaves d'archives pontificales du XIVe siècle, suite et fin", *Revue bénédictine*, 25.1, Desclée de Brouwer et Cie, 1908, pp. 19–47.

Ursmer BERLIÈRE, *Les élections abbatiales au Moyen Âge*, M. Lamertin, 1927.

Jules BESSON, "Dispensation", *The Catholic Encyclopedia*. Vol. 5. New York: Robert Appleton Company, 1909 (URL consulted 31 July 2021: http://www.newadvent.org/cathen/05041a.htm).

Jean-Noël BIRABEN, "Les maladies en Europe: équilibres et ruptures de la pathocénose", *in* Maria Laura BARDINET BROSO, Bernardino FANTINI and Mirko Drazen GRMEK (eds.), *Histoire de la pensée médicale en occident 1, Antiquité et Moyen Âge*, Éditions du Seuil, 1995, pp. 283–310.

Daniel BORNSTEIN, "How to Behave in Church and How to Become a Priest", *in* Miri RUBIN (ed.), *Medieval Christianity in Practice*, Princeton University Press, 2009.

Leonard E. BOYLE, *Pastoral Care, Clerical Education and Canon Law, 1200–1400*, Variorum reprints, 1981.

Michael BURGER, *Bishops, Clerks, and Diocesan Governance in Thirteenth-Century England: Reward and Punishment*, Cambridge University Press, 2012.

Pierre BUSER, *L'inconscient aux mille visages*, Jacob, 2005.

Bernard CHEVALIER, "Corporations, conflits politiques et paix sociale en France aux XIVe et XVe siècles", *Revue historique*, 268 (1982), pp. 18–44.

Peter D. CLARKE and Patrick N. R ZUTSHI, *Supplications from England and Wales in the Registers of the Apostolic Penitentiary, 1410–1503*, Boydell Press, 2012.

Lynda L. COON, *Dark Age Bodies: Gender and Monastic Practice in the Early Medieval West*, University of Pennsylvania Press, 2011.

Florent CYGLER, ""unité des cœurs" et "uniformité des mœurs" au défi de l'espace et du temps: les statuts des ordres religieux au Moyen Âge", *in* Isabelle HEULLANT-DONAT, Julie CLAUSTRE, Elisabeth LUSSET and Falk BRETSCHNEIDER (eds.), *Enfermements II. Règles et dérèglements en milieu clos, IV–XIXe siècle*, Publications de la Sorbonne, 2015, pp. 170–188.

Wipertus Rudt DE COLLENBERG, "Le choix des exécuteurs dans les bulles de provision au XIVe siècle (d'après les bulles accordées à Chypre par les papes d'Avignon)", *Mélanges de l'École française de Rome. Moyen-Âge, Temps modernes*, 92.2 (1980), pp. 393–440.

William J. DOHAR, "Medieval Ordination Lists: The Origins of a Record", *Archives (London)*, 20.87 (1992), pp. 17–35.

William J. DOHAR, "*Sufficienter litteratus:* Clerical Examination and Instruction for the Cure of Souls", *in* Jacqueline BROWN and William P. STONEMAN (eds.), *A Distinct Voice: Medieval Studies in Honor of Leonard E. Boyle*, University of Notre Dame Press, 1997, pp. 305–321.

Charles DONAHUE, *Law, Marriage, and Society in the Later Middle Ages: Arguments about Marriage in Five Courts*, Cambridge University Press, 2008.

Ninon DUBOURG, "Un/Acceptable Disability? *Defectus Corporis, Scandalum*, and Pontifical Grace", in Teodora ARTIMON and Andrea-Bianka ZNOROVSZKY (eds.), *Materializing Ugliness and Deformity in the Middle Ages*, Trivent Publishing, forthcoming.

Ninon DUBOURG, "*Deformitas* et célébration de l'eucharistie dans le droit canon médiéval", in Ida Gilda MASTROROSA, *Deformitas e diritto* (forthcoming).

Pierre GASNAULT, "L'élaboration des lettres secrètes des papes d'Avignon: Chambre et Chancellerie", *Publications de l'École française de Rome*, 138.1 (1990), pp. 209–222.

Jean GAUDEMET, *Les élections dans l'Église latine des origines au XVIe siècle*, Fernand Lanore, 1979.

Arthur GIRY, *Manuel de diplomatique*, Hachette, 1894.

Robert S. GOTTFRIED, *The Black Death: Natural and Human Disaster in Medieval Europe*, 2nd edition, Simon and Schuster, 2010.

Gilbert GUAYDIER, *Les irrégularités "ex defectu corporis"*, Société Générale d'Imprimerie et d'Édition, 1933.

Jussi HANSKA and Kirsi SALONEN, *Entering a Clerical Career at the Roman Curia, 1458–1471*, Ashgate, 2013.

Anne-Marie HAYEZ, "La personnalité d'Urbain V d'après ses réponses aux suppliques", *in Aux origines de l'État moderne. Le fonctionnement administratif de la papauté d'Avignon. Actes de la table ronde d'Avignon (22–24 janvier 1988)*, École française de Rome, 1991, pp. 7–31.

Monica-Elena HEREGHLEGIU, *Reservatio Papalis: A Study on the Application of a Legal Prescription According to the 1983 Code of Canon Law*, LIT, 2008.

Kerstin HITZBLECK, *Exekutoren: die ausserordentliche Kollatur von Benefizien im Pontifikat Johannes XXII*, Mohr Siebeck, 2009.

Jenni KUULIALA, "Infirmitas in Monastic Rules", *in* Christian LAES, Chris F. GOODEY and Martha Lynn ROSE (eds.), *Disabilities in Roman Antiquity: Disparate Bodies, a Capite ad Calcem*, Brill, 2013, pp. 342–356.

Jenni KUULIALA, "Nobility, Community and Physical Impairment in Later Medieval Canonization Processes", *in* Christian KRÖTZL, Katariina MUSTAKALLIO and Jenni KUULIALA (eds.), *Infirmity in Antiquity and the Middle Ages: Social and Cultural Approaches to Health, Weakness and Care*, Ashgate, 2015, pp. 67–82.

Jacques LE GOFF, "Métier et profession d'après les manuels de confesseurs au Moyen Âge", *Miscellanea Mediaevalia*, III: Beiträge zum Berufsbewufitsem des mittelaterlichen Menschen (1964), pp. 44–60.

Jacques LE GOFF, "Travail, techniques et artisans dans les systèmes de valeur du haut Moyen Âge (v[e]–xe siècle)", *in Artigianato e Tecnica nella società dell'alto Medioevo occidentale, Setimane di studio del Centro italiano di studi sull'alto medioevo 18*, Centro Italiano di Studi sull'Alto Medioevo, 1971, pp. 239–266.

Bruno LEMESLE, *La société aristocratique dans le Haut-Maine: XIe–XIIe siècles*, Presses universitaires de Rennes, 2015.

Clément LENOBLE, *L'exercice de la pauvreté. Économie et religion chez les franciscains d'Avignon (XIIIe–XVe siècle)*, Presses Universitaires de Rennes, 2013.

Catharina LIS and Hugo SOLY, *Worthy Efforts: Attitudes to Work and Workers in Pre-Industrial Europe*, Brill, 2012.

Joseph H. LYNCH, *Simoniacal Entry into Religious Life from 1000 to 1260: A Social, Economic, and Legal Study*, Ohio State University Press, 1976.

Monique MAILLARD-LUYPAERT and Jean-Marie CAUCHIES, *Papauté, clercs et laïcs: le diocèse de Cambrai à l'épreuve du Grand Schisme d'Occident (1378–1417)*, Publications des Facultés universitaires Saint-Louis, 2001.

René METZ, "L'entrée des mineurs dans la vie religieuse", *Studia Gratiana*, 20 (1976), pp. 187–200.

Irina METZLER, *A Social History of Disability in the Middle Ages: Cultural Considerations of Physical Impairment*, Routledge, 2013.

Charles de MIRAMON, *Les "donnés" au Moyen Âge*, Cerf, 1999.

Pascal MONTAUBIN, "L'administration pontificale de la grâce au XIIIe siècle, l'exemple de la politique bénéficiale", *in* Hélène MILLET (ed.), *Suppliques et requêtes: le gouvernement par la grâce en Occident, XIIe–XVe siècle*, École française de Rome, 2003, pp. 321–342.

Pascal MONTAUBIN, "L'opposition des clercs et des laïcs du royaume de France à la centralisation pontificale: l'exemple de la politique bénéficiale (1225–1303)", *in* Bernard BARBICHE and Rolf GROSS (eds.), *Schismes, dissidences, oppositions. La France et le Siège apostolique avant Boniface VIII*, École des chartes-Institut historique allemand, 2012, pp. 225–252.

Angela MONTFORD, "Fit to Preach and Pray: Considerations of Occupational Health in the Mendicant Orders", *in* R. N. SWANSON (ed.), *The Use and Abuse of Time in Christian History*, Boydell & Brewer, 2002, pp. 95–106.

Colin MORRIS, *The Papal Monarchy: The Western Church from 1050 to 1250*, Oxford University Press, 1989.

Michèle MULCHAHEY, *"First the Bow is Bent in Study ...": Dominican Education Before 1350*, Pontifical Institute for Medieval Studies, 2000.

Jacqueline MURRAY, "Masculinizing Religious Life: Sexual Prowess, the Battle for Chastity and Monastic Identity", *in* Katherine Jane LEWIS and Patricia H. CULLUM (eds.), *Holiness and Masculinity in the Middle Ages*, University of Wales press, 2004, pp. 24–42.

Franz NEISKE, "Les enfants dans les monastères du Moyen Âge", *Mémoires de la Société pour l'histoire du droit et des institutions des anciens pays bourguignons, comtois et romands*, 58 (2001), pp. 229–244.

Krijn PANSTERS, "Norm and Form: Virtues as Constituents of Identity in Medieval Religious Communities", *in* Mirko BREITENSTEIN, Julia BURKHARDT, Stefan BURKHARDT and Jörg SONNTAG (eds.), *Identität und Gemeinschaft: vier Zugänge zu Eigengeschichten und Selbstbildern institutioneller Ordnungen*, Lit, 2015, pp. 99–124.

Brandon PARLOPIANO, "*Propter Deformitatem:* Towards a Concept of Disability in Medieval Canon Law", *Canadian Journal of Disability Studies*, 4.3 (2015), pp. 72–102.

Greg PETERS, "Offering Sons to God in the Monastery: Child Oblation, Monastic Benevolence, and the Cistercian Order in the Middle Ages", *Cistercian Studies Quarterly*, 38.3 (2003), pp. 285–295.

Greg PETERS, *A Companion to Priesthood and Holy Orders in the Middle Ages*, Brill, 2016.

Odette PONTAL, "Le rôle du synode diocésain et des statuts synodaux dans la formation du clergé", *in Les évêques, les clercs et le roi (1250–1300)*, cahier de Fanjeaux n° 7, Privat, 1972, pp. 337–359.

Francis RAPP, "Les synodes diocésains en France au Moyen Âge", *in* Marc AOUN and Jeanne-Marie TUFFERY-ANDRIEU (eds.), *Conciles provinciaux et synodes diocésains du concile de Trente à la Révolution française: Défis ecclésiaux et enjeux politiques?*, Presses universitaires de Strasbourg, 2010, pp. 19–30.

Katja ROST, Emil INAUEN, Margit OSTERLOH and Bruno S. FREY, "The Corporate Governance of Benedictine Abbeys: What Can Stock Corporations Learn from Monasteries?", *Journal of Management History*, 16.1 (2010), pp. 90–115.

Adeline RUCQUOI, "La formation culturelle du clergé en Castille à la fin du Moyen Âge", *Le clerc séculier au Moyen Âge. XXI*e *Congrès de la SHMESP (Amiens, juin 1991)*, 22.1 (1991), pp. 249–262.

Kirsi SALONEN and Ludwig SCHMUGGE, *A Sip from the "Well of Grace", Medieval Texts from the Apostolic Penitentiary*, Catholic University of America Press, 2009.

Thomas W. SMITH, "Papal Executors and the Veracity of Petitions from Thirteenth-Century England", *Revue d'Histoire Ecclésiastique*, 110.3–4 (2015), pp. 662–683.

Friederike STÖHR, *Körpermakel – Arbeits(un)fähigkeit – Kirchenrecht: Körperlich versehrte, kranke und alte Geistliche im spätmittelalterlichen Deutschen Reich und in Skandinavien*, Didymos-Verlag, 2020.

Robert Norman SWANSON, "Angel Incarnate: Clergy and Masculinity from Gregorian Reform to Reformation", *in* Dawn Marie HADLEY (ed.), *Masculinity in Medieval Europe*, Longman, 1999, pp. 160–178.

Vincent TABBAGH, "Effectifs et recrutement du clergé séculier français à la fin du Moyen Âge", *Le clerc séculier au Moyen Âge. XXI*e *Congrès de la SHMESP (Amiens, juin 1991)*, 22.1 (1991), pp. 181–190.

Romain TELLIEZ, *Les institutions de la France médiévale: XI*e*–XV*e *siècle*, 2e edition, Armand Colin, 2016.

Maud TERNON, *Juger les fous au Moyen Âge: dans les tribunaux royaux en France XIV*e*–XV*e *siècles*, Presses Universitaires de France, 2018.

Julien THÉRY, "*Atrocitas/enormitas*. Pour une histoire de la catégorie de "crime énorme" du Moyen Âge à l'époque moderne", *Clio@Themis. Revue en ligne d'histoire du droit*, 4, online http://www.cliothemis.com/Atrocitas-enormitas-Esquisse-pour, 2011.

Jennifer D. THIBODEAUX, "Introduction: Rethinking the Medieval Clergy and Masculinity", *in* Jennifer D. THIBODEAUX (ed.), *Negotiating Clerical Identities: Priests, Monks and Masculinity in the Middle Ages*, Palgrave Macmillan, 2010, pp. 1–15.

Richard C. TREXLER, "Introduction", *in* Richard C. TREXLER (ed.), *Persons in Groups: Social Behavior as Identity Formation in Medieval and Renaissance Europe*, Center for medieval and early Renaissance studies, 1985, pp. 3–16.

Victor Witter TURNER, *The Ritual Process: Structure and Anti-Structure*, Aldine Transaction publishers, 1969.

André VAUCHEZ and Cécile CABY, *L'histoire des moines, chanoines et religieux au Moyen Âge: guide de recherche et documents*, Brepols, 2003.

Xenia VON TIPPELSKIRCH, "Spiritualités en captivité et circulation d'écrits sur le cloître à l'époque moderne", *in* Isabelle HEULLANT-DONAT, Julie CLAUSTRE,

Élisabeth LUSSET and Falk BRETSCHNEIDER (eds.), *Enfermements III. Hommes et femmes en milieux clos, XIIIe–XXe siècle*, Publications de la Sorbonne, 2017, pp. 71–85.

Jérôme WILGAUX, "Ὑγιὴς καὶ ὁλόκλαρος. Le corps du prêtre en Grèce ancienne", *in* Pierre BRULÉ (ed.), *La norme en matière religieuse en Grèce ancienne: Actes du XIIe colloque international du CIERGA (Rennes, septembre 2007)*, Presses universitaires de Liège, 2013, pp. 231–242.

Patrick N. R. ZUTSHI, "Petitioners, Popes, Proctors: the Development of Curial Institutions, c. 1150–1250", *in Pensiero e sperimentazioni istituzionali nella societas Christiana (1046–1250)*, Vita e Pensiero, 2007, pp. 265–293.

4 Staying in the Clergy

Abstract
This chapter moves to examine the consequences of the 'failure' of such disability tests and of clerics' disclosures of impairment in petitions. In such cases, gracious papal letters sometimes allowed for the relaxation of ecclesiastical regulations to accommodate the disabled cleric's conditions, if he himself desired to remain in the clergy and was deemed capable enough. The process of supplication was used to improve clerics' lives by adapting existing statutes to their personal situations.

Keywords: Coadjutors; Monastic Rules; Transfers; Mobility

The cover of the book you have in your hands, reader, represents a sick bishop, bedridden, who dictates his wishes to a notary, located at the bottom of his bed, as close as possible to the viewer. Behind the sick man stands another bishop, who helps him to write the letter, and, on the right, the recipient of the letter, the Pope.[1] From this iconographic representation, and from the text that inspired the illustration, we can determine that the sick bishop is addressing a supplication to the Pope in order, no doubt, to delegate some (if not all) of his attributions to his colleague, who will become coadjutor or substitute bishop. Indeed, the preamble to cause 7 of Gratian's *Decree*, illustrated here, speaks of what a bishop overwhelmed by a long illness should do:

> When a bishop overwhelmed by a long illness begs to have another bishop substituted for him, the Pope responds favourably to his prayers and grants him what is requested.[2]

1 This image is quickly commented by Schmitt, "Les suppliques dans les images", p. 82.

2 *Decretus Gratiani*, edited in Friedberg (ed.), *Corpus iuris canonici,* causa 7: '*Quidam longa inualetudinem grauatus episcopus alium sibi substitui rogauit, cuius precibus summus Pontifex annuit, et quod rogauerat ei concessit*' (my translation).

Dubourg, N., *Disabled Clerics in the Late Middle Ages. Un/suitable for Divine Service?*
Taylor & Francis Group, 2023
DOI: 10.5117/9789463721561_CH04

The text continues with chapter 1, 'the pain of the body does not deprive the bishop of his honour', which is exemplified in the miniature since the bishop is depicted in his sickly state, certainly, but still wearing all the attributes worthy of his office.[3] Whether he is in the process of relinquishing some of his prerogatives or abdicating altogether, it is indeed the act of supplication of a sick bishop who seeks to adapt his duties to his physical condition that is depicted here.

This chapter expands on issues raised in earlier chapters, to consider in depth the accommodations offered and/or authorized by the pontifical institution that allowed impaired clerics to remain in the clergy. Through the supplication process, the Curia facilitated the inclusion of disabled petitioners, by adapting regulations to their personal situations.[4] Successful petitions, those that led to grants of pontifical grace, reveal that both supplicants and Church authorities were willing to make efforts to adapt. The relative degree of flexibility demonstrated by the parties involved in the petition process depended upon the specific context in which the supplicant's case was embedded, and the cleric's unique circumstances.[5] Petitioners were obliged to establish their continued usefulness to the Church, providing evidence of their ability to overcome the limitations imposed by their impairment(s) and/or their broader skillset. In return, the Papal Chancery offered modifications to the supplicant's existing role or transferred them to a new post which was more suitable for their current capacities. In both cases, the retention of impaired clerics within the Church community required the adaptation of canonical statutes by the Curia.

Permission to adapt canonical legislation to respond to individual cases depended upon three main factors. The first consideration was the supplicant's ability to perform clerical work, the core duties associated with a given role. The Papal Chancery was particularly concerned about supplicants' job performance in benefices with *cura animarum*. Generally, in such situations, the typical ecclesiastical workload stipulated in canonical law was modified, and the supplicant was appointed an assistant. The latter, termed a 'coadjutor', assumed responsibility for the tasks that the impaired cleric could not perform – usually, all priestly duties. The second consideration pertained to monastic rules, strict regulations governing the institutional 'home' life of monastics. Close study of the lives of disabled

3 Op. cit., causa 7, questio 1, chapter 1: '*Pro molesti corporis suo honore non priuetur episcopus*'.
4 See Kuttner, *Harmony from Dissonance*.
5 Mellor and Shilling, *Re-forming the Body*, p. 70.

monks, abbots, nuns, and abbesses reveals the ways in which it was possible to soften the rigours of monastic life. The study of papal letters reveals that the enclosure did not, in fact, equate to a hermetic separation of monastics from the outside world. Rather, it operated as a symbolic barrier that was fundamentally permeable. The third consideration was supplicants' mobility, or lack thereof. The Church compromised on this issue more than on any other. The ability to move around with relative ease was, it seems, a prerequisite for the professional clerical life. Indeed, they needed to be able to attend to the administrative business in their benefice(s) and to the many ecclesiastical gatherings. After careful analysis of these three factors, the pontifical institution formulated modifications to allow petitioners to circumvent canonical law, according to their degree of physical or mental disability.

The Nomination of Coadjutors

Secular and regular clerics, from monks to priests, were all responsible for the salvation of Christian souls. It could be assumed that they had the dogmatic or liturgical knowledge, alongside the requisite physical and mental capacity, to fulfil their mission. After all, clerics undertook a long period of training in which they were prepared for the role and demonstrated their comprehensive suitability for the urgent task at hand. Clerics were thus highly qualified ecclesiastical specialists, irreplaceable in their mastery of the office and in the management of their benefice. It is for this reason, then, that the Church sought to offer adaptations in response to clerical impairment: clerics, even impaired men, were a valuable resource.[6] Moreover, the pontifical institution could not force clerics to resign (or could not make them redundant).[7] Thus, when impaired clerics wished to remain in office, the Church was obliged to offer appropriate accommodations. Impaired clerics were routinely assigned additional support, with the appointment of procurators, coadjutors, or vicars – individuals who assumed responsibility for tasks that impaired clerics could not perform. Indeed, some 25% of the cases in the corpus contain such a dispensation. On the one hand, this process allowed impaired clerics to maintain their professional and social

6 See Williams, "Understanding Incapacity".

7 Rodes, *Ecclesiastical Administration*, pp. 97–98. On the issue of resignation and redundancy, see Chapter 5.

identity.[8] Yet such procedures equally diminished their authority: as core functions of their office were reallocated, they risked being progressively sidelined. Such professional marginalization rendered clerics' existing need more visible, institutionally.

The Appointment of Auxiliaries

The pontifical institution relieved impaired clerics – secular and regular alike – of tasks they could no longer perform in order to ensure the fulfilment of daily pastoral duties.[9] Impaired clerics were authorized to hire an assistant to carry out certain well-defined tasks in the name of the 'public good' (*publica utilitas*).[10] Such appointments were permitted in canon law. Gratian's *Decree* notes, for example:

> Moreover, when someone, burdened by old age or impairment, is unable to administer his own office, and if he can ask a substitute to do so, let him do so in a rational manner.[11]

The clerical profession could be exhausting, both morally and physically. It required ceaseless rigour and a constant, high degree of preparedness which could cause various impairments, not the least (extreme) fatigue.[12] In theory, the decision to appoint an assistant depended on the cleric's relative ability to perform specific tasks. For example, a blind bishop could not perform Mass because he could not read. In practice, however, both physical and mental illnesses affected the administration of benefices in diffuse ways. For example, a bishop who could not walk without sticks was prevented from performing Mass in a non-obvious way, because of his appearance in the eyes of the flock. Impairment of any kind could thus be cause for the reduction of clerical duties and responsibilities, triggering the assignment of a coadjutor to take up the slack. The acceptance of such outside support was non-negotiable if the impaired cleric wished to remain in post.

In a letter dated 9 May 1217, for example, Honorius III was forced to interfere in local affairs because some clerics rebelled against the authority of the Bishop of Segovia due to his intermittent insanity:

8 Cochelin, "*In senectute bona*", p. 124.

9 Metzler, *A Social History*, p. 142.

10 Parlopiano, "*Propter Deformitatem*", p. 97.

11 *Decretum Gratiani*, edited in Friedberg (ed.), *Corpus iuris canonici*, second part, causa 7, chapter 11.

12 Montford, *Health, Sickness, Medicine*, p. 28.

> Our venerable brother the archbishop of Toledo has informed us that, our venerable bishop of Segovia, who has long been afflicted by a serious illness to the point that his mind is delirious, except during intervals of lucidity, authorized the master M. de Torogano to recovered in full the revenues of the canonical house, known for having belonged to S., the treasurer of Segovia. In this regard, the archbishop humbly begs us to authorize it, out of paternal solicitude, so that nothing prevents the aforementioned master to recover the revenues of the canonical house.[13]

The Archbishop of Toledo, the Bishop of Segovia's superior, had initiated the supplication process, probably on the bishop behalf, by sending a petition to the Chancery to address the situation. Honorius then addressed his letter to the deacon of Toledo and the archdeacon of Talavera de la Reina, probably the two people questioning the application of the bishop's decision to give the benefice to M. de Torogano. The bishop's intermittent delirium was evidently causing problems for the management of local financial affairs... Some seem to have used this argument to try to invalidate the appointments he made, even though he was presented by his superior as being able to have intervals of lucidity. It appears then that the decisions he made during those moments of clarity must be applied. It is noteworthy that the bishop was probably not deposed precisely because his mental impairment fluctuates; the kind of support he required would likely vary, according to the nature and frequency of his episodic symptoms.

Similarly, epilepsy is an illness structured by periods of lucidity and moments of complete incapacity during seizures. For this reason, cases featuring epileptic clerics are particularly illustrative in terms of the complexity of mandates to accommodate clerical impairment. Such cases necessitated the appointment of an assistant with a carefully defined remit, who was called upon only in certain prescribed circumstances. A letter from Alexander II

13 RV 9, f. 105 V – Honorius III to the deacon of Toledo and the archdeacon of Talavera de la Reina (Toledo), 9 May 1217. Letter analysed by Pressutti (ed.), *I regesti del pontefice Onorio III*, n° 567, for which I give the transcription according to the register: '*Venerabili fratre nostro archiepiscopo Toletano accepimus exponente, quod cum venerabili nostro Segobiensi episcopo gravi dudum esset infirmitate detentus, ita quod mentis alienationem absque intervallis dilucidis incurrisset canoniam mansionariam quas S. quondam Thesaurarius Segobiensis ecclesie habuisse dinoscitur, cum eiusdem ecclesie provisio sibi a nobis plenarie commissa fuisset magistro M. de Torogano clerico archiepiscopi memorati duxit integre concedendam. Unde nobis idem archiepiscopus humiliter supplicavit, ut ne idem magister supra ipsa canonia possit ab aliquo impediri providere sibi paterna sollicitudine dignaremus.*'

(1061–1073), addressed to Gebonardus, the Archbishop of Salzburg, discusses epilepsy and its consequences for the care of souls:

> One of the clerics presents himself to the presbyterate; but, as he suffers from the sickness languor (*caducus morbus*), as he has been recognized in our presence, we have decided not to allow him to celebrate Mass. It is true that this illness (*languor*) is not his fault, so we will have to deliberate on this matter in order to issue a decree with our authority. We therefore decide that, if the illness (*morbus*) strikes him frequently, he may not become an oblate and be prevented by all means from celebrating Mass. For he is considered unworthy, and it is dangerous that he should fall during the consecration of the Eucharist, a victim of an epileptic fit (*morbus epilenticus*). If God's mercy really allows him to recover (*convalesce*), as long as he is not guilty of his illness, but that it is indeed an illness (*infirmitas*), we do not forbid that he can offer sacrifices.[14]

The frequency of the episodic seizures that form epilepsy's primary symptomatic presentation are a central concern for the Pope, especially in terms of potential disruption to sacramental worship. The risk was simply too great. Epileptic men who experienced frequent seizures were prohibited from assuming an active role in the divine service. In the same letter, Alexander sketches protocols for epileptic clerics who had been allowed to become priests due to the relative mildness of their symptoms, yet later suffer seizures during the consecration of the Eucharist. If the priestly server drops Christ's body, the wafer, whilst seizing, he bears no fault: his illness is to blame. Although he is prohibited from the performance of sacramental rites thereafter, he can resume such duties if God cures his epilepsy. Is the epileptic priest strictly forbidden from serving Mass altogether, or does the injunction stand only when his symptoms are most severe? The temporal rhythm of seizures can vary widely; the time between episodes is not fixed. How, then, can Church authorities be sure that the priest is wholly cured and able to officiate once more, rather than experiencing a prolonged period of stability in between seizure episodes?[15]

According to the Council of Orange of 411, a bishop with a physical limitation (*infirmitas*, bodily defect), or suffering from a dullness of the

14 *Decretum Gratiani*, edited in Friedberg (ed.), *Corpus iuris canonici*, second part, causa 7, question 2, chapter 1.

15 Guaydier, *Les irrégularités*, p. 15. See also *Decretum Gratiani*, edited in Friedberg (ed.), *Corpus iuris canonici*, second part, causa 23, question 4, chapter 37.

senses (*hebetudo sensus*, defect of the mind), must delegate his role in the administration of the rites.[16] This statute is recapitulated in the 1094 *Decree* of Yvo of Chartres, and sets a baseline of expectation regarding the obligatory transferral of clerical duties in cases of impairment. It does not, however, take into account variable or episodic impairment. Herein lies the utility of the supplications and papal letters. They offer the means to handle practical issues relating to real-world examples of clerical impairment: the temporary exclusion of variably impaired clerics from certain aspects of their role in order to ensure the appropriate governance of Church affairs. In cases of fluctuating impairment, the Papal Chancery typically allowed priests to appoint a coadjutor to perform some of their duties on their behalf. However, the Curia did not wrest all responsibility away from such petitioners. Rather, it permitted supplicants to continue to undertake tasks within their capacity, likely adjusting their role to take into account the periods in which their impairment was more severe. The fact that such supplicants retained the requisite physical and mental capacities at certain times meant that the Church could grant graces for the allocation of support as and when necessary, as opposed to suggesting clerics' resignation. Coadjutors could be appointed on a strictly time-limited basis. Indeed, a quarter of the authorizations for the appointment of a coadjutor in the corpus are issued only for a fixed term, granted on average for a period of three years. Such measures allowed the Chancery to keep track of the replacements installed to support impaired clerics and facilitated its management of ecclesiastical benefices. The need for accommodations was nullified if the impaired cleric died or was cured. For this reason, the Chancery carefully monitored its files to verify the case for exemptions.

A series of letters studied by James R. King shows the local Church hierarchy's keen interest in the appointment of coadjutors, as a complement to the macro-level perspective offered in the papal corpus.[17] The documents also allow access to a more local level of decision-making than in the corpus for the present study. These missives concern the case of Thomas Chapel, rector of Bletchingdon in Oxfordshire, who was suffering from intermittent dementia, clearly linked to an illness. The Bishop of Sutton intervened in order to arrange appropriate accommodations, initiating correspondence

16 *Decree* of Yvo of Chartres, edited in Migne (ed.), *Patrologia Latina*, vol. 161, book 5, chapter 306, quoting canon 29 of the Council of Orange in 441. See Díez and Rodríguez (eds.), *Colección canónica hispana*, p. 95.

17 King, "The Mysterious Case of the 'Mad' Rector". The letters were published by Hill (ed.), *The Rolls and Register of Bishop Oliver Sutton*, vol. 3, p. 181; vol. 4, pp. 42, 124; and vol. 5, p. 206.

with Thomas himself on 22 January 1292 to direct him to employ a coadjutor. On 29 October of the same year, Thomas was reported missing, though he was later found, according to a letter dating to almost a year later (22 October 1293). Upon his return, the rector's illness appeared to be in remission, and he returned home. The bishop wrote to Thomas once more, ordering the cleric to appear before him and prove that he remained capable of performing his office. The matter ended on 8 February 1297, however, when the bishop formally appointed coadjutors for Thomas as his illness had returned in full force and he was once again of unsound mind. From that point onwards, the rector was prohibited from the performance of certain tasks associated with his role, and these responsibilities were entrusted to a coadjutor. Nevertheless, Thomas retained his title and continued to carry out the tasks of which he was capable. The allocation of an assistant appears to have afforded Thomas a partial 'retirement', before the severity of his impairment – or his death – necessitated his full retirement.

The Protection of Church Affairs

Benefice-holding clerics might be assigned a coadjutor as part of the petition process. This was a proactive measure to ensure that Church affairs were taken care of promptly. An assessor could be installed at the beginning of the pontifical investigation regarding a given case, to determine whether the supplicant was capable of managing his benefice. The assessor's main task was to oversee the care of souls. This entitled him to receive a portion of the assessed supplicant's benefice in order to live comfortably. A statute in Gregory IX's *Decretals* is clear on this issue.[18] If a priest cannot carry out his ministry – if he is leprous, or unable to speak, for example – he must be replaced by a coadjutor. In recognition of his work, the latter receives a share of the parish income, in a similar fashion to the sharing of assets with vicars.[19] The specific financial arrangements put in place varied, however. The petitions and papal letters reveal a distinction in how cases were treated, according to petitioners' relative wealth. Whilst subordinates of archbishops

18 *Decretales Gregory IX*, edited in Friedberg (ed.), *Corpus iuris canonici,* book III, title 6, '*De clerico aegrotante vel debilitato*' (About weak and infirm clerics), chapter 5, compiling a letter from Innocent III sent to the Archbishop of Arles concerning the Bishop of Orange and a letter from Honorius III wrote to the Bishop of Aversano.

19 Fossier, *Le travail au Moyen Âge*, p. 44: from Latin *vicarius*, 'who is in the place of'. Only three letters studied use this word, preferring '*coadjutor*' (coadjutor), the indefinite '*alium*' (another) or the vague formulation '*aliquam seu aliquas personas iidoneas*' (someone or another suitable persons).

and bishops had to pay their assessors themselves, if their supplication were successful, the institution paid for the assistance granted to archbishops and bishops.[20] Thus, withdrawal from active service depended upon relatively prosperous finances, as clerics had to employ their replacements from their own salary.[21]

Income disparity amongst the clergy impacted the consequences and hence the conceptualization of impairment itself. Indeed, for lower-ranked clerics, it might be difficult to pay for coadjutors on their low incomes. They might then prefer to leave the clergy to find another salary. However, for members of the high clergy with a substantial income, it was better to remain in office and continue to receive pensions. The case of Johannes, the elderly Bishop of Dol, is illustrative here. In a letter written by John XXII on 26 February 1322, we learn that the bishop lives with severe illness, alongside a variety of other 'perpetual impediments', including blindness:

> A short time ago, the dear sons of the chapter of the Church of Dol informed us by their special letters and nuncios that you, your body broken by the disease of old age, are suffering from a serious incurable illness and, notoriously, from blindness and other perpetual impediments. Your body is so ill from the aggressive properties of old age that you are incapable and useless in the exercise of the pastoral office. It is therefore permissible for you or the bishops and abbots around you to appoint one or more far-sighted and wise men to assume your office as coadjutors, and to care for your church which has been so neglected, through no fault of your own [...] the coadjutor or coadjutors are to assume the performance of both spiritual and temporal duties and assist you in the pastoral office.[22]

20 Shahar, *Growing Old*, p. 109.

21 Rosenthal, "Retirement and the Life Cycle", pp. 180–183.

22 RV 73, f. 203 R (RA 16, f. 360 R) – John XXII to Johannes, Bishop of Dol, 26 February 1322. Text analysed by Mollat (ed.), *Jean XXII*, n° 15 134, for which I give the transcription according to the register: '*Dudum siquidem dilectis filiis capitulo ecclesie Dolensis significantibus nobis per eorum litteras et nuncios speciales quod tu confractus senio valitudine corporali gavatus ac incurabili morbo videlibet notoria cecitate percussus et aliis perpetuis impedimentis que patiebatur in te tam infirmitatis corporalis quod infeste proprietas senectutis detentus impotens et inutilis eras effectus ad pastorale officium exercendum et quod licet per eos et quosdam tuos convicinos episcopos et abbates caritative hortatur fuisses ut unum vel duos viros providos et discretos assumeres in coadiutores tui officii memorati quare tamen hoc facere indebite recusaras carem ecclesiam propter hoc et alios defectus negligentiam et culpam tuam ut dicebant magna incomoda pertulerat et maiora preferre nisi littere hoc providere celeriter verisimiliter timebatur* [...] *ecclesie predicte pro facultatem tibi coadiutorem vel coadiutores assumere quatenus tam in spiritualibus quam in temporalibus circa executionem olim pastoralis assistant*'.

The Pope explicitly sets out the qualities required of coadjutors, demonstrating the fact that such appointees were not simply an extra pair of hands. Rather, they held the fate of souls, and the reputation of the Church, in their hands. Impaired clerics endangered the salvation of their parishioners, because their distribution of the sacraments could be imperfect. Above all, they risked disappointing their parishioners and damaging the status, and security, of their parish church through sub-standard management of its affairs. Johannes is described as impotent (*impotens*) and useless (*inutilis*), a standard comparison deployed in ecclesiastical texts, featuring often in the corpus of papal letters, miracle accounts, and canonization dossiers.[23] Such framing of the impaired body as a useless burden is a theme developed by both the clerical and secular elite, testifying to the shared conceptualization of non-normative embodiment at the highest echelons of medieval society.[24] For this reason, supplications and letters routinely evoke the embarrassment of petitioners and/or their relatives at the prospect of an individual becoming burden for the Church. The appointment of an assistant offered a workaround, allowing ecclesiastics of the highest ranks to enjoy their benefices, while delegating their effective management. For the Apostolic See, the appointment of assessors and assistants was essential in order to avoid the Church falling into ruin.

For bishops and priests who were likely be unable to perform Mass due to old age, disease and/or impairment, canon law favoured the appointment of coadjutors rather than offering the clerics to resign to elect a successor.[25] With support from assistants, some petitioners could feasibly remain in office until their death, the probable goal in Johannes' case.[26] Similarly, assistants could help older bishops to retain their benefices, even if succession was on the horizon, either through the bishop's resignation or imminent death. Such arrangements were not just advantageous for the impaired bishops. Indeed, the Pope may well have preferred to keep a trusted advisor in place in the episcopal see, or at the head of an abbey, even if he were elderly or sick, rather than appoint a strong and healthy successor whom he distrusted. Coadjutors were often recruited

23 Metzler, *Disability in Medieval Europe*, p. 162.

24 See Kuuliala, "Nobility, Community and Physical Impairment".

25 *Decretum Gratiani*, edited in Friedberg (ed.), *Corpus iuris canonici,* second part, causa 7, question 1, chapters 1 to 7 and 17–18. *Decree* of Yvo of Chartres, edited in Migne (ed.), *Patrologia Latina*, vol. 161, book 2, chapter 124, and book 5, chapter 352.

26 Orme, "Sufferings of the Clergy", p. 64.

from the supplicant's entourage, resident in his institution.[27] This meant that assistants had prior knowledge not just of the cleric for whom they deputized, but the specific regional and institutional contexts at play. At the same time, such appointments functioned as on-the-job instruction for coadjutors' future career progression. Indeed, *ante mortem* (before death) appointments allowed the coadjutor to be trained in the management of a benefice which he might inherit after the resignation or death of its holder. Suffragans and popes often preferred to elect the assistant who had been legally managing the benefice as successor, rather than appoint an external party: the coadjutor was usually the most capable in fulfilling the duties associated with this specific role, and more knowledgeable about local practices. The appointment of coadjutors, then, ultimately functioned as a smooth and effective 'power transfer scheme': the transferral of office between the outgoing bishop and his experienced former assistant risked the least damage to the benefice, which could result from mismanagement by ignorant external appointees.[28] In the 1298 *Liber Sextus*, Boniface VIII enacted major revisions to the law concerning the succession of coadjutors to the episcopal office. From then on, assistants had to be selected by the cathedral chapter, and authority for their appointment rested exclusively with the Pope.[29] Notwithstanding such changes, petitioners who wished neither to resign nor fully retire retained the option to enter a period of 'semi-retirement', by appointing an assistant to help them in the daily management of their church.[30]

Breaking Monastic Rules

Conventual enclosure was a founding principle of institutional life for monks and nuns in the Middle Ages.[31] Perpetual confinement, especially for women, was recommended by several Church councils, including at the Council of Epaone in 517.[32] The thirteenth century appeared as the

27 The popes settled the question of the resignation of benefice-holding clerics in much the same way as for regulars.

28 Cochelin, "*In senectute bona*", p. 126.

29 Jedin and Dolan, *History of the Church*, pp. 229–231. The author mentions the *Sexte* of Boniface VIII, especially book 2, title 19, *De procuratoribus*.

30 Cummins, "Attitudes to Old Age", p. 224.

31 Heullant-Donat, Claustre and Lusset (eds.), *Enfermements I – II – III*. Monasteries are used for masculine religious enclosure while convents are used for feminine communities.

32 Maassen (ed.), *Concilia aevi merovingici*, p. 28 (article 38).

'threshold' (*seuil*) of monastic confinement, with perpetual enclosure thenceforth remaining part of standard ecclesiastical regulations until the sixteenth-century Council of Trent.[33] Boniface VIII's *Periculoso* decree, promulgated in 1298, generalized statutes on enclosure, rearticulating and further concretizing earlier Council rulings. The decree proclaims that entering a convent is prohibited, unless authorization has been secured by the institution's competent superior and a legitimate reason has been provided.[34] From this point onwards, enclosure fell under the purview of general canon law, obliging all monastic communities to close their doors to outsiders and withdraw from the world. The universal application of legislation allowed the ecclesiastical institution to standardize practices across the entire Church, thereby solidifying its centralized authority. Grants of pontifical grace offered something of a loophole, however. Petitioners could receive permission to contravene religious vows, including those mandating enclosure, in cases in which, as Thomas Aquinas put it, 'the thing [vow] would become absolutely bad or useless'.[35] Only the Church's highest authority, the Pope, could take up the question of breaking such vows. Indeed, in these cases, so-called 'common' dispensations, permissions, and licences granted by lower-ranking prelates, were insufficient. Impairment, old age, or illness could provide a legitimate rationale for breaking vows (including enclosure), if the action was undertaken in order to avoid generating scandal or to remove the disabled supplicant from a dangerous situation.[36] Such dispensations relate to around 15% of cases in the corpus.

The contours of the monastic boundary, and the tensions catalyzed by its socio-cultural and spatial demarcation, are rendered in particularly fine detail in discussions of monastics' physical and mental impairment. Some impaired clerics might have been hidden from the gaze of their contemporaries. On the one hand, this functioned as a kind of ostracization. Yet, enclosure could also serve as a protective measure, safeguarding impaired monastics in institutions which supported their material needs. Impaired monks and nuns adapted to the demands of the pontifical institution, but also put in place strategies to facilitate their life as coenobites. The documents attest to the permeability of enclosure, for those in receipt of papal grace at least. 'Things from outside' (*exteriora*) were allowed to enter enclosed monastic

33 Dortel-Claudot, "La clôture des moniales", p. 66.

34 Makowski, *Canon Law and Cloistered Women*, p. 1.

35 Thomas Aquinas, *Summa Theologiae II–II*, q. 88, article 10: 'Whether a vow is subject to dispensation or commutation?' 11: 'Whether a dispensation can be granted in a solemn vow of continence?' 12: 'Whether the authority of a superior is required in a dispensation from a vow?'

36 See also Dubourg, "L'incapacité dans les lettres de dispenses pontificales".

institutions and encloistered monastics were permitted to re-enter the world for health reasons, either temporarily or permanently.[37] The Church could be surprisingly flexible in offering accommodations to the vow of enclosure. Ecclesiastical texts and the various rules, customs and statutes of the orders themselves demonstrate the relative porosity of conventual enclosure.[38]

The Relaxation of Rigorous Demands

For conventual institutions, accommodations were a fact of life. The monastic lifestyle was harsh: deprivation, confinement, and communal living could, and did, lead to physical and mental impairments.[39] As a practical measure, institutions had to provide accommodations for community members' physical weakness, to facilitate the smooth running of the facility whilst also making space for monastics with weaker health.[40] Monastic rules and instructions issued by Church councils routinely emphasized the need to lighten the workload allocated to weak or sick monastics. For example, the ninth-century Council of Chalons II recommended a less rigorous lifestyle for weak, elderly, or sick nuns:

> The nuns gathered in the monastery must study reading and singing, and celebrate the canonical hours together, and all of them, except those who suffer from an impairment (*infirmitas*), sleep in the dormitory, and come every day to the chapter and meeting and observe the rule affectionately drawn up by the Holy Fathers for them.[41]

Such guidance provided the grounds for monastics to petition for accommodations tailored to their needs. Following the Council's exhortations, the sisters of the Clarissian Convent of Montello in Beauvais, for example, received a dispensation from Clement VI in a letter dated 3 May 1345 to be excused from following all the canonical hours on account of their physical impairments.[42] Divided into eight offices, the canonical hours structured monastic time, with worship punctuating the monastic day in

37 Lauwers and Bottazzi, "*Interiora* et *exteriora*", p. 76 and following.

38 See Lehfeldt, *Religious Women in Golden Age Spain*.

39 Kerr, "Health and Safety", p. 4 and following.

40 Montford, "Fit to Preach and Pray", p. 96.

41 *Decree* of Yvo of Chartres, edited in Migne (ed.), *Patrologia Latina*, vol. 161, book 7, chapter 95 (my translation).

42 RV 165, f. 253 V – Clement VI to the abbess and sisters of the convent of Montello, order of St. Clare (diocese of Beauvais), 3 May 1345, for which I give the transcription according to the

a ceaseless, unforgiving rhythm. Following the hours assiduously could thus be difficult for weak or elderly nuns, even putting their health at risk. For this reason, Clement VI released old or senile nuns of this convent, monastics 'broken by impairment and old age', from the attendance of all daily Masses.

From as early as the eighth century, customary documents (specific to each monastery) were modified to add special provisions to monastic rules to take into account an institution's specific contexts, geographical and otherwise, and the risks it faced. Though first introduced in an informal manner, such tailored statues were taken as official regulations from the eleventh century onwards.[43] The 'Rules of Life', or 'Rules', governing monastic institutions illustrate the prevailing knowledge about the body and health in the Middle Ages. Notably, such texts eschew vocabulary linking ill health with sin, opting instead for metaphorical language.[44] These documents demonstrate the will of both Church authorities and monastic communities to care for impaired clerics, treating them with dignity and respect. The petition process allowed impaired monastics to request more specific, and more substantive, accommodations, through the relaxation of ecclesiastical legislation. For example, on 15 May 1289, Nicholas IV grants permission to the abbot and convent of Lindors in the diocese of St Andrew in Scotland for monks to be equipped with bonnets. Typically, the monks wore white silk vestments without hoods during processions. Without head coverings, they were left unprotected from the elements, a driver of illness in the community. The bonnets were a sensible prophylactic measure to fend off long-term sickness (*infirmitas longissimus*).[45] Similarly, sick monks and nuns were allowed dietary accommodations as a therapeutic intervention, with the aim of balancing their complexion.[46] For example, an undated letter from Alexander IV authorizes monks and friars languishing with sickness (*infirmitas*) in the infirmary to eat meat, whereas they would not have been allowed to eat

register: '*moniales antiqua adeo senio et debilitate confracte quod ordines suum et horas canonicas dicere nequeunt*'.

43 Consult Cygler, "Règles, coutumiers et statuts".

44 Studies reveal that medical language is used to deal with sins in general, and more specifically with rule-breaking and the 'infection' of sins as disease spreading. See Crisciani, "The Semantic Range of Medical Language".

45 RV 44, f. 132 R – Nicholas IV to the abbot and convent of Lindors (diocese of St Andrew), 15 May 1289. Text edited by Bliss (ed.), *Calendar of Entrie*, p. 528, and by Theiner (ed.), *Vetera monumenta*, letter n° 310, p. 142.

46 Coon, *Dark Age Bodies*, p. 89.

any normally.[47] In addition, sick monastics were effectively exempted from hygienic prescriptions (such as the right to bathe more frequently), as testified in the statutes and customs of religious orders.[48]

Monasteries and convent required external help for the specialist task of caring for their weakest members, and thus invited certain individuals from outside the community to traverse the 'permeable border' of enclosure.[49] Doctors and confessors, members of monastics' *familia*, servants, and visitors offering companionate support could all therefore enter institutions as helpers.[50] Individuals offering assistance of this kind tended to gravitate towards monasteries. Depending on the circumstances at hand, visitors might be granted permanent or temporary permission to enter the monastery for shorter or longer periods of time. With papal letters, the Chancery authorized and supervised the transgression of conventual enclosure. The infirmary was the locus of care-giving in the medieval monastery, and could be situated either outside of or within the bounds of enclosure. Even when nominally within enclosed space, the infirmary was a more explicitly inclusive space. In this site, monastic therapeutic knowledge was dispensed to the lay sick who passed through the region, as well as to suffering or elderly clerics and community members. Traditional monastic orders initiated the custom of employing physicians during the fourteenth century, as medicine became more professionalized, a move followed later by the mendicants. This was not necessarily a radical move; monastic rules already allowed a certain freedom when it came to medical treatment.[51] The Augustinian Rule, for example, allowed religious to break their vow of poverty and hire a doctor when the situation required.[52] Papal letters broadened such permissions, even allowing some convents to hire several physicians and surgeons. For example, a missive from Innocent IV dated 21 October 1252 allows the master and brothers of the hospital in Jerusalem to employ five doctors and three surgeons. These medics were hired to tend to sick clerics who came to the hospital seeking treatment, despite the fact that the presence of such

47 RV 24, f. 44 R – Alexander IV to the abbot and Cistercian convent of St. Anastasius in Rome. Text edited by Bourel de La Roncière, Loye, Canival and Coulon (eds.), *Les registres d'Alexandre IV*, n° 357.

48 Yearl, "Medieval Monastic Customaries", p. 175.

49 See Makowski, "L'enfermement des moniales".

50 Miramon, *Les "donnés"*, p. 72.

51 Montford, *Health, Sickness, Medicine*, p. 38 and following.

52 Verheijen (transl.), *La Règle de saint Augustin*, p. 35, chapter 5, article 35: 'If a sister declares herself ill, she must be believed; but if there is any doubt as to the remedies to be taken, a doctor must be consulted' (my translation).

'interlopers' was in direct contravention of the institution's governance, the Augustinian Rule.[53]

The issue of enclosure, and its transgression, was particularly acute for convents. Female communities had been subject to stricter mandates regarding the impenetrability of institutional space since the advent of monasticism itself.[54] It was essential that convents remained closed spaces. Hence the longstanding preoccupation of the pontifical institution with the division of the sexes in monastic communities, even if ecclesiastical regulations were only partially applied in practice. The Church sought to prevent men from traversing the boundary of conventual confinement in order to protect women.[55] Nevertheless, papal letters might allow men to enter the cloister for therapeutic reasons.[56] For example, a missive dated 29 October 1327 from John XXII allowed men – confessors and doctors – to enter a convent of women. The letter confirms that doctors and friars of the Order of Preachers are permitted to enter the Dominican monastery of Saint-Louis de Pissiaco to tend to seriously ill, bedbound nuns, both medically and spiritually:

> Consequently, this king [of France] has humbly begged us to respond favourably to your prayers, that doctors could be sent to visit the sick sisters and also that the friars of the order of preachers could be assigned to go and hear the confessions of the sisters of your monastery of Pissiaco, in the diocese of Chartres, in order to hear the confessions of the sisters of this monastery who are so ill that they cannot leave their beds to go to the confessional, and that the said doctors may enter the said monastery in a licit manner to visit the sisters and the confessors to hear their confession.[57]

53 AN, L 248, n° 215 (olim n° 216) – Innocent IV to the Master and the friars of the Hospital of Jerusalem, 21 October 1252. Text analysed by Barbiche, *Les actes pontificaux*, n° 704, p. 268, for which I give the transcription according to the original letter.

54 See Elliott, "Tertullian".

55 Lett, "Conclusions", p. 196.

56 Consult Soulard, "Le personnel masculin".

57 RV 85, f. 134 V – John XXII to the prioress and the convent of the Augustinian monastery of sisters of St. Louis of Pissiaco (Chartres), 29 October 1327. Text analysed by Mollat (ed.), *Jean XXII*, n° 30 224, for which I give the transcription according to the register: '*Ipsius igitur Regis, nobis super hoc humiliter supplicantis et vestris precibus favorabiliter annuentes ut medici ad visitandum egrotas sorores necnon et fratres ordinis predicatorum ad audiendum confessiones sororum monasterii vestri de Pissiaco Carnotensis diocesis deputati seu etiam deputandi pro audiendis confessionibus a sororibus eiusdem monasterii graviter egrotantibus que tamen in lectis propter egritudinem decumbentes accedere nequeant ad loca ad audiendas confessiones*

The contravention of strict enclosure was legitimate in this case, as following the normal rules would grossly endanger the nuns: they would be unshriven and go without medical treatment. The missive insists, however, that the male visitors should take every care to avoid causing scandal. In this way, it follows the canon 38 of Epaone already quoted before, that mandated that only older individuals of proven virtue could enter a female monastery, and only if they had a valid reason.[58] Moreover, John XXII also endorse the *Apostolic Constitutions* laid down by his predecessor Boniface VIII, more specifically the bull *Periculoso* issued by Boniface in 1298, which was subsequently incorporated into canon law in the *Liber Sextus*. It ordered strict enclosure for all nuns under penalty of scandal and excommunication, except in the case of serious illness.[59] In order to reinforce this control over the nuns, further clarifications were made by later canonists. It added stipulations regarding, for example, which professions – such as barbers and doctors – could enter the monastery, then pursuing the protection of the ill people.[60] As demonstrated by the case of the nuns of Saint-Louis de Pissiaco, the Chancery contravened the standard canonical, monastic and local rules, by allowing to put in place the foreseen exemptions, despite its broader distrust of unenclosed female monastics. In care-giving and therapeutic (monastic) spaces, men and women cohabited in order to guarantee effective treatment and secure good health, albeit with variations according to rank.[61] Papal favours licensing the mixing of the sexes were layered on top of monastic rules that already provided special facilities for people with impairments, the elderly, and the sick.

Beyond more formalized medical treatment, monastics could request the assistance of servants, intended as daily helpmates to improve their quality of life, from their direct superiors or the Pope. Servants likely hailed from the institution's *familia*, that is, the group of lay people materially and/or spiritually close to the monastic, fraternal or clerical community.[62] They worked alongside the *conversi* (lay brothers) on agricultural, craft and household tasks.[63] Servants remained part of the laity, and often lived

huiusmodi deputata, prefatum monasterium intrare licite dictique medici ipsas visitare sorores et confessores predicti ipsarum confessiones audire de licentia'.

58 Maassen (ed.), *Concilia aevi merovingici*, p. 28 (article 38).

59 *Liber sextus* from Boniface VIII, edited in Friedberg (ed.), *Corpus iuris canonici*, book III, article 16.

60 Makowski, *Canon Law and Cloistered Women*, pp. 124–126.

61 Hasquenoph, *Histoire des ordres*, p. 450.

62 Op. cit., p. 149.

63 Some decisions of the Carthusian chapter dated 1129 decreed that knights, damsels, old people or invalids could not be given to the monasteries of the order. See Miramon, *Les "donnés"*, p. 249.

outside enclosure, despite contributing directly to clerical and community life, and often being appointed by the papal institution. Arnulfus, former abbot and canon of the Augustinian abbey of Sainte-Geneviève in Paris, takes advantage of his resignation to secure the right to have additional help from Martin IV. The Pope's response is elucidating on the topic of servants and their typical duties:

> Thinking for a long time to take into account what is favourable for your health and after attention to the praiseworthy study of your consideration as, you, in the monastery of Sainte-Geneviève in Paris, of the order of Saint Augustine, under the immediate privilege of the church of Rome, exercising the government which you occupy, because of a heavy and troublesome illness which occurs, leaving you impotent, and unable to carry out the work and numerous cares which the office of government requires, you fear that the monastery will suffer from your impotence thus occasioned [...] therefore you spontaneously and freely resign the government of the monastery into our hands. [...] We concede by the authority of this letter that, in the said monastery of St. Genevieve you are permitted to have a suitable companion, taken from within the monastery, and two domestic servants in your house, and that you be given the necessities of human life, and in accordance with the harmony of the condition of your body. However, the aforementioned companions and familiars, like the other canons and servants, shall participate in the daily administration of the monastery. Furthermore, in addition to this, you shall receive each year one hundred Parisian pounds taken from the revenues of the monastery that you will recover on the day of St. Remi.[64]

64 RV 41, f. 38 V – Martin IV to Arnoulf, canon of the monastery of Saint Geneviève of Paris, 15 March 1282. Text edited by Olivier-Martin (ed.), *Les registres de Martin IV*, n° 127: '*Dudum siquidem salubri meditatione recogitans et studio laudando considerationis attendens quod tu ad monasterium Sancte Genovefe Parisiensis ad Romanam ecclesiam immediate spectantis, ordinis sancti Augustini, exercendum regimen cui preeras ob graves tibi supervenientis infirmitatis molestias impotens factus eras nec poteras labores et sollicitudines plurimas quas ejusdem cura regiminis exigit tolerare, ac verisimiliter metuens ut monasterium ipsum incommoda perpeti occasione hujusmodi tue impotentie cogeretur,* [...] *predicti monasterii regimen sponte ac libere in nostris manibus resignasti.* [...] *presentium tibi auctoritate concedimus ut in predicto monasterio Sancte Genovefe congruam pro te ac uno socio ydoneo de ipsius monasterii gremio assumendo et duobus famulis cameram habeas sive domum, ac ea que sustentationi humane vite necessaria esse noscuntur, pro te secundum tui conditionem corporis tibi competentia, et eisdem socio et famulis prout aliis canonicis et servientibus ipsius monasterii diebus singulis ministrantur, ac insuper centum libras parisiensium de proventibus ejusdem monasterii tibi in festo beati Remigii persolvendas quoad visceris* (*sic*) *percipias annuatim*'.

At heart, Arnulfus' request for the appointment of helpers is a question of dignity. Faced with 'many worries' as a result of his ailing body, he can no longer cope by himself. Outside support, in the form of servants, will allow him to live out his life with dignity. The Pope is receptive, topping up the financial compensation of his pension with more practical support, the permission to employ a suitable companion (*socius*) from the monastery of Sainte-Geneviève and two lay familiars (*famuli*) as assistants.[65] The latter are essentially domestic carers, responsible for servicing his accommodation and providing him with necessary daily support. Arnulfus' companion, by contrast, is to be selected from amongst the monks of his own community. All three auxiliaries must, however, substantively contribute to the smooth running of the monastery, like the other clerics and servants, on a daily basis. It is clear, then, that the *famuli* did not just assist Arnulfus, but served the entire monastery of which they were now quasi-members. In this way, they were situated similarly to *conversi*, and often adopted the same functions. The presence of *famuli* at the monastery was required daily. They were thus likely to live in a neighbouring village or, as with Arnulf, to remain at their master's side to provide round-the-clock care. In cases like Arnulf's, the monastic's body was no longer 'delegated to the use of the community', to quote Humbert of Romans, but instead relegated to the infirmary or the sick-bed.[66] This move was both isolating and supportive. Though the monk could no longer contribute productively to his institution, he was not entirely excluded from his community, and indeed received care from its members and within its bounds.

Transferral to Another Monastery or Order

Gratian insisted on the absolute necessity of enclosure for monks. Borrowing the metaphorical image of the 'monk-fish' from the *Life of Anthony* (written by Athanasius around 370), the canonist contended that, like a fish out of water, a monk cannot survive if displaced from his natural habitat, the monastery.[67] In this formulation, monastic living conditions – including enclosure – are a key component underpinning the identity of religious, who must aspire to *mansio quieta* (tranquillity at home).[68] The validity, and necessity, of enclosure is anchored in the three vows sworn upon the

65 A companion (*socius*) is obligatorily appointed for each beggar when an exit from the convent is required. See Hourlier and Le Bras, *Histoire du droit et des institutions*, p. 232.

66 Berthier (ed.), *Opera De vita regulari*, p. 391.

67 *Decretum Gratiani*, edited in Friedberg (ed.), *Corpus iuris canonici,* causa 16, chapter 1, question 8, 11, and 12.

68 Caby, "Comme un poisson dans l'eau", p. 118.

adoption of the religious lifestyle: chastity, poverty, and obedience. Enclosure cut monastics off from the outside world and its temptations, and thus facilitated chastity and poverty. At the same time, monks demonstrated their obedience by following the Rule to which their home institution was subject. Compliance with the strict regulations regarding enclosure could be difficult, and thus claustration itself proved a useful means to test, and prove, one's obedience.[69] The solemn and definitive monastic vow constituted a sacred contract 'made between God, the novice and the members of the chapter of the religious community'.[70] As such, the vow of obedience structured the relationship between a monastic and the specific order and house they joined. The supplication process, however, allowed for petitioners to secure permission from a higher authority – the Pope himself – to break the vow of obedience and transfer to another monastery or even another order.[71] The corpus demonstrates, for example, that the Papal Chancery permitted monastics to leave enclosure to transfer location, and thereby contravene the vow of *stabilitas loci* (stability of location), for reasons relating to ill health and incapacity (4 cases pertaining to religious communities; 13 cases relating to individuals). For similar reasons, the Chancery authorized a number of supplicants in the corpus to break their vows and transfer to another order (41 cases).

Through a series of reforms, the popes gradually redefined the regular clergy during the twelfth, thirteenth, and fourteenth centuries. They sought to promote the idea that monks should be dedicated solely to religion and, above all, follow the conventions of the monastic rule which governed their home monastery, including enclosure regulations.[72] This is evidenced by a letter of Urban II (1042–1099) written in 1099 to the abbot of Saint-Rufin, regarding the behaviour of regular canons – a bull that was later compiled in Yvo of Chartres' *Decree*.[73] In his *Decree*, Gratian subsequently broadened the focus of such earlier regulations, which had previously applied only to

69 In the mendicant orders, the monks were not bound to the enclosure, but they must take a vow of poverty before they could take the habit permanently. In addition, unlike the traditional orders, they must be able to preach, and therefore they must be more subject to idoneity since they must be able to give the sacraments and say Masses.

70 Hasquenoph, *Histoire des ordres*, p. 95 (my translation).

71 Impairment is also a 'just cause' for transferring from one monastery or order to another in petitions handled by the Apostolic Penitentiary. Fossier, *Le bureau des âmes*, pp. 350–355.

72 Maccarrone, "I Papi del secolo 12", p. 356.

73 Migne (ed.), *Patrologia Latina*, vol. 151, column 546 – Urban II to the abbot of Saint Rufin in 1099. *Decree* of Yvo of Chartres, edited in Migne (ed.), *Patrologia Latina*, vol. 161, book 6, chapter 411.

canons. He maintained that monks were also subject to enclosure.[74] In this way, the principle of *stabilitas loci* – the clerical obligation to remain in the institution in which, and to which, one had sworn vows – began to take shape. The petition process offered a means for supplicants to disobey this mandate. Petitioners wrote to the Chancery as individuals or in groups, requesting permission to transfer from one monastery to another. In certain instances, papal letters allowed the wholescale relocation of an entire congregation, an outcome that was much more likely if petitioners grounded their request in terms of a necessary intervention to preserve health. The Augustinian friars of Santa Eulalia del Campo, for example, resided outside of the city of Barcelona, in a marshy area next to the Nou Gate. Indeed, the stale air made them sick, according to the practical medical considerations mobilized in this missive. On 15 February 1295, Boniface VIII granted the friars permission to move into the city proper, transferring to a building formerly occupied by the Order of the Penance of Jesus Christ, which had been dissolved in 1274.[75] Similarly, a female community from St. Mary Vallis-Flogi (diocese of Nucera Umbria) in the Order of St. Damian was allowed to move location, as their original living conditions were deemed unhealthy, and they wished to build a convent within the city walls.[76] Such examples also illustrate monastic communities' attraction to urban centres during the thirteenth and fourteenth centuries.[77]

Individual petitioners could also invoke health reasons and the deleterious conditions in which they were living to obtain the right to move. For example, the monk Neukinus, born Arnaldus le Breissereal de Hodege, began his monastic career in the monastery of Saint-Jacques in Liège. He later petitioned the Pope to authorize his transfer to another institution, however:

> It was brought to our attention by the petition of the said Neukinus which contained that, residing in the aforementioned monastery [Saint-Jacques of Liège], his complexion does not agree with the air of this place, as long as his body is sick and cannot regain health. He therefore wishes

74 *Decretum Gratiani*, edited in Friedberg (ed.), *Corpus iuris canonici*, causa 3, chapter 19, question 3.

75 RV 47, f. 22 V – Boniface VIII to the Bishop of Barcelona, 15 February 1295. Text edited by Digard, Fawtier, Faucon, and Thomas (eds.), *Les registres de Boniface VIII*, n° 93. On this ancient monastery, see Feliu, "El monestir de frares".

76 *Autographo Conventu S. Francisci civitatis Nuceriae in Umbria* – Alexander IV to the nuns and the abbess of the convent of St. Mary Vallis-Flogis, Order of St. Damian (diocese of Nucere), 15 May 1256. Text edited by Sbaraglia (ed.), *Bullarium Franciscanum, Tomus* 2, letter 190, p. 132.

77 Gilli, *Villes et sociétés urbaines*, pp. 235–239.

> to transfer himself from the said monastery in the diocese of Liège to the monastery of Saint-Hubert in the Ardennes, which belongs to the same diocese and the same order. We wish to respond favourably to this request of Neukinus, and therefore we ask by apostolic writings at your discretion, that you or someone else accept Neukinus in the monastery, if it is so and notwithstanding the other canons.[78]

The letter emphasizes that Neukinus' desire for a transfer lies not in any dissatisfaction with his current institution or his order, but his chronic illness. Whilst the environment at the monastery of Saint-Jacques is not beneficial to his constitution, he has no qualms about the Benedictine Order of which he is a member. For this reason, he does not seek to secure a transfer of order, only institution, wishing to join a monastery in the mountainous Ardennes region. Neukinus seems to believe that the mountain air will be purer, and thus this change of environment will help him to regain his health (*sanitas*). With such a move, Neukinus intends to violate his vow of *stabilitas loci*, and thereby break the juridical bond between a monk and his monastery that was supposedly permanent. Indeed, theoretically, 'the religious was professed in one and only monastery, to which he belongs wherever he may be'.[79] Nevertheless, permission to transfer between houses in the same order, if necessitated by ill health and other legitimate circumstances, was easy enough to obtain, if the petitioner had the good fortune of belonging to an order with several monasteries. In such cases, vows of *stabilitas loci* could, in practice, be broken without any negative consequences, as long as the abbots of the two communities had come to prior agreement on the transfer. Institutional transfers were sometimes even expressly permitted, as in the Rule of St. Benedict from the sixth century (chapter 61) or explicitly anticipated, as in the *Carta Caritatis* (Charter of Charity and Unanimity) written in the twelfth century for the Cistercian Order.[80] Neukinus, however, had to seek the Pope's consent: the question

78 RA 180, f. 308 V – Gregory XI to Neukinus, monk of the monastery of Saint James in Liege, 17 December 1371. Text analysed by Hayez, Mathieu and Yvan (eds.), *Grégoire XI*, n° 15 056, for which I give the transcription according to the register: '*Cum itaque sicut exhibita nobis pro parte dicti Neukinum petitio continebat ipso in monasterio antedicto residendo tam propter aerem illius loci sue complexionis nullatenus congruentem quam corporis sui debilitate nequeat sanitate gaudere cupiatque propterea de dicto monasterio ad monasterium sancti Huberti in Ardenia dicti ordini Leodiensis diocesis se transfere, nos volentes ipsius Neukinumi votis annuere favorabiliter in hac parte, discretioni vestre, per apostolica scripta mandamus quatenus, vos vel duo aut unus vestrum per vos vel alium seu alios eundem Neukinum, si est ita, et aliud canonicati non obstante.*'

79 Hourlier and Le Bras, *Histoire du droit*, p. 215 (my translation).

80 Op. cit., p. 244.

is, why? His petition speaks, perhaps, to a conflict between the monk and his superiors, who either refused to let him leave or wanted to send him elsewhere. Tellingly, Neukinus' direct superior, the abbot of the monastery of Saint-Jacques, does not figure as an intermediary in, or direct addressee of, the correspondence, as would be typical.[81] Rather, the monk's request was forwarded to the Curia by three deacons from the churches of St. Paul, St. Martin, and the Holy Cross, in Liège.

If transferal between houses in the same order was relatively easy, changing order entirely was another story. The issue emerged in the tenth century, with the foundation of monastic orders that were intended to be more severe than pre-existing offerings (Cistercian, Dominican and Franciscan Orders). Instances of ordinal transfers (*transitus*, i.e., a monk's transfer to another religious congregation), became ever more frequent in the eleventh century, particularly in the context of the so-called Gregorian reform as monks moved to the new orders. In fact, in a letter preserved in Gregory IX's *Decretals*, Innocent III authorized all requests for transfer to stricter orders, even without the consent of the supplicant's superior.[82] Nevertheless, Thomas Aquinas maintained that switching order was not praiseworthy, and the person who attempted it risked exposing himself to scandal. Aquinas allowed only three scenarios in which changing orders could, on the contrary, be deemed an honourable act: in the search for a more perfect religious life; to join a stricter order; or because of impairment or ill health.[83] Ordinal transfers became so commonplace in the thirteenth and fourteenth century that the papacy felt compelled to intervene to ensure that they were carried out in accordance with the rules.[84] Transferring to a more severe order was usually not a problem. Yet impaired petitioners desired the reverse trajectory, transferal to an order with a more flexible, or lenient, rule. For this reason, many Cistercian, Dominican, and Franciscan religious in the corpus wished to join Benedictine monasteries. Such transfers were, however, viewed in a dim light at best. Not only did such requests require weighty justification, according to

81 It appears that of the thirteen individual requests for a change of house, eight were issued by a third party (61%), seven of which were foreign to the monastery to which the monk belonged at the time of his petition. This proportion appears to be much higher than the average (see Introduction), revealing that external intercession plays a crucial role in breaking the vow of *stabilitas loci*. On standard protocols for correspondence, including choice of intermediary and addressee, see Chapter 1.

82 *Decretals of Gregory IX*, book III, title 31, chapter 18.

83 Thomas Aquinas, *Summa Theologiae II-II*, q. 189, article 8.

84 Hasquenoph, *Histoire des ordres*, p. 50.

Aquinas, they also had to be authorized both by the petitioner's superior and the Pope himself.

The case of Robertus Belagent, a friar of the Order of Preachers, is exemplary. The friar seeks permission from Clement VI to be transferred to a Benedictine monastery, as his impairment renders him unable to abide by the harsh precepts of the Dominican Rule any longer:

> Read to us, your petition contains that, while you have persevered in the order of friars preachers for many years, you have always been accustomed to read as a lector and have always been recognized for your good and honest life, reputation and conversation. But, nevertheless and for rational causes, among which is the serious illness from which you have long suffered and which has persevered in this order for years, you desire to be transferred to the order of St. Benedict and to wear the regular vestments of that order, for the safety of your life and mind. You therefore humbly beg us to provide for your request by giving you a gracious dispensation with mercy. We therefore authorize you, according to your requests, to move from the Order of Preachers to the Order of St. Benedict, into which you must be received voluntarily and, after being received, you may have a voice and take part in the chapter and be admitted to all the legitimate acts of that Order, contrary to what was decided by Pope Clement V at the Council of Vienna, notwithstanding all the apostolic constitutions and the statutes and customs of the aforementioned orders and monasteries, we dispense by apostolic authority by giving a special grace.[85]

85 RV 162, f. 106 R – Clement VI to Robertus Belagent, a monk of the preaching order, 7 November 1343, for which I give the transcription according to the register: *'Lecte nobis pro parte tua petitionis series continebat quod licet tu in ordine fratrem Predicatorum multis annis perseverans in pluribus facultatibus qui in dicto ordine legi solent lector extitens ac semper bone vite ac fame et conversationis honeste tamen ex certis et rationabilibus causis tam ex parte infirmitatum gravium quare alter ad persevendum ulterius in dicto ordine nequis tuum annuum inclinare ac pro securitate vite et conscientie tue desideras ad ordinem sancti Benedicti transferri et ipsius ordinis viduere habitum regularem. Quare nobis humiliter supplicasti ut providere super hiis de oportune dispensationis gracia misericorditer dignaremur. Nos itaque tuis supplicationibus inclinari tecum ut de dicto ordine Predicatorum ad dicti sancti Benedicti ordinem libere tansire et in illo monasterio sancti Benedicti, dicti ordini in quo inveneris voluntarium receptionem recipi et quod postquam fueris in monasterio ipsi receptis in eo et in ipso ordine sancti Benedicti vocem et locum in capitulo habere et ad omnis actus legitimos dicti ordinis sancti Benedicti admitti valeas felicis recordationis Clementis pape V, predecessoris nostri, super hoc in concilio Viennensis et qualibet alia constitutione apostolica in contrarium edita necnon quibuscumque privilegiis statutis et consuetudinibus ordinum et monasterii predictorum contrariis nequaquam obstantibus auctoritate apostolica de specialis dono gracie dispensamus'.*

Robertus' decision to transfer to a Benedictine institution is eminently practical: the order's rule allowed elderly and/or sick monks to benefit from special consideration (such as permission to eat meat, bathe more frequently or wear warmer clothes). No matter how resolved supplicants themselves were to obey by monastic rules, the rigorous lifestyle of the mendicant orders, and the chronic nature of certain illnesses, rendered many unfit, or unable, to remain in the most ascetic coenobite communities.[86] In much modern scholarship, such as the work of Ursmer Berlière, there seems to be a presumption that the invocation of impairment to legitimize *transitus* was widely exploited as a means for monastics to escape 'fraudulently' from ordinal rules that they either considered to be overly harsh, or simply could no longer abide.[87] It is, of course, impossible to know for sure. But pretext or not, the criterion of invalidity was taken into account by the Chancery. Moreover, its potential use by supplicants as a 'catch-all' justification, if not an outright excuse, testifies to its currency in terms of successfully influencing decisions about the dispensation of papal grace. The transferral of mendicant friars to more lenient orders became strictly regulated in the fourteenth century, after widespread abuse of the *transitus* system.

Moreover, supplications and letters allowed the Curia to determine many aspects of conventual life in the petitioner's new institution. For example, Clement VI does not just permit Robertus Belagent's transfer to the Benedictines, but explicitly allows the newcomer to exercise his agency by having a voice in the chapter – that is, Robertus was treated as a full member of his new order. Indeed, whilst canon law suggests that you could transfer, it would mean you were not treated as a full member of the new order, as you would not have a voice in chapter (i.e., agency in terms of the direction/management of the order). Thus, the Pope directly contravenes the provisions of the Council of Vienna in 1312 and other papal precedents.[88] Indeed, this proscription is found in the *Liber Septimus* written as early as 1317 by Pope Clement V (1264–1314), subsequently published in 1322 by his successor John XXII. Moreover, when they allow for a transfer because of illness for example, such texts prohibit the full participation of mendicant friars in their new, more lax order, denying them a voice in chapter.[89] Transfers from a strict to a more flexible order, for which the

86 See Montford, "Fit to Preach and Pray".

87 Berlière, *Épaves d'archives pontificales*, p. 59.

88 Other papal precedents include, for example, an ordinance of 4 July 1335 issued by Benedict XII, which prohibited the transfer of mendicant friars to more lax orders.

89 *Clementines* of Clément V, edited in Friedberg (ed.), *Corpus iuris canonici,* book III, title 9, 'On the regulars', chapter 1.

papacy, according to some historians, 'showed great complacency', did not survived against the affirmation of apostolic omnipotence.[90] Indeed, the Council of Trent put an end to this practice in its fourteenth session on 25 November 1551, legislating that 'those transferred to another order shall remain under obedience in enclosure, and shall be incapable of secular benefices'.[91]

Clerical Mobility

Many impairments cause, or are associated with, a reduction in mobility. About 40% of all supplications in the corpus cite mobility limitation to justify requests to disobey regulations regarding clerical travel. Mobility appears to be vital for clerics to undertake necessary ecclesiastical work, and thereby fulfil the Church's mission to spread God's glory and care for souls across Christendom. Members of the clergy were obliged to travel in their local region, in order to undertake pastoral duties. Secular clerics in particular had to be able to traverse their own benefices with relative ease (to visit parishioners and take care of other clerical duties). Clerics of higher rank, tasked with more institutional management – such as bishops, abbots, and priors – were obliged to make trips throughout their entire diocese, and even visit its dependencies. Beyond such local travel, ecclesiastical business trips to distant locales were par for the course for many. For example, the most prominent clerics were called upon to travel to ecclesiastical gatherings, and/or to carry out diplomatic missions for the Apostolic See. The petition process provided both secular and regular clerics with reduced mobility the opportunity to secure exemptions to such notionally obligatory travel, albeit only in certain circumstances.

Residency and Local Travel Requirements

Secular clerics were required to reside in the territory to which their benefice was attached, just as regular clerics were obliged to remain in their monastery.[92] Alongside ignorance, moral decay, and concubinage, disobedience of this strict residency policy topped the list of the worst 'vices'

90 Hasquenoph, *Histoire des ordres,* p. 50.

91 Waterworth (transl.), "The Council of Trent", pp. 92–121.

92 This residency requirement refers collectively to the fact that secular clerics had to live in their benefice and that they had to undertake routine local travel.

afflicting the secular clergy.[93] Some clerics took the liberty of entrusting small tasks to their vicars before absconding from their benefice entirely, though they continued to receive the income from the ecclesiastical office they had effectively abandoned. Typically, such clerics left their assigned homes to relocate to the Avignon court or join the entourage of a prince or influential prelate. Popes were routinely put in the rather awkward position of ordering the departure of clerics who had turned up at their court without an invitation, stipulating a set timeframe for their return to their benefices. Timescales varied according to the individual pontiff's tolerance, with clerics given a departure deadline of a week, a fortnight, a month, and sometimes even a year hence.[94] Some clerics, however, encountered genuine difficulties in traversing the territory covered by their benefice, travelling from one prebend to another if they had several to their name, or in recovering their income from distant and/or spread-out communities (as they sometimes had to recover it in person and did not have any vicar to do that for them). More than 150 clerics in the corpus requested permission to delegate such tasks due to their mobility limitations.

According to canon law, clerics could not change their geographical location at will. Regulars were attached to their monastery, under a vow of enclosure; seculars could not move away from their prebend, unless they were ill, travelling, or studying. The situation was even more oppressive for secular canons, as they had to secure the agreement of the chapter for travel and study that took them away from their home institution. Notwithstanding any superficial similarity, the prohibition of free clerical movement is anchored in different concerns for seculars and regulars, and the different roles they played in the Church. Regulars lived in the stasis of enclosure, whilst seculars had to be mobile. In the *Liber Sextus*, Boniface VIII directed clerics to collect the income attached to their ecclesiastical office in person, on a daily basis. Excuses were granted only to three groups: clerics with impairments (*Infirmus*); those who were rendered physically unable to undertake the task by 'just and rational' causes; and those who were busy elsewhere, hard at work for the benefit of their church.[95] Gregory XI revisited this provision in the *Liber Extra*, confirming that if clerics did not establish residency in the territory they would lose all financial privileges associated with their benefice, for a period of no less than six months. Again,

93 Fossier and Verger, *Histoire du Moyen Âge*, p. 145.

94 Hayez, "La personnalité d'Urbain V", p. 21.

95 *Liber Sextus* from Boniface VIII, edited in Friedberg (ed.), *Corpus iuris canonici*, book III, title 3, chapter 1.

exemptions were granted only to select groups: impaired clerics (*infirmus*), and those undertaking study or travel whilst in the service of the Curia.[96] Sick clerics (*aegritudo*) could be not resident in the territory for a relatively short period of time, because they need to seek treatment elsewhere (for example) or unable to travel across the territory to visit all requisite local sites. In those cases, they were allowed to continue to receive the income from their benefice, provided that someone suitable (*sanus*) person could celebrate their offices in their place, at times when they were unable to do so themselves (in case of leave of absence).[97]

Although canon law provided the means to relax residency and travel requirements for impaired clerics, papal favours could allow them even greater freedoms. With grants of papal grace, the Chancery could extend a cleric's leave of absence or release him for residency and travel requirements altogether, on a temporary or definitive notice, depending on the cases. This is demonstrated, for example, in a case in which King John II of France acted as an intercessor. The king petitions Innocent VI to (temporarily) waive the relevant requirements of not being able to move from one benefice to another for Johannes, canon of Senlis, without the cleric forfeiting any income:

> It is considered worthy of pardon that the master Johannes, who resides in another of his ecclesiastical benefices which he has already obtained or will later obtain for his trouble in the service of the king via a temporal transaction, so much so that his body is ill and disproportionately afflicted frequently and heavily by a large arthritic gout, in such a way that he is not able to serve faithfully by remaining personally in our service. But also he has in turn to resided personally in the aforementioned benefice, or, for taking care and preserve is health, residing in Paris, where there is an abundance of doctors and other experts, for which reason he asks to be exempted from having to receive daily the fruits of his aforementioned ecclesiastical benefices, on behalf of our benevolent generosity for his life and salvation, for five years, so that he may nevertheless receive the revenues of his benefices as if he lived there personally. Done for three years.[98]

96 *Decretales Gregory IX*, edited in Friedberg (ed.), *Corpus iuris canonici,* book III, title 4, chapter 15.

97 Op. cit., title 6, chapter 1.

98 RS 28, f. 26 V – King John II of France to Innocent VI, 7 February 1355, for which I give the transcription according to the register: '*Magistrer Johanni concedere dignemini, quod ipse residendo in altero beneficiorum suorum ecclesiorum que nunc obtinet vel imposterum obtinebit cum propter labores quos in serviciis regiis subire haberent transactis temporibus adeo*

With his body weakened by arthritic gout, Johannes is no longer able to manage his multiple benefices as stipulated by regulations, visiting each every day to collect income.[99] Apparently, the canon of Senlis now resides in Paris and wants to remain there full-time, so he asks the Pope to allow him to not have to visit his other benefices himself, but still retain their income. The accumulation of prebends became an increasingly common practice during the period of the Avignon papacy. This created something of a supply problem: the Curia saw an ever-increasing number of requests from ecclesiastics in search of benefices.[100] From the thirteenth century onwards, the popes had been trying to regain control of clerical benefices that had fallen into the hands of lay collators, that is, members of the laity who had the authority to confer benefices upon individuals of their choosing. Johannes' intercessor, the king, was a notable lay collator, and indeed had awarded the canon, or planned to award him, with a benefice under his purview.[101] This provides crucial context for the Apostolic See's response to the petition. The Church seeks to curry favour with the royal collator, by allowing Johannes to remain in Paris on the pretext that the best doctors and experts were in the city. At the same time, however, the Chancery does not agree to the request in full: Johannes is authorized to receive the income from his other benefices for three years, two years short of the term requested in the original supplication.[102] One might ask: why would they shorten the term? Is this so that, after three years, they can reassign these other benefices to other clerics? Or is it because, by then, Johannes could survive on the benefice collated by the king alone – the one in Paris?

Johannes' case is just one of many in the corpus that demonstrate that residency and travel requirements for secular clerics were not necessarily as strict as they first appeared. They could be modified when impairment,

sit iuris sui corporis debilitatus et maxime gucte arthetice, oculeis, quibus graviter et frequenter affligitur, sic quod in nostris serviciis personaliter insistendo non potest amplius deservire. Sed necnon deinceps habet residere personaliter in dicta predicta sua, aut pro sanitate corporis sui procuranda et conservandi residendo Paris ubi est copia medicorum, aliorum expertorum super hoc fructus dictorum suorum beneficiorum ecclesiasticorum ex benigna largitate nostra ad eius vitam vel salutem ad quiquennium, cum ea integritate percipere possit cotidianis distributionibus dumtaxat exceptis, cum qua illos perciperet si in eisdem beneficiis personaliter resideret. Fiat ad triennium'.

99 See Miramon, "La place d'Hugues de Saint-Cher".

100 Chevalier-Boyer, "Les sermons de Guillaume de Sauqueville", p. 158.

101 Guillemain, *La politique bénéficiale du pape Benoît XII*, p. 21.

102 Graces were generally granted for a limited time, ranging from two months to five years, passing through the vague mention of 'as long as the illness lasts', with a median duration of two and a half years (out of 45 letters that mention it).

illness, or old age was invoked in requests for grace. The Pope took into account the supplicant's unique circumstances, and their physical incapacity, when making decisions as to where he should live, as long as a fixed place of residence could be established. Clerics, even ones with impairments, could not adopt a transitory lifestyle, flitting from one abode to another. Whilst the petition process offered advantages for supplicants with mobility limitations, it was equally expedient for the Church: it permitted the institution to regulate more strictly the management and the accumulation of benefices.

The general requirement for clerics to reside in their benefices full time was coupled, for bishops, with the mandate to undertake regular travel. Bishops were obliged to make annual inspections of their diocese, known as 'pastoral visits', or nominate a representative in their stead, usually an archdeacon. Initially, such tours were a privilege, and not obligatory. In Gratian's *Decree* (*Cleros* canon), bishops were accorded the 'right of visitation' to all parishes in their diocese, as part of their duty of providing pastoral care to the faithful.[103] With the sixth canon of the Fourth Lateran Council, however, this right became an annual obligation.[104] These visits served several purposes. On the one hand, they allowed Church authorities, and clerics high up in the ecclesiastical hierarchy, to solidify their power base by exerting greater control over clergy at the local level. At the same time, the visits reflected the Church's desire to promote the reformist ethics of the Fourth Lateran Council and subsequent progressive assemblies, with bishops tasked with spreading the word by preaching and training local clergy. Bishops with physical or mental impairments could, however, receive exemptions from such obligatory travel. Indeed, in his *Decree*, Gratian leveraged a decision made during the Fourth Council of Toledo in 633 to proclaim that a bishop prevented from visiting his diocese by illness could send another person in his place.[105] Whilst exemptions were thus canonically permissible, Gratian underscored that such waivers are not 'automatic', but must be authorized by dispensations of papal grace on a case-by-case basis. It is for this reason, then, that Helias, the Bishop of Autun, writes to Clement V to ask permission for the appointment of a procurator to visit his bishopric on his behalf.

In a letter dated 15 July 1312, the Pope issues his decision on Helias' case:

103 *Decretum Gratiani*, edited in Friedberg (ed.), *Corpus iuris canonici,* first part, distinctio 21, chapter 1.

104 See Coulet, *Les visites pastorales*.

105 *Decretum Gratiani*, edited in Friedberg (ed.), *Corpus iuris canonici,* first part, question 1, chapter 11.

> Thus, you confirm that you are not able to exercise your office of visiting the churches, monasteries and other places, nor the ecclesiastical persons of your population and diocese, because of your own body weighed down by illness. You beg us to grant you, by the present indulgence, the possibility of freeing yourself from the custom and right of your office of visiting the churches, monasteries and other ecclesiastical places and persons, so that you may have it assumed by someone or other suitable persons who may fulfil this duty of visitation for three years, provided that they recover your money in moderation, no more than a hundred currency, notwithstanding in any case the rules issued in this matter.[106]

The bishop's ill health prevents him from undertaking the requisite inspections of ecclesiastical personnel and institutions under his governance. For Clement V, this provides ample justification for exempting Helias from his touring duties. The Pope authorizes the use of a suitable proxy or proxies for a period of three years, with the procurators also permitted to recover Helias' income. A portion of that income, however, had to be paid to the procurator. Moreover, Helias had to pay the Chancery in order to receive this letter... With the strengthening of the papal administration during the Avignon period, this kind of procuratorial arrangement became a means of funnelling money to the papacy. Such financial agreements, alongside revenue from the local taxation of benefices, meant that the Chancery was the pontificate's biggest profit centre, generating up to three quarters of its income.[107] Elderly and impaired bishops might also be excused from performing other tasks involving diocesan travel. Gout and arthritis (*podagre ac ciragre infirmitatibus*) rendered Gerardus, Bishop of Soissons, frequently unable to attend the reconciliation of churches and cemeteries in his territory. John XXII formally permitted such absences in a letter

106 RV 59, f. 103V – Clement V to Helias, Bishop of Autun, 15 July 1312. Text analysed by Benedictine monks (eds.), *Registres de Clément V*, n° 8 169, for which I give the transcription according to the register: '*Cum itaque tu sicut asseris proprii corporis debilitate gravatus nequeas in ecclesiis monasteriis locis et personis ecclesiasticis tue civitatis et diocese visitationis officium exercere. Nos tuis supplicationibus inclinati tibi auctoritate presentium indulgemus ut ecclesias monasteria ceteraque loca et personas ecclesiastica supradicta in quibus tibi visitationis officium competit de consuetudine vel de iure possis libere per aliquam seu aliquas personas iidoneas quam vel quas ad hoc duxeris assumendas usque ad triennium quotiens tempus visitationis ingruerit visitare et procurationes que centum numerum non excedunt recipere moderatas in pecunia numerata quacumque constitutione contraria super hoc edita non obstante.*'

107 Vincent, *Église et société*, p. 94.

dated 24 November 1325.[108] Similarly, Guillelmus, Cardinal of St. Stephen of Celiomonte, suffered with such physical weakness (*debilitas*) – and such a heavy workload – that, on 16 May 1353, Innocent VI authorized his nonattendance at a notionally mandatory meeting to examine heretics outside his diocese.[109] Canon law enshrined the right for clerics to be exempted from pastoral missions on health grounds, in theory at least. But this right was actualized only through grants of papal grace, allowing popes to regulate closely the circumstances in which exemptions were practically awarded.

Work-related Travel: Trips Further Afield

The residency requirement was not the only challenge faced by seculars with limited mobility. Business travel was a routine part of life for many secular clerics, with journeys taking them far from home. This could include, for example, trips to councils and ecclesiastical assemblies, or missions undertaken at the request of the Holy See, whether diplomatic or personal in nature. Such work-related travel was a major issue for impaired clerics. Indeed, the corpus contains petitions from more than 150 impaired clerics who were unable to make frequent trips, or who faced insurmountable barriers in undertaking the travel involved in the missions assigned to them.[110]

Both secular and regular clerics were subject to mandatory convocation to ecclesiastical council and assemblies. The Pope summoned clerics in vast numbers for such occasions. For example, Alexander III convoked more than 300 bishops for the Third Lateran Council in 1179. Similarly, the Fourth Lateran Council of 1215 assembled more than 412 bishops with 800 abbots, priors, and patriarchs from all over Christendom.[111] Clerics who did not heed the papal summons and absented themselves from synods without informing the Pope of their situation faced excommunication. Canon law explicitly provided the means to mitigate such harsh sentencing, however. Illness (*infirmitas*) offered just cause for the absence of metropolitan bishops and bishops from synods, according to Gratian's *Decree*, quoting chapter 35 of the Council of Agde (506).[112] Numerous councils enacted these rules, revealing

108 For an example, see RV 80, f. 142 V (RA 24, f. 252 V) – John XXII to Gerardus, Bishop of Soissons, 24 November 1325. Text analysed by Mollat (ed.), *Jean XXII*, n° 23 908.

109 For an example, see RV 224, f. 485 V – Innocent VI to Guillelmus, Cardinal of St. Stephen of Celiomonte, 16 May 1353.

110 Metzler, *A Social History*, p. 142.

111 Baldwin, "Paris et Rome en 1215", p. 107.

112 *Decretum Gratiani*, edited in Friedberg (ed.), *Corpus iuris canonici*, first part, distinctio 18, canon 1.

the importance that the Apostolic See attached to widespread clerical turn-out at these gatherings but also how they took illness seriously.[113] Diocesan assemblies followed the same rules. These were meetings that, following the Fourth Lateran Council, were scheduled annually, at least in theory.[114] Clerics who could not attend the synod had to present a valid excuse to the Pope in advance, and send a cleric or chaplain in their place.[115] The Apostolic See deemed old age, ill health and impairment, or genuine danger posed by travel to be acceptable excuses for clerics' nonattendance.

The case of Johannes, Bishop of Lincoln exemplifies the handling of such absences. The elderly Johannes had written to Clement V to alert the Pope that he was physically unable to travel to attend the Council of Vienna, scheduled to last from October 1311 to May 1312. Clement responds in July of the same year:

> In truth it is permitted, as you have explained to us, that you, with your body broken by old age, are not able to come personally to the aforementioned council. Although your absence on this account is excused by a procurator or by your nuncio; nevertheless, several persons consider your proffered excuse to be untruthful and deem it to be false. You were therefore judged in absentia and declared guilty by our ecclesiastical sentence and judgment, and [we judge] that therefore you are able to attend the aforementioned council without risking your constitution or vigour, especially as it was reported that you had previously ridden in the kingdom of England; We kindly wish to be able to give you an indemnity for your absence, whether you were able to come or not, by special grace, and that you may not be accused or bound to the sentence and judgment given.[116]

113 *Decree* of Yvo of Chartres edited in Migne (ed.), *Patrologia Latina*, vol. 161. The councils of Arles (chapter 18) and Orleans under Childeric (chapter 1), reported by Yvo of Chartres at the end of Book IV (unnumbered chapters), and the councils of Auvergne (chapter 15), Meaux (chapter 3), Laodicea (chapter 40), or Agde (chapter 36), compiled in Book 5 of his *Decree*, chapters 155, 156, 157, and 159, return to this dispensation for impaired clerics to go to synods or councils.

114 Jedin and Alberigo (eds.), *Conciliorum oecumenicorum decreta*, Fourth Lateran Council, canon 6.

115 Pontal, "Le rôle du synode diocésain", p. 340.

116 RV 59, f. 223 V – Clement V to Johannes, Bishop of Lincoln, 26 July 1312. Text edited by Benedictine monks, *Registres de Clément V*, n° 8 742: '*Verum licet sicut ex parte tua fuit propositum coram nobis, tu proprii corporis senectute confractus, ad concilium venire personaliter nequiveris antedictum, ac huiusmodi absentiam tuam ex premissa causa per procuratorem seu nuntium tuum nisus fueris excusare; quia tamen a pluribus dicebatur excusationem huiusmodi veritate carere, quodque ea tanquam falsa nequaquam obstante, eras contumax reputandus, ac pronuntiandus in*

Johannes followed protocol by notifying the Pope of his inability to attend to Council on account of his age. The Chancery accepts the bishop's excuse, and authorizes him to send a procurator or nuncio in his place. However, Johannes has been accused of fraud: unknown individuals have witnessed the bishop riding a horse in England.[117] If true, this means that he could feasibly have travelled to Vienna on horseback, without risking his health. On 3 April 1312, during the Council itself, Clement had issued the bull *Vox in excelso* against the Templars. This decree licensed the absence of clerics who had been summoned to the meeting, if they suffered from ill health and therefore could not travel by horse.[118] Subject to accusations of his equestrian prowess, Johannes thus risks the sentence of excommunication. The bishop escapes this fate, however, thanks to a pontifical grace. The letter reveals that citing a mobility impairment in itself was sufficient to grant grace and forgive non-attendance of an ecclesiastical assembly. It was not just bishops who could receive convocation waivers. The corpus also features cases relating to abbots and priors, such as Robertus Joli, a Hospitaller prior, whose attendance at the Order's assembly and general chapter was excused on account of his sickness (*infirmitas*), despite his own 'great desire' to participate.[119]

In certain cases, supplicants were called to travel in person to the Apostolic See in order to undergo examinations. Beyond the accommodations they sought in their supplications, impaired petitioners with mobility limitations could also request papal graces from such summons. Trips to the Apostolic See could be physically challenging, even dangerous, and costly for less well-off clerics. Gradually, such disadvantages were recognized, and general legal protections were introduced with the aim of supporting individuals who encountered problems related to such visits. For example, canon 37 of the Fourth Lateran Council allowed for cases involving plaintiffs who lived

sententias et processus per nos contra illos ex prelatis eisdem, qui ad ipsum concilium, ut premictitur, venire contumaciter non curarunt latas et habitos incidisse, presertim cum per regnum Anglie equitare sicut antea dicereris; nos indempnitati tue providere salubriter intendentes, huiusmodi absentiam tuam tibi, sive venire potueris, sive non, ex speciali gratia nolumus imputari, nec te ligari sententiis vel processibus antedictis'.

117 Impaired clerics often used horses as mobility aids. This is demonstrated, for example, in the constitution of the Friars Preachers (Chapter 22), enacted between 1215 and 1237, which forbids monks and abbots to travel on horseback, except those who obtain permission or who were in great need, such as the impaired. See Thomas, *De oudste constituties van de Dominicanen*.

118 Bull *Vox in exelsio* of Pope Clement V, published in Prutz (ed.), *Geheimlehre und Geheimstatuten*, p. 175.

119 RA 191, f. 386 V – Gregory XI to Robertus Joli, prior of the Hospitaller Order in France, 13 September 1373. Text analysed by Hayez, Mathieu, and Yvan (eds.), *Grégoire XI*, n° 28 201.

more than two days' journey from the Curia to be brought in local courts, rather than in Rome.[120] Similarly, in the *Decretals*, Gregory X confirmed that certain supplicants – the dying, the impaired (*infirmus*), the elderly, and the poor – were not obliged to go to Rome to receive their grace in person.[121] In such cases, a representative from the Curia could be appointed to conduct the examination near to the supplicant's location.

This is the case, for example, for Witkus Hiltprandi of Eldagessen, a priest canon of the church of Bramberg in the Bavarian lands. In a petition processed by the Chancery on 25 February 1364, Witkus requests a third-party examination (*ad partes*):

> Whereas recently, your holiness, Witkus Hiltprandi of Eldagessen, prebendal canon priest of the church of Bramberg, on the advice of the emperor's advocate-general in Bavaria, was judged sufficiently worthy of being examined *ad partes* by the bishop of Avignon in order to receive the canonry of the said church of Bramberg, as he suffers from a very serious foot disease, which prevents him from conveniently visiting the Roman Curia, and moreover he is not able to ride due to the severity of his illness, he must now have an examination *ad partibus* as it has been long postponed.[122]

Witkus suffers from a serious foot disease that prevents him from attending the Apostolic See, and undergoing examination there as is standard. Indeed, travel to Rome endangers his health. Consequently, the examination must take place *ad partes*, outside the Curia, and be conducted by individuals delegated by the Pope, Urban V. The corpus contains other examples demonstrating the different ways requests to disobey papal summons were handled.

120 Jedin and Alberigo (eds.), *Conciliorum oecumenicorum decreta*, Fourth Lateran Council, canon 37. See also the *Decree* of Yvo of Chartres, edited in Migne (ed.), *Patrologia Latina*, vol. 161, book 5, chapter 292.

121 *Decretales of Gregory IX*, edited in Friedberg (ed.), *Corpus iuris canonici*, book 5, title 39, chapter 26.

122 RS 42, f. 4 V – Witkus Hiltprandi of Eldagessen, priest canon of the church of Bramberg (Bavaria) to Urban V, 25 February 1364. Text analysed by Hayez, Mathieu and Yvan (eds.), *Urbain V*, n° 20, for which I give the transcription according to the register: '*Cum nuper sanctitas vestra Witkoni Hiltprandi de Eldagessen, presbytero canonico prebendato ecclesie Bambergensis, consiliario advocato generali domini imperator terre sue in Bavaria de canonicatu eiusdem ecclesie Bambergensis duxerit providendum dignetur sanctitas vestra examen ipsius committere ad partes quia sufficienter ipsius alia coram domino episcopo Avinionensi sufficienter est probata et gravissimum morbum in pedibus patitur, quod Romanam curiam commode visitare non potest, sicut etiam in partibus tam eiusdem morbi in equis ambulare nequivit iam multe tempore retroacto*'.

For instance, the Archbishop of Brindisi, Peregrinus, received a letter dated 4 August 1273, for which the *vidimus* (the 'we have seen' (implicitly: 'the act to be certified') is preserved. Gregory X had launched an enquiry procedure against the archbishop, summoning him to the Curia. Peregrinus, however, cites ill health as a justification for his inability to attend.[123] In contrast to Witkus' supplication, Peregrinus' letter contains a medical certificate. It was drawn up by a panel of two royal judges and two abbots at the archbishop's own request, and he presented the document to the Pope to evidence his inability to travel to the Apostolic See. The certificate states that the bishop has long suffered from asthma and strangury and is now senile, and thus cannot journey to the Curia on horseback. Despite the pontificate's immense authority, such documents demonstrate that illness, impairment, and old age were seen as valid reasons for disobeying a papal summons.

Bouts of sickness and accidents were impossible to avoid, even for clerics invested with papal authority as delegates on diplomatic missions. These papal proxies could find themselves unable to continue their journey, or even embark upon it in the first place. The majority of missions preserved in the pontifical registers were peace delegations, dispatched to calm relations between France and England. Diplomatic assignments were fairly routine in the period, as the Church frequently sent out missions. On occasion, impaired clerics were permitted to decline outright the mission they had been assigned, or otherwise they were authorized to return to the Curia before planned due to exigent circumstances.

For instance, John XXII had commissioned a trio of delegates – Hugues Aimery, the Bishop of Orange, Willelmus, the Archbishop of Vienna, and Johannes of Grandisson, chaplain of the pope – to undertake a diplomatic mission for the French king, Charles IV, by visiting England a few days before the abdication of King Edward II. Hugues, however, was struck down with a terrible illness, and obliged to turn back:

> Not without great compassion, we know that you are so weighed down by a serious and interminable illness, that you are not even be able to travel to England without peril to your body. We do not wish to expose you to any danger of this kind and, we do not wish that prelates and clerics remain in vain and inconveniently in France, so we want and command that only, and fully once you have recovered your vigour through a moderate diet, you can return without detours to the Curia, and the meantime, that you

123 De Leo and Monti (eds.), *Codice diplomatico Brindisino*, pp. 169–172, translated into French by Théry and Gilli, "Le Siège apostolique", doc. 38, p. 411.

> may have one or other of your colleagues as a substitute to undertake this mission. Therefore, may our dear and illustrious son in Christ Charles, King of France and Navarre, by favourable letters, give you the right to return to the Curia.[124]

In this letter, dated 23 December 1326, the Pope relieves Hugues from his mission, and authorizes his slow return to the Apostolic See in a series of smaller trips, as his chronic illness prevents a sea-crossing. At the same time, the Pope writes to the French king, Charles IV, for which Hugues was travelling to advise him of the situation and to ask him to release the petitioner from his duty.[125] Hugues Aimery was subsequently replaced in his mission by Hugh of Angoulême, archdeacon of Canterbury, allowing the bishop time to rest and recover from his illness.[126] The role of papal legate proved risky: it obliged clerics to cross warring territories, to travel long distances and, in Hugues' case, to cross the English Channel. It is clear that the prospect of the Channel-crossing prompted the bishop to abort his mission, signaled by Hugues' reference to his inability to visit England, as it is explained specifically later in the letter. The bishop's ill health placed the entire diplomatic mission in jeopardy. The Chancery had to act quickly to appoint another nuncio in Hugues' stead to ensure the delegation's continued viability and contact the French king directly to smooth things over. The care with which delegates, and their replacements, were selected demonstrates that these clerics were not merely letter carriers, but rather genuine diplomats, skilful negotiators who were authorized to plead for peace on behalf of the Apostolic See.

124 RV 114, f. 107 V – John XXII to Hugonus, Bishop of Orange, Apostolic Nuncio, 23 December 1326. Text analysed by Coulon and Clemencet (eds.), *Lettres secrètes et curiales du pape Jean XXII*, n° 3 105, for which I give the transcription according to the register: '*Non sine magna compassione, percepto adeo te gravi et diutina infirmitate fore gravatum quod absque tui corporis periculo nequires in Angliam transfretare. Nos nolentes quod huiusmodi periculis te exponas nec etiam quod in partibus France in gravamen prelatorum et personarum ecclesiasticarum inutiliter remaneas intendentes volumus et tue fraternitati mandamus quatenus nisi plene convalueris, ita quod imposita per nos prosequi una cum aliis collegis tuis valeres commode, moderatis dietis prout vires tuas ad hoc sufficere cognoveris redire ad curiam non postponas. Nos enim carissimo in Christo filio nostro Carolo Regi France et Navarre illustri ut tuum regressum gratum habeat, litteras dirigimus oportunas*'.

125 RV 114, f. 107 V – John XXII to King Charles IV of France, 23 December 1326. Text edited in op. cit., n° 3 106.

126 RV 114, f. 107 V – John XXII to Johannes Cerchamont, deacon of Poitiers and chancellor to the king of France, 28 December 1326. Text edited in op. cit., n° 3 110.

Conclusion

The pontifical institution demonstrated great capacity and notable commitment in adapting its underlying structures and regulations to adapt to clerics' physical and mental disabilities. Canonical legislation laid the groundwork for the personal difficulties encountered by impaired petitioners to be taken into account in pontifical judgments on their requests. The Chancery went even further, granting pardons that were more expansive in their remit than the established canonical provisions. In this way, the petition process was a mechanism by which the Church could selectively implement or soften the rules to which all clerics were subject, offering adaptations tailored to the ability and disability of each individual supplicant.

The Apostolic See permitted impaired supplicants to remain in office, providing the means to mitigate the negative impact of impairments on their job performance. Leveraging various pieces of ecclesiastical legislations and the dispensation of papal grace, the Curia allowed clerics to appoint a coadjutor as a proxy, to whom all activities they themselves could not carry out were delegated. This arrangement meant that impaired supplicants retained their function, their income and social status, even if they no longer undertook the routine duties associated with a particular clerical role and now occupied a less influential position than before. Indeed, impaired clerics were professionally sidelined by the appointment of a coadjutor: they could forget any hope of further career development. Over half (51%) of clerics in this position in the corpus presented themselves as elderly (*senes*) in their petitions, and probably did not expect to be promoted in any case. Following the appointment of an assistant, resignation was often seen as the logical next step, if not outright inevitable. Some clerics, on the other hand, may well have wished to pursue an ecclesiastical career, but were prevented in doing so by their impairment. For them, the employment of an assistant led to professional marginalization, as it was an insurmountable impediment to any further career progression. The inability to fulfil the demands of the job without assistance set impaired clerics apart from their able-bodied colleagues, even though they continued to receive a part of the income from their benefice and retained their ecclesiastical title.

The Church's willingness to offer adjustments is particularly evident within cases dealing with monastic enclosure. Over centuries of canonical legislation, enclosure was presented as a fundamental element of the monastic lifestyle, and even monastic identity. In such texts, enclosure gradually concretized as an impermeable barrier separating monastics from the earthly world. And yet, the corpus reveals that, in cases of physical or mental impairment, enclosure could be a very porous barrier indeed. With the right justification, entrance to and exit from the convent, be that for short visits or long-term trips, could be fairly easily arranged. Above all, transgressing enclosure was justified in the need to offer care and support for monastics. This concern for the well-being of monks and nuns reveals that enclosure was more theoretical construct than everyday reality. This also shows that the Church sought to manage the monastic life as effectively as possible. Certain groups, including servants and doctors, were routinely allowed to pierce enclosure. Even recluses were allowed visitors. Similarly, clerics could transfer between institutions, or even change order entirely, whilst monastic institutions relied for their continued existence on strong links with the lay world. In particular, the Chancery needed to keep tight control over monastic transferrals to more lenient orders. Such accommodations could, in theory, be exploited by otherwise capable, able-bodied clerics who merely wanted to join another congregation out of laziness. This would amount to an unforgiveable breach of religious vows, in particular those relating to residential stability and obedience to ecclesiastical superiors. For this reason, then, accommodations secured through grants of papal grace were not value-neutral. The receipt of such assistance placed impaired clerics outside the bounds of the 'normal' or normative clergy, and forever tainted their career prospects. Whether they were forced to relax the monastic rigour that had likely structured their lives to date, or they were compelled to transfer to an unfamiliar house or new order, impaired monks and nuns lost a part of their identity. Once accommodations were in place, monastics had to redefine their place in the ecclesiastical community, carving out an identity that matched their new circumstances.

A reduction in mobility was, and is, one of the most common consequences of impairment. Such limitations forced supplicants to change both their relationship with the world beyond their home institution and the way they inhabited more familiar spaces. With supplications, clerics with impaired mobility sought to alter the nature of their work in order to maintain an active role in the Church. This included, for example, requests for a lightened or modified workload, or for different duties entirely. Mobility was a basic requirement for secular and regular clerics. Clergymen had to be able get around with relative ease. So many fundamental duties depended upon clerics' ability to travel, whether it was to carry out their parish duties, fulfil their ecclesiastical obligations, or to respond to papal requests. Yet many clerics simply could not undertake such trips; the situation necessitated an institutional, administrative response. With canon law and grants of papal grace, the Curia regulated the circumstances in which impaired clerics were permitted to eschew the travel typically required by pastoral missions. The Church proposed alternative solutions for disabled clerics to handle the challenges posed by their involuntary immobility. In this way, everything was done to ensure that supplicants did not have to suffer on account of their lack of mobility – at least as far as their relationship with the pontifical institution was concerned.

The Apostolic See offered a diverse range of institutional responses to the various scenarios laid out in impaired clerics' supplications. It was not always possible, however, to formulate a response that was either suitable for, or desired by, all petitioners. In such cases, clerics might ask to leave the clergy entirely.

Bibliography

Primary Sources

BENEDICTINE MONKS (eds.), *Registres de Clément V*, E. de Boccard, 1948.

Joachim-Joseph BERTHIER, (ed.), *Opera De vita regulari*, Typis A. Befani, 1888.

William Henry BLISS (ed.), *Calendar of Entries in the Papal Registers Relating to Great Britain and Ireland: Papal Letters, Volume I, A.D. 1198–1304*, Tanner Ritchie Pub., 2005.

Charles BOUREL DE LA RONCIÈRE, Joseph de LOYE, Pierre de CANIVAL and Auguste COULON (eds.), *Les registres d'Alexandre IV (1254–1261): recueil des bulles de ce pape*, Boccard, 1902.

Auguste COULON and Suzanne CLEMENCET (eds.), *Lettres secrètes et curiales du pape Jean XXII (1316–1334) relatives à la France*, Boccard, 1961.

Annibale DE LEO and Gennaro Maria MONTI (eds.), *Codice diplomatico Brindisino. Volume primo*, Trani, Vecchi & C., 1940.

Gonzalo Martínez DÍEZ and Félix RODRÍGUEZ (eds.), *Colección canónica hispana, Concilios galos, Concilios hispanos (primera parte)*, Vol. IV, Editorial CSIC-CSIC Press, 1984.

Robert DIGARD, Antoine FAWTIER, Maurice FAUCON and Antoine THOMAS (eds.), *Les registres de Boniface VIII: recueil des bulles de ce Pape publiées ou analysées d'après les manuscrits originaux des Archives du Vatican*, Bibliothèque des Écoles françaises d'Athènes et de Rome, 1884.

FRIEDBERG (ed.), *Corpus iuris canonici*, Akademische Druck- u. Verlagsanstalt, 1959.

Anne-Marie HAYEZ, Janine MATHIEU and Marie-France YVAN (eds.), *Urbain V: suppliques de 1362 à 1365 (années I à IV)*, [electronic version: Ut per litteras apostolicas], Brepols, 1978.

Anne-Marie HAYEZ, Janine MATHIEU et Marie-France YVAN (eds.), *Grégoire XI (1370–1378): lettres communes analysées d'après les registres dits d'Avignon et du Vatican*, École française de Rome, 1992.

Hubert JEDIN and Giuseppe ALBERIGO (eds.), *Conciliorum oecumenicorum decreta*, Istituto per le scienze religiose, 1973.

Friedrich MAASSEN (ed.), *Concilia aevi merovingici*, Impensis Bibliopolii Hahniani, 1893.

Jacques Paul MIGNE (ed.), *Patrologiae Cursus Completus, Series Latina*, Migne, 1844–1855.

Guillaume MOLLAT (ed.), *Jean XXII (1316–1334): Lettres communes analysées d'après les registres dits d'Avignon et du Vatican*, Albert Fontemoing, 1923.

François OLIVIER-MARTIN (ed.), *Les registres de Martin IV recueil des bulles de ce pape*, Fontemoing, 1901.

Pietro PRESSUTTI (ed.), *I regesti del pontefice Onorio III dall'anno 1216 all'anno 1227*, Tipogr. A. Befani, 1884.

Hans PRUTZ (ed.), *Geheimlehre und Geheimstatuten des Tempelherren-Ordens: eine kritische Untersuchung*, Mittler, 1879.

Giovanni G. SBARAGLIA (ed.), *Bullarium Franciscanum, Tomus 2. Referens ea, quae Alexandri et Urbani VIII sunt*, typis Archangeli Casaletti in Aedibus de Maximis, 1761.

Augustin THEINER (ed.), *Vetera monumenta Hibernorum et Scotorum historiam illustrantia: ab Honorio PP. III. usque ad Paulum PP. III, 1216–1547*, Typis Vaticanis, 1864.

THOMAS AQUINAS, *Summa Theologiae II–II*, ed. By The Aquinas Institute and transl. by Fr. Laurence SHAPCOTE, URL consulted on 31 July 2021: https://aquinas.cc/.

Luc VERHEIJEN (transl.), *La Règle de saint Augustin*, Études augustiniennes, 1967.

James WATERWORTH (transl.), "The Council of Trent", in *The canons and decrees of the sacred and oecumenical Council of Trent*, Dolman, 1848.

Secondary Sources

John W. BALDWIN, "Paris et Rome en 1215: les réformes du IVe concile de Latran", *Journal des savants*, 1.1 (1997), pp. 99–124.

Bernard BARBICHE, *Les actes pontificaux originaux des archives nationales de Paris 1, 1198–1261*, Biblioteca Apostolica Vaticana, 1975.

Ursmer BERLIÈRE, *Épaves d'archives pontificales du XIVe siècle*, Desclée de Brouwer et Cie, 1908.

Cécile CABY, "Comme un poisson dans l'eau …: "*propositum vitae*" et lieux de vie monastique (XIe–XIIIe siècle)", *in* Michel LAUWERS (ed.), *Monastères et espace social. Genèse et transformation d'un système de lieux dans l'Occident médiéval*, Brepols, 2014, pp. 111–146.

Christine CHEVALIER-BOYER, "Les sermons de Guillaume de Sauqueville: l'activité d'un prédicateur dominicain à la fin du règne de Philippe le Bel", History thesis, University Lyon 2, 2007.

Isabelle COCHELIN, "*In senectute bona*: pour une typologie de la vieillesse dans l'hagiographie monastique des XIIe et XIIIe siècles", *in* Henri DUBOIS and Michel ZINK (eds.), *Les âges de la vie au Moyen Âge*, Presses de l'Université de Paris-Sorbonne, 1992, pp. 119–138.

Lynda L. COON, *Dark Age Bodies: Gender and Monastic Practice in the Early Medieval West*, University of Pennsylvania Press, 2011.

Noël COULET, *Les visites pastorales*, Brepols, 1977.

Riccardo CRISCIANI, "The Semantic Range of Medical Language in the Rule of Benedict", *American Benedictine Review*, 54 (2003), pp. 20–29.

Josephine M. CUMMINS, "Attitudes to Old Age and Ageing in Medieval Society", Philosophy thesis, University of Glasgow, Department of History, (Medieval) Faculty of Arts, 2000.

Florent CYGLER, "Règles, coutumiers et statuts (V^e^–XIIIe siècles). Brèves considérations historico-typologiques", *in* Marek DERWICH (ed.), *La vie quotidienne des moines et chanoines réguliers au Moyen Âge*, Institut d'Histoire de l'Université de Wrocław, 1995, pp. 31–49.

Michel DORTEL-CLAUDOT, "La clôture des moniales, des origines au code de droit canonique", *in* Colette FRIEDLANDER (ed.), *La clôture des moniales*, Vie consacrée, 1997, pp. 65–79.

Ninon DUBOURG, "L'incapacité dans les lettres de dispenses pontificales: aller à l'encontre de la réglementation ecclésiastique médiévale pour franchir la clôture", in Albrecht BURKARDT and Alexandra ROGER, *L'exception et la Règle, les pratiques d'entrée et de sortie des couvents, de la fin du Moyen Âge au XIXe siècle*, Presse universitaire de Limoges, 2022, pp. 41–54;

Dyan H. ELLIOTT, "Tertullian, the Angelic Life, and the Bride of Christ", *in* Lisa M BITEL and Felice LIFSHITZ (eds.), *Gender and Christianity in Medieval Europe New Perspectives*, University of Pennsylvania Press, 2013, pp. 15–33.

Lluís G. FELIU, "El monestir de frares de la Penitència de Jesucrist de Barcelona", *Analecta Sacra Tarraconensia*, 10 (1934), 45–51.

Arnaud FOSSIER, *Le bureau des âmes. Écritures et pratiques administratives de la Pénitencerie apostolique (XIIIe–XIVe siècle)*, École française de Rome, 2018.

Robert FOSSIER and Jacques VERGER, *Histoire du Moyen Âge: XIIIe–XVe siècle*, Éditions Complexe, 2005.

Robert FOSSIER, *Le travail au Moyen Âge*, Pluriel, 2012.

Patrick GILLI, *Villes et sociétés urbaines en Italie: milieu XIIe–milieu XIVe siècle*, Sedes, 2005.

Gilbert GUAYDIER, *Les irrégularités "ex defectu corporis"*, Société Générale d'Imprimerie et d'Édition, 1933.

Bernard GUILLEMAIN, *La politique bénéficiale du pape Benoît XII, 1334–1342*, H. Champion, 1952.

Sophie HASQUENOPH, *Histoire des ordres et congrégations religieuses en France du Moyen Âge à nos jours*, Éditions Champ Vallon, 2013.

Anne-Marie HAYEZ, "La personnalité d'Urbain V d'après ses réponses aux suppliques", *in Aux origines de l'État moderne. Le fonctionnement administratif de la papauté d'Avignon*, École française de Rome, 1991, pp. 7–31.

Isabelle HEULLANT-DONAT, Julie CLAUSTRE and Élisabeth LUSSET (eds.), *Enfermements I. le cloître et la prison, VIe–XVIIIe siècle*, Publications de la Sorbonne, 2011.

Isabelle HEULLANT-DONAT, Julie CLAUSTRE, Élisabeth LUSSET and Falk BRETSCHNEIDER (eds.), *Enfermements II. Règles et dérèglements en milieu clos, IVe–XIXe siècle*, Publications de la Sorbonne, 2015.

Isabelle HEULLANT-DONAT, Julie CLAUSTRE, Élisabeth LUSSET and Falk BRETSCHNEIDER (eds.), *Enfermements III. Hommes et femmes en milieux clos, XIIIe–XXe siècle*, Publications de la Sorbonne, 2017.

Rosalind M. T. HILL (ed.), *The Rolls and Register of Bishop Oliver Sutton*, Lincoln Record Society by the Hereford Times, 1948–1965.

Jacques HOURLIER and Gabriel LE BRAS, *Histoire du droit et des institutions de l'Église en Occident. Les religieux, tome X, L'âge classique, 1140–1378*, Éditions Cujas, 1971.

Hubert JEDIN and John Patrick DOLAN, *History of the Church: From the High Middle Ages to the Eve of the Reformation*, Burns & Oates, 1980.

Julie KERR, "Health and Safety in the Medieval Monasteries of Britain", *History*, 93.309 (2008), pp. 3–19.

James R. KING, "The Mysterious Case of the 'Mad' Rector of Bletchingdon: The Treatment of Mentally Ill Clergy in Late Thirteenth Century England", *in* Wendy J TURNER (ed.), *Madness in Medieval Law and Custom*, Leiden, Brill, 2010, pp. 57–80.

Stephan KUTTNER, *Harmony from Dissonance: An Interpretation of Medieval Canon Law*, The Archabbey Press, 1960.

Jenni KUULIALA, "Nobility, Community and Physical Impairment in Later Medieval Canonization Processes", *in* Christian KRÖTZL, Katariina MUSTAKALLIO and Jenni KUULIALA (eds.), *Infirmity in Antiquity and the Middle Ages: Social and Cultural Approaches to Health, Weakness and Care*, Ashgate, 2015, pp. 67–82.

Michel LAUWERS and Marialuisa BOTTAZZI, "*Interiora* et *exteriora*, ou la construction monastique d'un espace social en Occident entre le Ve et le XIIe siècle", *in* Paolo BUFFO, Caterina CICCOPIEDI, Luciana FURBETTA and Thomas GRANIER (eds.), *La società monastica nei secoli VI–XII. Sentieri di ricerca*, Rome, École française de Rome, 2016, pp. 59–88.

Elizabeth A. LEHFELDT, *Religious Women in Golden Age Spain: the Permeable Cloister*, Routledge, 2017.

Didier LETT, "Conclusions. La différence des sexes est-elle soluble dans un milieu clos?", *in* Isabelle HEULLANT-DONAT, Julie CLAUSTRE and Falk BRETSCHNEIDER (eds.), *Enfermements III. Hommes et femmes en milieux clos,* XIIIe– XXe *siècle*, Publication de la Sorbonne, 2017, pp. 193–202.

Michele MACCARRONE, "I Papi del secolo 12. e la vita comune e regolare del clero", *in La vita comune del clero nei secoli 11. e 12.*, Vita e pensiero, 1962, pp. 349–398.

Elizabeth M. MAKOWSKI, *Canon Law and Cloistered Women: Periculoso and Its Commentators, 1298–1545*, Catholic University of America Press, 1997.

Elizabeth M. MAKOWSKI, "L'enfermement des moniales au Moyen Âge. Débats autour de l'application de la décrétale Periculoso", *in* Isabelle HEULLANT-DONAT, Julie CLAUSTRE and Élisabeth LUSSET (eds.), *Enfermements I. le cloître et la prison,* VIe–XVIIIe *siècle*, Paris, Publications de la Sorbonne, 2011, pp. 107–117.

Philip A. MELLOR and Chris SHILLING, *Re-forming the Body. Religion, Community and Modernity*, Sage, 1997.

Irina METZLER, *Disability in Medieval Europe: Thinking about Physical Impairment during the High Middle Ages, c. 1100–1400*, Routledge, 2006.

Irina METZLER, *A Social History of Disability in the Middle Ages: Cultural Considerations of Physical Impairment*, Routledge, 2013.

Charles de MIRAMON, *Les "donnés" au Moyen Âge*, Cerf, 1999.

Charles De MIRAMON, "La place d'Hugues de Saint-Cher dans les débats sur la pluralité des bénéfices (1230–1240)", *in* Louis-Jacques BATAILLON, Gilbert DAHAN and Pierre-Marie GY (eds.), *Hugues de Saint-Cher. Bibliste et théologien*, Brepols, 2000, pp. 341–386.

Angela MONTFORD, "Fit to Preach and Pray: Considerations of Occupational Health in the Mendicant Orders", *in* R. N. SWANSON (ed.), *The Use and Abuse of Time in Christian History*, Boydell & Brewer, 2002, pp. 95–106.

Angela MONTFORD, *Health, Sickness, Medicine and the Friars in the Thirteenth and Fourteenth Centuries*, Ashgate, 2004.

Nicholas ORME, "Sufferings of the Clergy: Illness and Old Age in Exeter Diocese, 1300–1540", *in* Margaret PELLING and Richard M. SMITH (eds.), *Life, Death, and the Elderly: Historical Perspectives*, Routledge, 1991, pp. 62–73.

Brandon PARLOPIANO, "*Propter Deformitatem*: Towards a Concept of Disability in Medieval Canon Law", *Canadian Journal of Disability Studies*, 4.3, 2015, pp. 72–102.

Odette PONTAL, "Le rôle du synode diocésain et des statuts synodaux dans la formation du clergé", *in Les évêques, les clercs et le roi (1250–1300)*, cahier de Fanjeaux n° 7, Privat, 1972, pp. 337–359.

Robert E. RODES, *Ecclesiastical Administration in Medieval England: The Anglo-Saxons to the Reformation*, University of Notre Dame Press, 1977.

Joel T. ROSENTHAL, "Retirement and the Life Cycle in Fifteenth-Century England", *in* Michael M. SHEEHAN (ed.), *Aging and the Aged in Medieval Europe*, Pontifical Institute for Medieval Studies, 1990, pp. 173–188.

Jean-Claude SCHMITT, "Les suppliques dans les images", in Hélène MILLET (ed.), *Suppliques et requêtes: le gouvernement par la grâce en Occident, XIIe–XVe siècle*, Rome, École française de Rome, 2003, pp. 77–87.

Shulamith SHAHAR, *Growing Old in the Middle Ages "Winter Clothes Us in Shadow and Pain"*, Routledge, 1997.

Thierry SOULARD, "Le personnel masculin au service des religieuses de l'abbaye Notre-Dame de La Règle de Limoges à la fin du Moyen Âge", *in* Nicole BOUTER (ed.), *Les religieuses dans le cloître et dans le monde des origines à nos jours*, Publications de l'Université de Saint-Étienne, 1994, pp. 379–391.

Julien THÉRY and Patrick GILLI, "Le Siège apostolique et la hiérarchie ecclésiastique en Italie", *in* Patrick GILLI (ed.), *Le gouvernement pontifical et l'Italie des villes au temps de la théocratie (fin XIIe–mi XIVe s.)*, Presses universitaires de la Méditerranée, 2010, pp. 367–427.

Antoninus H. THOMAS, *De oudste constituties van de Dominicanen: voorgeschiedenis, tekst, bronnen, ontstaan en ontwikkeling (1215–1237)*, Leuvense universitaire uitgaven, 1965.

Catherine VINCENT, *Église et société en occident: XIIIe –XVe siècle*, A. Colin, 2009.

Gareth H. WILLIAMS, "Understanding Incapacity", *in* Graham SCAMBLER and Sasha Jane SCAMBLER (eds.), *New Directions in the Sociology of Chronic and Disabling Conditions: Assaults on the Lifeworld*, Palgrave Macmillan, 2010, pp. 180–204.

Mary K. K. YEARL, "Medieval Monastic Customaries on Minuti and Infirmi", *in* Barbara S. BOWERS (ed.), *The Medieval Hospital and Medical Practice*, Ashgate Publishing, 2007, pp. 175–194.

5 Leaving the Clergy

Abstract
This chapter probes the fate of the disabled men who were less fortunate: those who had to leave the clergy entirely, either of their own volition or due to the severity of their disability. At times, poor health or impairment forced clerics to resign from their positions as they became unable to perform their rights and duties. Often, they were forced to find care and support outside of their clerical community. Case studies demonstrate, however, that petitions and pontifical letters sometimes allowed for the adaptation, even contravention, of existing rules so that the disabled former clerics could live out their days with dignity.

Keywords: Resignation: Retirement; Transfers; Leprosaria

Invoking the sixth-century Pope Gregory the Great, Gratian sets out a roster of unsuitable candidates for the priestly office in his *Decree*, written between 1140 and 1150. He cites the usual suspects – men who have been married twice, simoniacs, usurers, and so on – before seizing upon the least desirable of all: the mad, or as Gratian puts it, men 'rendered frantic or possessed by the devil' (*forssenez ou travaillez del deable*).[1] It seems clear, then, that an individual with *defectus mentis* is prohibited from entering the priesthood, and certainly from giving the sacraments. Yet, in a letter sent to Bishop Eleutherius of Tournai and later compiled by Gratian, Gregory the Great asserts that bouts of madness or the loss of one's senses do not always provide grounds for the expulsion of a recently ordained cleric: 'for that which prevents entry into orders does not always entail the deposition of a cleric already ordained'.[2] Gratian relies directly on this letter to draw his own conclusions: a bishop overcome by passion (*passio*) leading to insanity (*mente alienate*) could not be forced to resign, as he had already

1 *Decretum Gratiani*, edited in Friedberg (ed.), *Corpus iuris canonici*, first part, distinctio 33, chapter 2. Anonymous French translation edited in Löfstedt (ed.), *Gratiani decretum*, p. 73.
2 *Decretum Gratiani*, edited in Friedberg (ed.), *Corpus iuris canonici*, first part, distinctio 50, chapter 4.

Dubourg, N., *Disabled Clerics in the Late Middle Ages. Un/suitable for Divine Service?*
Taylor & Francis Group, 2023
DOI: 10.5117/9789463721561_CH05

been ordained. On one hand, the *Decree* rules that a cleric, who, weighed down by old age or illness (*defectus corporis*), is prevented from performing his office, is authorized to substitute a person in his place.[3] In those cases, assessors were nominated, implying that such well-off clerics continued to receive the income associated with their office until their death.[4] On another hand, the *Decretals* of Gregory IX highlight the link between old age and lack of vigour, both of which can provoke a cleric's resignation.[5] In both cases, whether the bodily and/or mental incapacity was caused by illness or age conditions, no distinction was made between in the adjudication of clerics' requests for assistance and/or resignation, because the conditions had similar effects.[6] Impairment then involved either the rapid appointment of an assistant to ensure that the petitioner's benefices were appropriately managed and remained intact, or, if in case of resignation, the endowment of special benefits to support him in his new life.

The Church's central aim was to prevent resigners from falling into poverty – by giving them help to keep their benefices or by allocating them a pension. The institution sought to support impaired clerics who had toiled in its service by keeping them in the broad ecclesiastical fold, albeit situating them on its outskirts. The loss of benefices, and the social status attached to such sources of income, served to cast impaired resigners on the margins of society. The petitions and papal letters highlight, however, that such marginalization was neither automatic nor entirely negative. Analysis of the sources shows that the Church's procedures functioned, above all, to protect impaired individuals. Retirees could, for example, benefit from financial compensation to stave off destitution and build a relatively good life for themselves after the end of their clerical career. Even clerics who lost their rank, or those without a sufficient pension, were taken care of by the Church. Many such clerics were cared for in hospices, monasteries, and even private houses, for the remainder of their lives.[7]

Leaving the Workforce

There were no regulations – in canon law, customary legislation, or monastic rules – that governed the replacement of bishops or abbots who resigned their

3 Op. cit., second part, causa 7, chapter 11.

4 Lewin, *Pensions and Insurance*, p. 23.

5 *Decretales Gregory IX*, edited in Friedberg (ed.), *Corpus iuris canonici*, book I, title 9, chapter 1.

6 Op. cit., chapter 10.

7 Shahar, *Growing Old*, p. 111.

office.[8] The procedure was thus highly flexible. In some cases, for example, the petitioner's assistant might allow him to remain in charge until his last breath, with no clear plan to install a replacement before it was absolutely necessary.[9] It is possible that such practical arrangements went unspoken in letters, put in place by the petitioners without seeking pontifical permission. After the petitioner's death, it was natural for his appointed assistant to receive a promotion and formally take over the role for which he had previously deputized. Despite the availability of such informal provisions, however, some clerics wished to formally resign their office. This required them to petition the Pope for permission to leave the Church's workforce. In these circumstances, the Pope was called upon to resolve issues that impacted both the ecclesiastical institution and the resigner himself.

The petition process offered a means for impaired clerics to resign, and in so doing, often provided them with a valuable opportunity to secure a pension in order to live comfortably thereafter. Resignation entailed the loss of all income associated with the cleric's (former) benefices, hence the need for additional financial support. The petitions and papal letters allow us to distinguish between 'resignation' and 'retirement', even though, in reality, the two states often overlapped. Resignation refers simply to leaving one's office. Retirement, by contrast, denotes that one has left one's office and is in receipt of a pension. Analysis of documents in the corpus reveals that the clerics who wrote to the Apostolic See to abdicate their office were among the aristocratic elite. Clerics of lower social status, on the other hand, typically offered their resignation to their superiors, unless there were local institutional conflicts with which to contend. Aristocratic petitioners could obtain a pension from the pontifical institution, though this was not automatic. If successful, these supplicants became 'pensioners', whose existence is attested to as early as the thirteenth century.[10] In these cases, retirees used the allowance to cover their expenses until death.

Resignation: Letters of Revocation

Petitions and papal letters which detail a cleric's resignation are called 'letters of revocation'. With these missives, the Pope officially retracted

8 See Trembinski, "An Infirm Man".

9 Orme, "Sufferings of the Clergy", p. 64.

10 Gonzales, "L'heure de la retraite a sonné"; Mattéoni, *Servir le prince*, p. 385; Sommé, *Isabelle de Portugal*, pp. 622–625; Lachaud and Penman, *Établir et abolir les normes*, p. 235; Cummins, "Attitudes to Old Age", pp. 220–221.

the authority that he had previously entrusted to the petitioner.[11] However, letters of revocation were neither letters of dismissal nor of deposition, as these formats were based on the presumption that the supplicant was at fault and would need to perform penance. Rather, these functioned as letters of absolution, allowing the petitioners to relinquish their office without any stain on their spiritual record. Examples of letters written to popes requesting resignation dating to the early Middle Ages remain extant, revealing that impairment, illness and/or old age were cited as conditions motivating clerics' resignation. Alcuin (735–804) and Raban Maur (780–856), for example, abdicated their offices as they became physically unable to perform their duties.[12] However, following the reign of Innocent III (1161–1216), the Pope's right of review was asserted. It became obligatory to receive a missive of grace in which the cleric or his superior detailed a reason for the supplicant's resignation that the Church authority deemed to be legitimate. The supplications and papal letters bear witness to the fact that both physical and mental incapacity were accepted as grounds for resignation by the pontificate. Indeed, the majority of letters of revocation dating to the thirteenth century stipulate such impairment as the motivator for the supplicant's departure (58%). Strikingly, this figure declines sharply in the following century: only 14% of fourteenth-century letters and 12% of petitions provide this explanation. This drop tallies with the fact that the concerns of ecclesiastical authorities were broadening during the fourteenth century, a period in which the Chancery dealt with fewer clerical matters overall, and therefore processed fewer renunciations.

The papacy could not force clerics to resign if they did not wish to. However, if clerics decided to leave their office, they were obliged to abide by the formal resignation procedure and follow through on their intent. Canon 28 of the Fourth Lateran Council mandates that '[h]e who has requested and obtained permission to leave his benefice shall be bound and even compelled to leave it, since he has taken this resolution only for the utility of his church or for his own interests'.[13] Figure 5.1 demonstrates that the vast majority of petitioners who appealed to the Pope to resign their offices were at the top of the ecclesiastical hierarchy: abbots, priors, rectors, bishops, and archbishops.

This is relatively unsurprising, as the benefices under discussion must have had to possess a certain notability for the petition to be sent to the head

11 Durand de Maillane, *Dictionnaire de droit canonique*, tome V, article 'révocation', p. 220.

12 Metzler, *A Social History*, p. 141.

13 Riguaud (ed.), *Acta conciliorum*, vol. 1, col. 42 (my translation).

of the Church. What's more, lesser-ranked clerics were not obliged to apply to the Pope to withdraw from their office, only to their local hierarchy though they retained the right to petition the pontiff if so desired.[14] Secular clerics seemed to write progressively less to the Chancery regarding abdication during the fourteenth century. This decrease highlights the attenuation of the role of the Apostolic See in the renunciation of seculars, while the number of resignations of regular clerics remains constant. Figure 5.2 offers a breakdown of the data relating to the causes cited for resignation in the corpus.

Figure 5.1 Recipients of resignation letters

Resignees	**Letters from the 13th c.**	**Letters from the 14th c.**	**Petitions (1342–1366)**
Regular clerics	44 (31%)	43 (61%)	10 (56%)
Men	*41*	*36*	*8*
Women	*3*	*7*	*2*
Secular clerics	97 (69%)	27 (39%)	8 (44%)
Higher ranks	*95*	*25*	*8*
Lower ranks	*2*	*2*	*0*
Total	141	70	18

Figure 5.2 Reasons for resignation in papal letters and petitions (when the reason is known)

	Old age and impairment(s)	**Old age alone**	**Impairment alone**
Letters from the 13th c. (141)	59 (42%)	15 (11%)	67 (48%)
Letters from the 14th c. (70)	30 (43%)	15 (21%)	25 (36%)
Petitions (1342–1366) (18)	10 (56%)	3 (17%)	5 (28%)
Total	101	35	98

Physical or mental impairment was a major driver (including explicitly permanent conditions such as blindness, paralysis, incurable disease), closely associated with old age.[15] The majority of letters mention advanced age, an effective criterion to garner pontifical favour that would be hard to

14 Rosenthal, "Retirement and the Life Cycle", pp. 173–188.

15 The same conditions are found in the 'retirements' allowed by the coroner (the official charged by the crown with investigating deaths to protect human life, in Anglo-Saxon countries). See Gilchrist, *Medieval Life*, p. 146 or I. Metzler, *A Social History*, pp. 122–135.

challenge. By looking at the text of the letters, it seems that all supplicants seeking to resign were over 60 years old.[16] This age appears to be the lower bound for abdication, since the highest-ranked members of the clergy were elected to their esteemed office from 22 (subdiaconate) to 30 years old (bishopric).[17] Nevertheless, old age alone does not explain the large number of resignations granted: illness and other impairments also justified requests for resignation in 48% of thirteenth-century letters, alongside 36% of fourteenth-century letters and 28% of petitions (see Figure 5.2). The resulting physical disability was considered a legitimate reason for leaving the clergy, in the same way as in noble careers, where capacity took precedence.[18] Indeed, following the Gregorian reform, a bishop wishing to resign was obliged to supply one of the reasons that the Pope, Innocent III, considered to be valid for leaving his office. In a letter sent to the Bishop of Cagliari and preserved in the *Decretals* of Gregory XI, Innocent envisages that clerics who are weak (*debilis*), ignorant, of bad conscience, irregular, or who risk causing scandal might ask for a resignation.[19]

Similarly, in his *Summa Theologiae*, Thomas Aquinas asks '[w]hether he who has vowed to enter religion is bound to remain in religion in perpetuity?'. He furnishes the following response:

> A man who has entered religion gives neither scandal nor bad example by leaving, especially if he does so for a reasonable motive; and if others are scandalized, it will be passive scandal on their part, and not active scandal on the part of the person leaving, since in doing so, he has done what was lawful, and expedient on account of some reasonable motive, such as sickness (*infirmitas*), weakness (*debilitas*), and the like.[20]

Aquinas certifies that monks and nuns might leave enclosure if they had a 'good reason', such as illness or bodily weakness, in an effort to avoid generating scandal. This contention is reiterated in monastic rules regarding the resignation of a useless abbot. The general chapters of the Cistercian order state that an abbot must ask his superior for permission to resign

16 This age at which incapacity appears to emerge is very close to that of current retirement. Its delimitation in medieval times is studied by Cummins, *Attitudes to Old Age*, pp. 32–39.

17 Shahar, *Growing Old*, p. 107.

18 Mornet, "Âge et pouvoir", p. 149.

19 *Decretales Gregory IX*, edited in Friedberg (ed.), *Corpus iuris canonici*, book I, title 9 – *De renunciatione* (chapters I; III; IX; X; XI; XV).

20 Thomas Aquinas, *Summa Theologiae II–II*, q. 189, article 4.

before abdicating.[21] The latter was then responsible for judging the legitimacy of the request and verifying the reason given by the petitioner. Letters of grace confirming a supplicant's resignation were therefore often sent directly to the superior of the would-be resigner. This kind of resignation was considered 'express': it formally and imperatively manifested the Pope's will to the superiors and colleagues of the resigning cleric.[22] Moreover, a considerable number of letters include a comminatory clause during the thirteenth and fourteenth centuries – that is, a clause that stipulated punishments that would be levelled against individuals that did not obey the papal mandate or who had lied in their original petition. Approximately one in three letters with such clauses were sent to individuals charged with enforcing the papal decision, or conducting an investigation on its behalf to verify the legitimacy of the grace the missive offered.[23] Even men at the top of the Church hierarchy, vested with substantial ecclesiastical power, could not resign as and when they liked. On the contrary, they remained subject to pontifical authority, which obliged them to provide a legitimate justification for their resignation that could be verified by the institution. This was especially important in cases in which resigners had been awarded a pension.

Retirement: Pensions and Other Financial Support

In England and Germany, some impaired royal servants and officers were eligible to receive *corrodies*, a kind of pension paid by monasteries, religious communities or the Crown in some contexts, as soon as the thirteenth century.[24] Similarly, the petitions and papal letters demonstrate that the papacy granted certain clerics a pension that allowed them to enter, and enjoy, 'full retirement', with sufficient funds to live out the rest of their lives in relative comfort.[25] Although the term 'retirement' was not yet coined, evidence for such financial arrangements dates to as early as the beginning of the thirteenth century.[26] It was not necessarily commonplace, however. In the corpus, pensions are awarded in less than half of resignation cases:

21 Marilier (ed.), *Chartes et documents*, *Charte de charité et d'unanimité*, statut 23.

22 Durand de Maillane, *Dictionnaire de droit canonique*, tome II, article 'demission', p. 88.

23 See Introduction.

24 Metzler, *A Social History*, p. 129; Cummins, *Attitudes to Old Age*, p. 221; and Harvey, *Living and Dying*, p. 179.

25 Salonen, "What Happened to Aged Priests", p. 185.

26 Gonzales, "L'heure de la retraite a sonné", p. 258.

49% of thirteenth-century letters, 39% of fourteenth-century letters, and 44% of petitions.

The men with the most power in the Church hierarchy – namely archbishops, bishops, wealthy rectors and vicars – left their benefices without fear of economic problems. They had capitalized on the considerable income they had received throughout their careers, endowing them with significant personal wealth.[27] Moreover, they often belonged to aristocratic families on which they could rely for financial and other support. Pensions were not 'means tested', however: clerics with access to such resources could still petition for a pension, which was supposed to provide for their needs after they left office.

Figure 5.3 Resigners in receipt of a pension

		Resigners (all)	Resigners with pension
Letters from the 13th c. (141)		Secular (44)	21 (47 %)
		Regular (97)	48 (49 %)
Letters from the 14th c. (70)		Secular (27)	10 (37 %)
		Regular (43)	17 (39 %)
Petitions (1342–1366) (18)		Secular (8)	3 (37 %)
		Regular (10)	5 (50 %)
Total		229	104

Figure 5.3 demonstrates that regular clerics were somewhat more likely to receive a pension than their secular colleagues. This is almost certainly due to their living arrangements: former abbots remained resident in the monastery for which they were previously responsible, and the institution paid them directly. The highest-ranked secular clerics, chiefly bishops, enjoyed the same salary as abbots of the largest convents, and therefore also received a generous income.[28] All clergymen had, in principle, the right to receive a pension. If a cleric fell into poverty after resigning his office, this could taint the reputation of the office itself, and the Church as an institution – hence, the need to selectively award financial support to resigners. A similar logic is evident in the construction of special hospices for clergymen, a topic discussed in depth below.[29] Despite this rationale, pensions were not, it seems, awarded on the basis of need. In fact, the majority of petitioners

27 Shahar, *Growing Old*, p. 31.
28 Cummins, *Attitudes to Old age*, p. 222.
29 Shahar, *Growing Old*, p. 110.

writing directly to the Pope were illustrious ecclesiastical dignitaries. It is possible that smaller allowances granted to minor clerics did not merit the attention of the pontiff. It is also possible that such clerics were left entirely empty-handed by the Apostolic See, and, without a pension, were forced to live off charity, or even take up begging. Indeed, some were left to fend for themselves when they become too old to fulfil their office. In such cases, deprived clerics could sometimes find ways to finance their pension from secular powers, as some institutions founded by kings and dukes, for example, also offered care for elderly clergymen.[30] In their letters and petitions some clerics appealed to the Pope explicitly for permission to leave their posts and receive an income to allow them to survive in retirement.[31] According to the documents, the papacy could provide a subsidiary income for their retirement.

At a basic level, pensions offered by the Chancery had to be sufficient to allow retired clerics to live comfortably, or at least without lacking necessities. The precise value of the pension varied in each case. It appears that the sum was usually equivalent to approximately one third of the income previously accrued by the petitioner from his benefices.[32] The raw figures are rarely explicitly disclosed in the corpus, though the highest award for which we have such data amounted to 100 florins per year (equal to 350 grams of gold).[33] Whilst the Church awarded pensions, the institution was not responsible for their payment: the funds came instead from the revenues of the diocese or monastery to which the supplicant belonged.[34] In fact, letters always state where the funds are supposed to be drawn from.

The case of Nicolaus, abbot of the Benedictine convent of St Stephen in the Ligurian city, is illuminating here. A missive from Boniface VIII, addressed to the Archbishop of Genoa on 23 August 1295, details the allocation of a pension to the ailing abbot:

30 Metzler, *A Social History*, p. 135-137

31 Gonzales, "L'heure de la retraite a sonné", p. 262.

32 Orme, "Sufferings of the Clergy", pp. 62–73.

33 Letter RV 49, f. 36 V concerns friar Philipus, formerly Bishop of Fiesole, who is 'old and weighed down by infirmities' and who resigns before the Pope. He is authorised on 26 April 1298 by Boniface VIII to receive 100 gold florins a year as long as he lives. In this case, the Pope obliges the Bishop of Spoleto to pay Philipus' pension on the eighth day of October, Ascension Day, to the house of the Friars Minor in Perugia. The mention of this date perhaps indicates that Philipus returned as a brother to this monastery. Text edited by Digard, Fawtier, Faucon, and Thomas (eds.), *Les registres de Boniface VIII*, n° 2 558.

34 Elderly religious may face financial difficulties. The granting or not of a pension may lead to disparities among the clergy. See Rosenthal, "Retirement and the Life", pp. 180–183.

> It has been stated before us by the dear son Nicolaus, abbot of the monastery of St Stephen of Genoa, Order of St Benedict, that, already broken by his illness and the weakness of his own aged body, he has become unable to ensure the government of his monastery, and therefore he wishes to resign (freely) from his abbacy. Thus, this abbot has humbly begged us to take care of his resignation. Therefore, we order your brotherhood [the Archbishop of Genoa] by apostolic writings that, if this is so, this abbot be released from his abbacy, rights and belonging by your authority when receiving his resignation. If he ever suffers from the lack of certain necessities, let him receive a stipend from the goods of this monastery in order to be able to feed himself sufficiently according to what may be assigned by the monastery and for as long as you deem it appropriate.[35]

Nicolaus, broken by illness and old age, is no longer able to run his monastery. His resignation, authorized by the Pope, was the result of impairment. Nevertheless, Nicolaus will receive material support after his abdication in the form of a pension from the abbey, paid thanks to the abbacy's property. The exact amount is unknown, as the Chancery simply specifies that the allowance should enable Nicolaus 'to feed himself sufficiently'. Furthermore, the Pope mandates that the monks should take care of the former abbot as long as he lives. Resignation is characterized as a positive action, a mechanism by which a cleric could be offered additional support, not as a negative consequence of physical or mental impairment. This is equally illustrated by the famous example of Francis of Assisi, who withdrew from his order, leaving it in the hands of his followers, from as early as 1219, as a result of a leprosy-like disease that scarred his body and made him visually impaired.[36] Moreover, Francis is not a unique example of a 'retiree' saint. Various hagiographic accounts and monastery chronicles present similar

35 RV 47, f. 142 V – Boniface VIII to the Archbishop of Genoa, 23 August 1295. Text analysed by Digard, Fawtier, Faucon, and Thomas (eds.), *Les registres de Boniface VIII*, n° 639, for which I give the transcription according to the register: '*Ex parte dilecti filii Nicole abbatis monasterii sancti Stephani de Janua, ordinis sancti Benedicti, fuit expositum coram nobis quod ipse debilitate, infirmitate ac senio proprii corporis iam confractus ad gerendum ipsius monasterii regimen inhabilis est effectus propter quod intendit abbatiam ipsius monasterii* [*libere*] *resignare. Quare idem abbas nobis humiliter supplicavit ut cessionem eius recipere curaremus. Quocirca fraternitate tue, per apostolica scripta mandamus quatenus, si est ita, libera ab eodem abbate auctoritate vestra predicte abbatie ac iurium et pertinentiarum ipsius resignatione recepta ei ne defectum in neccessariis patiatur de bonis dicti monasterii pro substentatione sua sufficientes redditus percipiendos ab eo quamdiu vixerit studeas assignare prout prefatis facultatibus eiusdem monasterii videris expedire*'.

36 See Trembinski, *Illness and Authority*.

accounts of other holy men and women entering retirement in a highly positive light.[37] In these cases, which necessarily inspired clerics' writing to the popes, the saint's decision to renounce their office was applauded: it prevented the ruin of ecclesiastical goods and affairs.

Clerics at the top of the ecclesiastical hierarchy, seculars and regulars alike, were thus endowed with the same kind of privileges in 'retirement' as they had held in post. This is therefore probable that the highest-ranking clergy did not resign their office without compensation, even if we do not have all their graces registered.[38] On the other hand, lower-ranked clerics, who had not amassed enough resources to capitalize on their ecclesiastical income in post, and who were not generally members of wealthy families, did not benefit from these pensions. In some instances, disadvantaged clerics chose to retire to a monastery without seeking a pontifical pardon, thereby disappearing from our records. At other times, however, patrons provided destitute retirees with secular pensions, or they transferred to hospitals for the remainder of their lives, leaving traces in the papal archives.

Transferral to Specialist Institutions

Diagnosis, or at least acknowledgment, of an impairment was crucial in terms of practical care arrangements. Once diagnosed, an impairment could perhaps be cured, whether by doctors, surgeons, barbers, or by the adoption of a healthier diet. In such cases, clerical patients with notionally curable conditions were sometimes temporarily transferred to special facilities for treatment. By contrast, if their impairment was untreatable – for example, a condition or disease that was incurable (e.g., blindness) or fixed (e.g., old age, limb loss) – clerics had to formally resign their duties and move to a place that offered them adequate care. From the twelfth century onwards, the convent is portrayed in medieval texts as a kind of 'retirement home' for elderly nobles and clerics.[39] The existence of such places, which were mostly run by ecclesiastical institutions before the thirteenth century, reveals the integration of sick and impaired individuals in the fabric of the medieval community. Originally, the purpose of hospitals was not to cure patients, as is the case today, but rather to take care of them in a more generalized sense. Staff worked to restore the health of hospital residents through a balanced

37 Cochelin, "*In senectute bona*", p. 126.

38 Shahar, *Growing Old.*, p. 103.

39 Irsigler and Lassotta, *Bettler und Gaukler*, pp. 18–20.

diet and the provision of temporary accommodation.[40] This functioned more as a social solution to the 'problem' of sickness, rather than offering substantive medical care for sick patients. The petitions and pontifical letters reflect this reality, while highlighting the progressive medicalization of these places of refuge between the thirteenth and fourteenth centuries, in parallel with the medicalization of medieval society more generally.[41] Analysis of documents in the corpus further supports the contention that such institutions gradually became places of care that specialized according to the publics that they served.[42]

As the *Decree* of Yvo of Chartres testifies, the Church's mission was to support widows, adolescents, and the 'weak of body' (*corporis debilis*).[43] Thus, hospitals provided care for certain conditions in the name of the common good, under the umbrella of 'general health measures'.[44] The establishment of secular charity from the thirteenth century onwards led to the secularization of such care-giving institutions. At the same time, it propelled the specialization of institutions according to the populations to which they provided care – hospitals dedicated to treating clerics, for example – and/or the type of impairment for which they offered treatment, such as in the case of leprosaria.

Clerical Hospitals

From the fourteenth century onwards, hospitals specialized in the type of care they offered and/or the type of patients they admitted, following their founders' wishes.[45] Previously, the ecclesiastical model of charity was dominant: support was provided to any and all poor people, free of charge. As hospitals gradually became financed and administered by municipalities, institutions offering ecclesiastical charity became specialist endeavours, rather than standard. This shift was also linked to changing attitudes towards the poor. During the fourteenth and fifteenth centuries, ever more attention was paid to moral taxonomies of poverty: a distinction was made between the deserving poor, who were genuinely incapable of working, and the fraudulent poor who were not worthy of any social aid, as

40 See Crislip, *From Monastery to Hospital*.
41 See Dubourg, "*Deo iudicio percusset*".
42 Metzler, "Liminality and Disability", p. 284.
43 *Decree* of Yvo of Chartres, edited in Migne (ed.), *Patrologia Latina*, vol. 161, book 8, chapter 326.
44 See Grmek, "Le concept d'infection".
45 Brodman, *Charity and Welfare*, p. 73.

they could help themselves, if only they made the effort.[46] At the same time, the institutionalization of assistance meant that financial support, which had previously chiefly taken the form of donations to specific individuals, now more often took the form of bequests to communities that took direct care of the poor, acting on donors' wishes and thereby structurally displacing them.

Patrons or founders of hospitals laid down general sanitation measures to which 'their' institution had to conform. The form and function of hospitals derived from their aspirations, their family ties, or the needs of the community.[47] The foundation of a hospital allowed individuals to demonstrate, and concretize, their elevated social status, which was reflected in the number of poor people admitted, the size of the premises, or the particular type of needy souls that it served. A letter written by Clement VI, in response to Joan, Queen of Sicily, concerning her late husband Robert's desire to build a chapel in Naples, attests to this.[48] The chapel was intended to feed and house a hundred people who would otherwise go hungry, chosen from among the king's familiars or their heirs, whether they were knights, squires, or of inferior status, on the condition that they suffered from old age or other 'legitimate' impediments that rendered them incapable of working to support themselves.[49] This letter reflects a shift occurring throughout Christendom: alongside its increasing institutionalization, Christian mercy was becoming more geographically limited, typically concentrated on the donor's home diocese, or even just on their entourage.[50] It also illustrates the existence of a classification of 'good reasons' for seeking assistance, a hierarchy of the poor that emerged as early as the eleventh century, and that remained operative in the fourteenth century.[51]

Institutions offering care were discriminating in terms of which patients they would admit for treatment. Some physical and mental conditions were deemed permissible, whilst others rendered the patient ineligible for admission.[52] For example, the 1144 founding charter of St John's Hospital in Oxford stated that lepers, paralytics, people suffering from dropsy, ulcers, or chronic diseases, lunatics, and epileptics were not to be admitted to the

46 Metzler, *A Social History*, p. 185.
47 Sweetinburgh, *The Role of the Hospital*, p. 19.
48 RV 162, f. 95 R – Clement VI to Joan, Queen of Sicily, 20 September 1343.
49 Metzler, *A Social History*, p. 158.
50 Rawcliffe, *The Hospitals of Medieval Norwich*, p. 11.
51 Agrimi and Crisciani, "Charité et assistance", p. 158.
52 Rubin, *Charity and Community*, p. 158.

hospital.[53] The chronically ill were often excluded from care facilities, as they took up valuable hospital resources that could be better used for the cure of patients with acute (i.e., temporary) conditions.[54] By consequence, from the thirteenth century onwards, founders began to designate the specific purposes for which their institutions had been established.[55] A letter written by Alexander IV to the Bishop of Norwich on 10 March 1255 offers insightful testimony:

> Your serial petition which we have heard contains that you [...], out of your own property and acquisitions through your activities, you build of your own will, in the city of Norwich, a hospital in honour of the Blessed Virgin Mary and St Giles, for the service of priests who, sick (*debilis*) or broken down by old age, cannot celebrate divine Mass or cannot or will not sustenance themselves, and also for the service of a number of poor students who study in this city, as well as thirteen poor and sick people, in order to help them daily, and that the master, the brothers and the ministers of this hospital make the necessary arrangements for the above.[56]

In this letter, the Pope authorizes the bishop to found the hospital of St Mary and St Giles. This facility was to offer care for ailing or elderly priests who could no longer perform divine services or feed themselves, the needy schoolchildren of Norwich, and thirteen poor or sick people per day. These were amongst the city's most vulnerable, the destitute and the socially marginalized. The foundation is likely authorized in recognition of the lack of care available for elderly or sick priests in the bishop's diocese. As residents of the hospital, disadvantaged clerics in Norwich received care in a safe location, whilst remaining integrated in the community's social fabric.

53 The example of St John's Hospital in Oxford is discussed by Buhrer, "'But What is to Be Said of a Fool'".

54 Metzler, "Liminality and Disability", p. 284.

55 Sweetinburgh, *The Role of the Hospital*, p. 112.

56 RV 24, f. 28 V – Alexander IV to the Bishop of Norwich, 10 March 1255. Text edited by Bourel de La Roncière, de Loye, Canival, and Coulon (eds.), *Les registres d'Alexandre IV*, n° 254: '*Sane petitionis tue seriem audivimus continentem quod tu* [...] *in proprio fundo tuo in civitate Norwicensi de bonis per tuam industriam acquisitis, quoddam hospitale in honorem beate Marie Virginis ac sancti Egidii ad opus sacerdotum qui debilitate vel senectute confracti divina celebrare non possunt seu non habeant unde valeant sustentari, et etiam ad opus certi numeri pauperum scolarium in civitate predicta studentium ac tredecim pauperum reficiendorum ibidem cotidie necnon infirmorum illuc declinare volentium construxisti, magistro, fratribus et ministris in eodem hospitali ad executionem premissorum necessariis nichilominus institutis*'.

Alexander IV's decision in this case follows in the wake of several pieces of legislation that emphasized the need to provide ongoing care to elderly or impaired priests. As early as 816, at the Aix-la-Chapelle assembly, the pontifical institution had authorized a bishop to make a house available to elderly and sick canons.[57] Priests, in theory at least, had no children of their own to take care of them, and thus could not always, or even often, rely on family members for support in later life. Likewise, if priests suffered from incurable conditions, including age-related impairment, they were refused entry to the public hospital the same as anyone else. Without access to care, they were at substantial risk of marginalization.[58] Consequently, a second provision made at the Council of Mainz in 1261 decided to release funds to create or maintain hospices for elderly priests.[59] Places of refuge for vulnerable clerics thus became institutionalized from the thirteenth century onwards.[60] Above all, the Church aimed to prevent resignees from resorting to begging, an activity that jeopardized their ecclesiastical dignity.[61] For this reason, resignees who were not fortunate enough to receive a sufficient pension were accepted by specialist hospitals catering to clerics. Created by the Church, these institutions bear witness to the pontificate's recognition that retirees without a large, or any, pension, could find themselves in dire straits.[62] Such open reception arrangements, which guaranteed care for impaired clerics, spread in the thirteenth century to encompass entrance to 'hostels of God' (hôtels-Dieu) operated by religious and lay congregations, and subsequently to hospitals in cities in the fourteenth century.[63]

Then, in the fourteenth century, papal authority was frequently invoked to allow for the construction of new care facilities of various types, including hospitals, hospices, and houses of charity. Founders wished to secure papal protection for their institution, contributing to its prestige and their own. Thus, the papal institution played a fundamental role in the construction and set up of certain care institutions, though their day-to-day running and management was later entrusted to ecclesiastics or lay confraternities. The papacy also directly advanced the standardization of charitable practices, in particular through the injunction that all hospitals and leprosaria were

57 Shahar, *Growing Old*, p. 110.

58 Cummins, "Attitudes to Old Age", p. 225.

59 See Bertram (ed.), *The Chrodegang Rules*.

60 The hospital for elderly priests in Tournai is the first we know of; see Albou, *L'image des personnes âgées*, p. 76.

61 Minois, *Histoire de la vieillesse*, p. 259.

62 Shahar, *Growing Old*, p. 110.

63 Agrimi and Crisciani, "Charité et assistance", p. 169.

obliged to follow the rule of St Augustine that was first issued in the Council of Paris in 1212.[64] With the foundation of care facilities, the Church likewise contributed substantially to the development of the European therapeutic sector between the thirteenth and fifteenth centuries.[65] Indeed, popes also founded their own hospitals, such as the hospital of the Holy Spirit in Rome, evidencing the rapid expansion of medical activity in the medieval era.[66]

Leprosaria

Leprous clerics appear to have had two choices: either they could enter enclosure in a private house, or they could join a leper hospital (*leprosarium*). In certain cases, clerics were allowed to split the difference and were given permission to live as recluses outside leprosaria. This is the fate, for instance, of the leper Rogerius (known as Renardus), a priest and rector of the church of Cormelles in the diocese of Bayeux. In a letter dated from the 23 October 1256, Alexander IV allows Rogerius to retain the income from his rectory to obviate any need for begging.[67] He is also permitted to live in a house built by his own hand, as long as it is at minimum a stone's throw away from other buildings. The distance was necessary to avoid the creation of any scandal owing to his presence outside the leprosaria.[68] In other cases, clerics were obliged to transfer to leprosaria, and were thus subject to broader social exclusion. Such examples illustrate the relative degree to which impaired resignees faced marginalization. The issue was especially acute for clerics with leprosy: the figure of a leprous cleric raised the potential for immense *scandalum*, and a diagnosis of leprosy typically separated an individual from his community forever. The supplications and papal letters indicate, however, that the social exclusion of lepers, even residents of leprosaria, was not necessarily total. The sources confirm the porous nature of the boundary between the leprosarium and the world, both secular and ecclesiastical, beyond its confines.[69] Nevertheless, the Chancery functionally arranged for the relative ostracization of leprous clerics, by taking an active role in the endowment and regulation of leprosaria on occasion.

64 The obligation to follow the rule of St. Augustine is found in the Councils of Paris in 1212, Rouen in 1214, and Lateran IV in 1215.

65 Brodman, *Charity and Welfare*, p. 93.

66 Lazard, "L'Ospedale di Santo Spirito", p. 202.

67 This example can be found in length in Dubourg, "Being a Leprous Cleric".

68 Shahar, *Growing Old*, p. 104.

69 See Tabuteau, *Lépreux et sociabilité*; Brenner and Touati (eds), *Leprosy and Identity*.

In the few cases in which the Apostolic See directed retirees to enter leprosaria, all clerics transferred of their own free will. A diagnosis of leprosy placed individuals at the margins of medieval social space, yet equally accorded them a well-defined role within it. Lepers were routinely indigent, owing to the severity of the condition and the stigma it carried. In this context, begging became an organized activity for lepers, managed by the communities that derived income from lepers' mendicancy, alongside legislation enacted by public authorities.[70] The latter wanted to curb the number of vagrants by determining which recipients of charity were 'good paupers' and thus deserved to be supported, achieved in part through the introduction of *matriculae*.[71] It makes sense, then, that transferral to a leprosarium, a relatively welcoming institution in which they would receive care, was the preferable choice for some clerics. By appealing to the Pope for transfer to a leper hospital, leprous clerics retained agency, inasmuch as they subjected *themselves* to the ostracization of the leprosarium. In this context, the Chancery's approval of such transfers demonstrates its respect for supplicants' wishes.

In a petition dated 8 May 1342, for example, we learn that Johannes de Peredo, a married cleric with leprosy from Pauillac in the diocese of Auxerre, apparently made this kind of calculation:

> The devoted cleric, Johannes de Peredo, stricken with the disease of leprosy, a native of Pauillac sur Loire, in the diocese of Auxerre, where his wife and offspring remain, who for sixteen years was a teacher and notary for the king of France, asks out of mercy and with a benevolent and godly eye to join a house of St Lazare, in the city of Béziers, in order to, in his own words, endure the divine scourging patiently, [...] and because his last day approaches, he wishes to receive his chair quickly. Done. R.

The postscript to the previous block quote and pontifical 'fiat' states that:

> He may transfer himself, by the grace pious attention of God, and notwithstanding the customs of this house [of St Lazare], which is done in such circumstances thanks to contrary grace. Done, R.[72]

70 Metzler, *A Social History*, p. 175.

71 Consult Rouche, "La matricule des pauvres".

72 RS 6, f. 341 R – Johannes de Peredo, cleric of the diocese of Auxerre to Clement VI on 8 May 1342, for which I give the transcription according to the register: '*Devote Johannes de Peredo clericus morbo lepre percussit, oriundus commorans apud Poilliacum super Ligerem in Autissiodiorensis diocesis, huius uxore et liberis qui quidem Johannes ibidem scolas regit tabellio*

Johannes' request to enter a leprosarium in order to 'endure the divine scourge with patience' was approved by Clement VI, and the Curia sprang into action to ensure that his transfer was successful. The Chancery sent the reply letter to multiple addressees – the unnamed Archbishop of Béziers; Arnaldus Eronget, canon of Béziers; and an anonymous official of the same church – to ensure that Johannes would be provided with all 'necessary things' (*neccessaria*) to join the local leprosarium, including food and clothing, and that he would receive appropriate care once installed:

> With paternal piety and sense of duty, we ask [you] to provide for his needs, since he is stricken with leprosy by divine will. Therefore, we accept [the request] of our dear son Johannes de Peredo, a married cleric from the diocese of Auxerre, where he is originally from and where he has a wife and offspring in Pauillac sur Loire, in the same diocese, where he practised as a teacher and public notary for sixteen years according to his own words, because he is stricken with this disease with divine assent. […] We undertake and mandate at your discretion by apostolic letter that, the aforementioned Johannes be assigned by you or another man to live at the house of St Lazare of Béziers and be considered suitable to receive food, clothing and all other necessary things.[73]

The recipients of the letter were thus responsible for Johannes' care, financially and more practically. Entrance into a leprosarium came at a cost. Generally, lepers did not enter the community empty-handed, but were obliged to bring with them the necessary items to establish their new lives. According to the statutes of the leprosarium of Nîmes, for example, new

quare domini Regis Francie fuit per spacium sexdecim annorum quatenus intuitu misericordie ipsum instituere dignemini oculo pietatis eidem Johannem mansionem in domo sancti Lazarii, civitas Bitericensis misericorditer impendendo ut ibidem verbera suum Creator pati valeat patienter […] *ut cum diem extremum clausit cum superis, valeat celeriter cathedraris. Fiat. R. Transeat gratis pro Deo intuitu pietatis non obstante consuetudinibus pro dicta domo hunc gracie contrariis si que fuit. Fiat. R*'.

73 RV 162, f. 218 R – Clement VI to the Archbishop of Béziers, to Arnaldus Eronget, canon, and to the official of the same church, 8 May 1342, for which I give the transcription according to the register: '*Paterne pietatis officium tunc diligenter exequimur cum morbo lepre beneplacito Divino percussis mandamus in suis necessitatibus subveniri. Cum itaque sicut accepimus dilectus filius Johannes de Peredo, clericus coniugatus in diocese Autissiodorensis, commorans habens uxorem et liberos qui apud Poylliacum super Ligerem, dicte diocese, scolas rexisse et officium tabellionatus per sexdecim annos exercuisse dicitur, sit nutu Divino, dicto morbo percussus.* […] *discretioni vestre per apostolica scripta committimus et mandamus quatenus vos vel duo aut unus vestrum per vos alter alium seu alios dicto Johanni in domo beati Lazari, Bituricensis, auctoritate nostra mansionem assignari congruam faciatis sibique in ea victum et vestitum et alia necessaria*'.

residents should arrive with a trousseau consisting of 'a bed, a mattress, a cushion, 6 sheets, 2 blankets, 6 bowls, 2 pewter dishes'.[74] In this respect, entry into a leprosarium was similar to entry into the orders. For example, the residents of the Dover leper-hospital were tonsured like monks, visually affirming their cloistered identity.[75] In the documents studied, supplicants might choose to enter a leper community rather than be isolated. The fraternity that arose from the common life of men, and sometimes women, brought together in sickness might offer a better social bond than the alternative: partial integration into the orders, considering that some lepers were authorized to live in individual houses.

In this letter, Johannes de Peredo was authorized by Clement VI to join the leper hospital of St Lazare in Béziers. By his own testimony, he preferred to leave his wife and children in Pauillac and enter the leper community alone. This raises the thorny issue of marital relationships for lepers and, more specifically, wretched matches – marriages in which one spouse is leprous – though the topic is not broached explicitly in the missive. Initially, the Church held that marriage was indissoluble, including in cases of spousal illness. A diagnosis of leprosy for one spouse was not grounds for the dissolution of the union. However, the rules evolved during the fourteenth century, gradually becoming more lenient and moving towards the annulment of 'mixed' marriages between healthy and leprous partners. Entry into a leprosarium became a legitimate reason for breaking off a marriage. If one spouse joined a cloistered institution, the other could annul the union by going before the bishop's tribunal.[76] Johannes' desire to be taken care of exclusively by the leprosarium suggests, perhaps, that he had broken all family ties. No longer able to rely on his wife and children for support, he turned to his ecclesiastical family and the pontifical institution for care. Entry into the leprosarium served as a rite of passage for new members, a symbolic break from the world beyond the institution's bounds and residents' previous lives. This included, for example, an initiation that marked an individual's arrival in the fraternity, which had much in common with the monastery.[77] At the end of the medieval period, entrance rites sometimes took the form of mock funerals for new residents conducted by the bishop. Such services are documented in at least thirty-six European dioceses, although it is impossible to know if

74 Le Blévec, "Les lépreux peuvent-ils vivre en société?", p. 289.

75 Rawcliffe, *Leprosy in Medieval England*, p. 303.

76 Le Blévec, "Les lépreux peuvent-ils vivre en société?", p. 283.

77 Bériou and Touati, *Voluntate dei leprosus*, p. 65.

the rites actually took place.[78] In any case, analysis of petitions and papal letters shows that a small number of clerics chose to join the leprosarium, rather than to remain within the monastery, perpetually isolated from other residents and ostracized by clergymen. Whilst transferral to the leper hospital led to a relative social exclusion, within the marginalized space of the institution, retirees could find meaningful fellowship with others in the community and flourish in the relationship it developed within its social fabric.

A diagnosis of leprosy was required for an individual to join a leper hospital.[79] Numerous rules were applied in such institutions in order to control lepers, but also to protect the healthy population from the risk of contagion.[80] This included, for example, strict enclosure, which functioned as a kind of quarantine. Leprosaria demanded almost monastic discipline of their residents, allowing municipal authorities to reinforce the isolation system from the thirteenth century onwards.[81] Then, the whole system of leprosaria was set up to mandate that residents were highly obedient to regulations, so municipal authorities could exert ever greater control over lepers. The Pope, however, had the authority to contravene or modify such rules, if an alternative was permitted by the statutes of a given institution. Another letter written by Clement VI is illustrative on this point. On 30 April 1343, Clement writes to Robertus de Bours, known as Peuboin, a cleric of the diocese of Thérouanne, to discuss the matter of the cleric's marital arrangements:

> Since dear brother Robertus de Bours, known as Peuboin, a married cleric of the diocese of Thérouanne, is stricken with the disease of leprosy, and together with the dear daughter of Christ Margareta Dailly, his wife, they live separated because of this, and reside in the hospital of the poor St Mary's of Reims among the brothers and sisters, submitting themselves to the service of God with the sick and the poor. We desire, with regard to her praiseworthy request to live together, and we ask at your discretion by apostolic letter that Margareta can be authorized by you, or another people, to join the service of the sick and the poor and be received among the brothers and sisters in this hospital.[82]

78 Bériac, *Histoire des lépreux*, p. 215.

79 The most recent research shows the medicalization of leprosaria. See Hermann, "Lépreux et maladières dans l'ancien diocèse de Genève".

80 Agrimi and Crisciani, "Charité et assistance", p. 171.

81 Tabuteau, "Historical Research Developments on Leprosy", p. 44.

82 RV 151, f. 30 R – Clement VI to Robertus de Bours, clerics of the diocese of Thérouanne, 30 April 1343, for which I give the transcription according to the register: '*Cum dilectus filius*

After contracting leprosy, Robertus joined the hospital for the poor of St Mary's of Reims with his wife. He petitions the Pope to request that his healthy wife, Margareta Dailly, be allowed to enter service at the same institution as a sister serving the poor and the impaired. For this reason, the letter was registered in the category *de religionis ingressu* ('on entering religion'). Clement authorizes Robertus' request, and, in another letter, registered under the same category but addressed to the abbots of the monasteries of St Nicaise and St Denys in Reims, and the official of Reims, allowed his transfer to the leprosarium of St Lazar in Reims. This raises fundamental questions about the presence of the healthy (or minimally, non-leprous) laity in hospitals and leprosarium as carers for leprous and non-leprous residents. Indeed, from the earliest days of leprosaria, healthy lay people had entered communities in order to serve lepers.[83] This activity was spiritually beneficial: lepers were considered to be privileged intermediaries between God and man from the eleventh to the twelfth century.[84] However, Margareta might have chosen to join the service of the ill and poor of St Mary's hospital to live near her husband and yet not alone in celibacy, with little consideration of the positive religious implications. For Robertus, joining a leper hospital functioned to ostracize him from broader society, but at the same time, it allowed him to stay in the same city as Margareta and build a new life within a supportive community inside the leprosarium, but also in the network of care institutions in Reims. Moreover, the latest research minimizes the marginalization of these institutions, insisting more on their preponderant place in the social fabric. For example, it was long imagined that lepers used rattles and other noisy instruments to signal their presence and repel other road users. Yet, in fact, such noise-makers were used to indicate the presence of beggars, leprous and non-leprous alike.[85]

Robertus de Bours, dictus Peuboin clericus coniugatus Morinensis diocesis sit morbo lepre percussus et ob hoc dilecta in christo filia Margareta Dailly eius uxor ab eius consorcio separari et in hospitali pauperum beate Marie Remensis in quo fratres et sorores existunt cupiat in infirmis et pauperibus Domino famulari. Nos volentes ipsam in huiusmodi suo laudabili proposito consovere, discretioni vestre per apostolica scripta mandamus quatenus vos vel duo aut unus vestrum per vos vel alium seu alios prefatam Margaretam in eodem hospitali ad servicium infirmorum et pauperum recipi faciatis in fratrem et sororem'. Another letter was issued on the same day to allow Robertus to enter the leprosarium. See RV 151, f. 31 R – Clement VI to the abbots of the monastery of St Nicaise and St Denys of Reims and the official of Reims.

83 Saint Margaret's leprosarium in Barcelona is a good example of the links between the urban context, the city's network of hospitals, and the role of carers in everyday life. The issues of mobility that these links reveal are developed extensively by Jáuregui, "Inside the Leprosarium".

84 See Schelberg, "Leprosen in der mittelalterlichen".

85 See Tabuteau, "Vingt mille léproseries au Moyen Âge?".

Similarly, leprosaria were not closed off from the rest of the city or village community, but were instead open to the world – which may have allowed Robertus and Margareta to continue to see each other.[86] As with monastic enclosure, the claustration of the leprosarium was not absolute. Whilst the petitions and papal letters show that residents of leprosaria were always subject to some degree of spatial segregation, they also indicate that this did not necessarily lead to residents' social ostracization. Clerical resignees who entered leprosaria retained links to broader society and to the wider clerical community, both spheres in which they continued to participate through the porous walls of their living quarters. The petition process, and the accommodations secured by engaging with it, directly contributed to this sense of inclusion, by ensuring that all clerics, even those who had technically left the clergy, could receive care and support.

Monasteries as Retirement Homes

In the papal letters, numerous impaired clerics ask to end their days by retiring to a monastery. Even so, the corpus likely offers only a partial glimpse of what is almost certainly an even broader phenomenon. In thirteenth-century letters, 4% of supplicants were explicitly allowed to enter conventual life after their resignation, and 16% in fourteenth-century missives. However, 44% of supplicants asking for letters of permission to resign announced their desire to join monastic orders in their petitions, an issue which was never spoken of again in their case documents. We can therefore legitimately assume that details regarding supplicants' transfer of institution after resignation were not always included in the letters, or that later letters following up on this topic were not conserved. We can also suspect that, given that they were allowed to resign by the popes, the request of retiring in the monastery was also granted. The focus of petitions was squarely on resignation; the post-resignation adoption of monastic status was a secondary issue, and, in any case, such arrangements might have been settled at the local level. The Pope might have chosen to elide all discussion of such transfers to focus instead on the core components of the petition, which all related to supplicants' ecclesiastical status: whether they were regular or secular clergy, and whether they sought to enter, or remain, in monastic spaces.

86 This is the thesis of Brenner, *Leprosy and Charity*.

Staying in the Monastery

The majority of cases in which supplicants requested permission to quit their functions in the monastery or the convent feature monks or nuns who, overwhelmed by their physical or mental incapacity, were obliged to resign their office. Monastic resignees from both male and female convents often obtained a pension that replaced their benefice, but they remained resident in their 'home' monastery, unless other arrangements were put in place. After resignation, abbots essentially received a demotion, and thereafter lived as monks in their own community or in a neighbouring convent. Indeed, 85% of the petitions and letters on impaired regular clerics that wished to stay in the conventual life concern abbots who asked to remain in their home community as monks. The exemplary case of the elderly Augerius, former abbot of the community of St Mary of Lagrasse, sheds light on such arrangements. On 15 April 1309, Clement V writes a letter summarizing Augerius' circumstances to Guillelmus, Augerius' chosen successor, a candidate selected with the help of the Bishop of Agde:

> You [Guillelmus] proposed before us that, while our beloved son Brother Augerius, formerly abbot of your monastery of Lagrasse, is known to have reached a decrepit age, seeing that the monastery benefited from his prudent government and has increased its temporal and spiritual benefits, and, wishing to please him by this special gift of kindness, we were inclined by your supplications to grant and depute, to the said brother Augerius, as long as he will lived, a share of the fruits, revenues and products of the aforementioned monastery, up to the sum you judge necessary, that is to say, enough to feed him properly, in recognition of his service to the monastery of Lagrasse and to the Benedictine order.[87]

87 RV 56, f. 110 V – Clement V to Guillelmus, abbot of the monastery of St Mary of Lagrasse (Carcassone), 15 April 1309. Text analysed by Benedictine monks (eds.), *Regestum Clementis papae V*, n° 4 250, for which I give the transcription according to the register: '*Cum dilectus filius frater Augerius, dudum abbas tui monasterii Crassensis, sicut ex parte tua fuit propositum coram nobis ad decrepitam etatem pervenisse noscatur, nos attendentes quod monasterium ipsum dum eiusdem regimini profuit sue prudentie studiis spiritualis et temporalis comodi suscepit augmentum ac volentes personam suam propre hoc dono specialis benivolentie pervenire tuis supplicationibus inclinati concedendi et deputandi dicto fratri Augerio quoad vixerit aliquos fructus, redditibus et proventibus dicti monasteri, usque ad summam que tue discretioni videbitur, de quibus detentus valeat sustentari quibuscumque ipsius monasteri et ordinis sancti Benedicti qui in dicto monasterio servari dinoscitur*'.

Guillelmus asks to award a 'retirement pension' to Augerius, paid by the coenobitic community of which the former abbot was a faithful steward during his abbacy. The Chancery concurs, permitting Augerius a 'pension' as compensation for services previously rendered to the monastery, and authorizes Guillelmus to determine a sum that would be sufficient to support him appropriately. However, the framing of the payment makes it clear that this allowance is not a legal obligation, but rather a goodwill gesture by the institution.[88] In the sixth century, the last lines of the Rule of the Master, a collection of monastic regulations, settled the question of individual housing, stating that: 'for two brothers who have become decrepit with age, a dwelling shall be built within the gates of the monastery and near them'.[89] These elderly monastics were given the task of interviewing visitors: they were set aside and permitted separate lodging by virtue of their wisdom. In contrast, in the Rule of St Benedict, the elderly were given better access to communal and individual facilities because of their physical weakness (such as bath, private rooms, etc.). In the provisions of the Council of Vienna of 1312, monastics were prohibited from living alone outside the monastery. Indeed, religious were not permitted to live independently, but were obliged to share their dwelling with at least one other person if they must stay outside the monastery.[90] The monastic life remained communal, even after retirement. No mention is made of any financial allowance granted to retired abbots in canon law, meaning that they, theoretically, had to live like their brothers, albeit according to a modified (easiest) rule of life. Similarly, canons had to remain in their convent until death, though they were exempted from attending Matins after they reached the age of 70.[91] Augerius appears to have been a dynamic force during his abbacy. He made various advantageous arrangements for the abbey, and reformed the observance of the rule. In another letter, dated 22 February 1310 and written also to Guillelmus, Clement V recapitulates certain decisions Augerius had made during his time as abbot. This second letter begins with a reference to the former abbot's retirement, with his departure motivated by his advanced age which had rendered him useless, unable to govern the monastery adequately.[92] Strikingly, this second letter, written almost

88 Shahar, *Growing Old*, p. 105.

89 Minois, *Histoire de la vieillesse*, p. 187.

90 Hourlier and Le Bras, *Histoire du droit et des institutions de l'Église*, p. 223.

91 Gutton, *Naissance du vieillard*, p. 17.

92 RV 57, f. 222 V – Clement V to Guillelmus, abbot of the monastery of St Mary of Lagrasse (Carcassone), 22 February 1310. Text edited by Benedictine monks (eds.), *Regestum Clementis papae V*, n° 6 065.

a year after the letter expressly pertaining to Augerius' resignation, gives us more information than its predecessor about the circumstances of his abdication, including his physical and mental condition, even though its subject matter is quite different. However, this time, we are far from the hagiographic eulogy of the first letter, and much more in the lived reality of the problems that the great age of an abbot could have posed.

Equally, new retirees could enjoy special facilities that had some connection to their (former) home institution. The Benedictine abbess Elissandra de Noeriis of St Mary of Jocro, in the diocese of Meaux, requested such privileges from Clement VI:

> The petition that you brought to our attention contained that, now a nun, while you were until recently abbess of the Benedictine monastery of St Mary of Jocro, belonging to the Roman Church, in the diocese of Meaux, in the last moments of your life you ardently wished to devote your humble desires, all your actions and worldly concerns to God only, to submit yourself in quiet peace and conscious devotion, which was not possible when you were abbess, because of the abbatial dignity and administration of the monastery, tired by the difficulties and concerns of the aforementioned monastery and weighed down by old age. [...] In short, we wish, based on your merits, to respond favourably to your requests in this regard, so that you may live in the house or manor of Clareo, belonging to the Jocro estate of this monastery, with a portion of bread and wine for you and your four servants, and a pension of 300 *livres tournois* in the currency of the kingdom of France, to take care of you for the rest of your days.[93]

Elissandra freely relinquished her office in light of her advanced age and associated exhaustion. Rather than remaining within the convent proper,

93 RV 165, f. 27 V – Clement VI to Elissandra de Noeriis, from the Benedictine monastery of St Mary of Jocro, 9 May 1345, for which I give the transcription according to the register: '*Cum itaque sicut petitio tua pro parte nobis exhibita continebat nuper tu nunc monialis tunc abbatissa monasterii beate Marie de Jocro ad Romanam ecclesiam nullo medio pertinentis ordinis sancti Benedicti, Meledensis diocesis, utlimis temporibus vite tue cupiens ferventi desiderio abiectis omnibus actus et secularibus curis soli Deo adhaerere, et in tranquilitate pacis et conscientie devotionem reddere famulatum quod facere non posses quamdiu esses diversis oneribus et curis dicti monasterii fatigata et senectute gravata dignitati abbaciali et regimini eiusdem monasterii* [...] *Nos igitur volentes promissorum meritorum obtentu tibi super hoc quantum cum Deo possumus salubriter providere huiusmodi supplicationibus inclinati domum seu manerium de Clareio propre dictam villam de Iocro ad prefatum monasterium pertinentem ac portionem panis et vini de ipso monasterio pro te et quatuor servitoribus tuis necnon pensionem trecentarum librarum Turonensis parvorum fortis monete nunc in regno Francie curetis quod vixeris*'.

she preferred to move by herself to a residence near the village of Jocro that was owned by the institution. In theory, the former abbess was prohibited from living outside enclosure, hence the need to appeal for papal grace to authorize her transfer. Elissandra also asked to receive a pension of 300 *livres tournois* per year. She wished not only to break enclosure and the mandate to live communally, but also to retain the material support from which she benefited as a cloistered nun, including her portions of bread and wine. Moreover, she appealed for permission to appoint four servants to her household, who would care for her in her old age. Clement VI approves the retiree's request in full, which suggests both that Elissandra genuinely did leave enclosure, and that she maintained close links with her former monastic life at the convent and its current occupants. The petitions and letters again confirm the way in which monastic rules could be adapted to allow for the physical separation of impaired clerics from their various communities, whilst simultaneously minimizing their social exclusion.

Entering the Monastery

From the twelfth century onwards, the monastery became known as a 'retirement home' for elderly nobles and clerics. Many medieval commentators criticized the assumption of the habit late in life as a calculated move to secure a comfortable life and care in one's advanced years, rather than a reflection of any sincere vocation.[94] The late conversion movement began to spread from the middle of the eleventh century in parallel with the increase in lay donations to religious communities.[95] In the thirteenth century, hospitals transitioned from spaces of general care for the needy and vulnerable to hospices for patients with acute sickness, conditions that were both curable and time-limited. Consequently, these institutions often refused to accept long-term 'invalids', the chronically ill and elderly. Monasteries plugged this care gap, filling up with elderly people with varying degrees of impairment.[96] They accepted individuals excluded from other care institutions, offering care both for palliative patients at the end of life and for elderly residents on an ongoing basis.

Retirement to the convent was a complicated issue for priests with secular benefices. Nevertheless, many might have favoured joining orders

94 On the debate about the late assumption of the monastic habit, see Metzler, *A Social History*, p. 146.

95 Miramon, "Embrasser l'état monastique", p. 847.

96 Sweetinburgh, *The Role of the Hospital*, p. 60.

rather than transferring to a hospital.[97] Of the secular clergy seeking such arrangements in the corpus, bishops (i.e., clerics invested with a share of papal authority) are by far the most numerous. Indeed, of the 132 seculars requesting permission to retire to a monastery, only two held positions below the level of bishop: a prior and a chaplain. Clerics asked to leave the priesthood and enter the monastery because their impairments were likely to cause 'scandal' in the community.[98] In such cases, the Church took particularly good care of high-ranked elderly clerics: both Yvo of Chartres' and Gratian's *Decree* established that a bishop could not be ousted from his role, even if he were ill and incapable of satisfying the requirements of his office, unless and until he resigned.[99] This provision encouraged the pontifical institution to ask for the resignation of clerics who were perceived to be harming their benefices, owing to their disability. Thus, this could have opened up a negotiation that could be advantageous for the retiring bishop. Now, then, the bishop had leverage – he could ask for special privileges in his petition, requesting transfer to a specific monastic institution, receive some income, and so on.

The supplication addressed to Urban V on 22 August 1363 by Baldewinus, titular Bishop of Tripoli, affiliated to the Cistercians, demonstrates the negotiation that could take place:

> It is granted to him [Baldewinus], by special grace in order to relieve his insufficiency (*inopia*), for he is old and ill, a monk's prebend in the monastery of St Paul in Utrecht and another in the Benedictine monastery of Oestbroec outside Utrecht insofar as each of these are worth about sixty florins (guilders) if you consider him worthy of receiving them, notwithstanding his privileges or customs. Made again if he renounces the episcopate [*crossed out in the original*: and if he wishes to become a monk, B] without further reading. Done. B.[100]

97 Metzler, *A Social History*, p. 144 gives several examples of these defectors from the eleventh to the fifteenth century.

98 Fossier, "La contagion des péchés", p. 30.

99 *Decretum Gratiani*, edited in Friedberg (ed.), *Corpus iuris canonici,* second part, causa 7, canon 1. *Decree* of Yvo of Chartres, edited in Migne (ed.), *Patrologia Latina*, vol. 161, book 5, chapter 305 et 307.

100 RS 40 f. 43 V – Baldewinus, Bishop of Tripoli to Urban V, 22 August 1363. Text analysed by Hayez, Mathieu, and Yvan (eds.), *Urbain V*, n° 327, for which I give the transcription according to the register: '*Specialem graciam facientes ad relevandam inopiam suam cuius sit senex et valitudinarius eidem unius monachi prebenda in monasterii sancti Pauli Trajectensis et unam aliam in monasterio de Oestbroec extra muros Trajectensis, ordinis sancti Benedicti quarum quelibet ipsarum valet sexaginta florenum vel circa vester dignemini conferre quibuscumque*

The bishop petitions the Pope to ask for more income to support himself in old age, as he needs to live comfortably and pay for care etc. He then receives two monastic prebends, worth about 60 florins each. Urban V is happy to honour the cleric's request, on one critical condition: Baldewinus must resign his titular bishopric in exchange. Canonical support for such clerical transfers is found in Gratian's *Decree*. The text prescribes that a priest in a very weak condition may enter the regular clergy, if he had first resigned.[101] This was almost certainly what he had in mind when formulating his initial request, as his bishopric of Tripoli was only titular (without being in charge of a diocese). Strikingly, the original supplication featured another condition that was probably included when the text was read to the Pope, yet maybe subsequently removed by the Chancery. Urban V had requested explicit assurance that Baldewinus really did want to become a monk, or in other words, that he would transfer to the monastic orders at some point in the future. The elision of this prerequisite, and the supplicant's success in securing his desired prebends in and around Utrecht, suggests that Baldewinus' was in fact living there or at least want to return to the Netherlands from his posting (maybe in Avignon). Embracing the monastic life seemed like a practical – and lucrative – way to achieve this aim, rather than a purely spiritual endeavour. Transfer to monastic orders later in life was a sensible choice for secular clerics. Monasteries were well equipped to shelter and care for sick and impaired residents, thanks particularly to their infirmaries.[102] However, there was a risk that the community would refuse to accept a candidate who was judged to be too old, even if he were a secular cleric.[103] Point 60 of the Rule of St Benedict warns the chapter not to admit new members 'too quickly'.[104] Indeed, many religious orders expressly stipulated that old age, impairment, or illness rendered an applicant ineligible for entrance, as he would be unable to cope with the rigours of monastic life.[105]

Alongside secular clergymen transferring to monasteries, the corpus documents instances in which wealthy nobility, both men and women, were allowed to enter monastic institutions later in life, regardless of their

privilegiis seu consuetudinibus suis et aliis quibuscumque non obstante ut in forma, fiat in altero si renunties episcopatum B. [cassere in originali: et velis esse monachus B.], sine alia lectione, fiat, B.'.

101 *Decretum Gratiani*, edited in Friedberg (ed.), *Corpus iuris canonici*, second part, causa 17.

102 Orme, "Sufferings of the Clergy", p. 63.

103 Numerous examples of letters from the Penitentiary showing the fear of integrating an elderly petitioner are collected by Metzler, *A Social History*, p. 146.

104 Schmitz and Borias, *Règle de Saint Benoît*, chapter 60.

105 Metzler, *A Social History*, p. 147.

previous activities. The circumstances of Conradus de Marcha, a former knight and current lay brother of the Order of Friars Minor, is detailed in two letters written by Clement VI, dated 17 January 1342. This case allows us to address the question of lay 'retirement', especially in cases of professions *ad succurrendum* ('to the rescue', i.e., late in life):

> Because, therefore, as we have recently accepted from you that you, who are now a novice of the order of Friars Minor, formerly a secular knight, founded and endowed the nunnery of Clarenbergh of the order of St Clare with your own property, and now, appearing at a decrepit age, your supplications make us inclined to allow you to enter with six mature and aged brethren of your aforementioned order into the aforementioned nunnery, notwithstanding any statutes and customs of the nunnery and any contrary constitutions, however, we hereby authorize it through this letter that, when you will be able to enter lawfully, provided that you are the head of the aforementioned nunnery, it will be permitted that you enter, but the aforementioned brothers shall not be allowed to remain there to eat nor to stay there overnight.[106]

As a knight, Conradus had founded and endowed the Clarian monastery of Clarenbergh in the diocese of Cologne, a community of female religious. It made sense, then, after his adoption of the religious life and becoming a lay member of the Order of Friars Minor, the elderly Conradus would ask to transfer to Clarenbergh with six fellow friars and end his days in the comfort the profits from his secular life had provided. These documents demonstrate that the convent could also be used as something like a retirement home for powerful members of the laity, if they were no longer able to work due to illness or impairment. What is more, they emphasize the role of professions *ad succurrendum* in terms of elevating the status of a monastic retiree's family, signalled by the high-profile location in which family members

106 RV 172, f. 159 V – Clement VI to Conradus de Marcha lay brother of the order of Friars Minor, 17 January 1342. Text edited by Volbert Sauerland (ed.), *Urkunden und Regesten*, n° 478, p. 188: '*Cum itaque, sicut ex parte tua nuper accepimus, tu, qui nunc es in ordine fratrum minorum novitius, olim miles secularis existens monasterium monialium in Clarenbergh ordinis sancte Clare Coloniensis diocese, de bonis tuis propriis fundaveris et dotaveris et nunc in etate decrepita constitutus existas, nos tuis supplicationibus inclinati, ut cum sex provectis et honestis fratribus tui predicti ordinis dictum monasterium monialium quibuscumque ipsius monasterius statutis et consuetudinibus ac quibuslibet constitutionibus contrariis nequaquam obstantibus libere ingredi, quando tibi videbitur, licite valeas, dummodo illi*[*us*]*, que ipsi monasterio prefuerit, ad id accedat assensus et tu dictique fratres ibidem non comedatis nec etiam pernoctetis, tenore tibi presentium indulgemus*'.

were buried.[107] Conradus benefitted from papal grace by being allowed to live amongst the nuns of Clarenbergh, even if his friar companions were allowed only to visit, rather than reside there. In a second letter, Clement VI even permitted his burial in a suitable place in the abbey.[108] Then, we can imagine that he had in mind the transformation of the community he had founded out of personal devotion to constitute a family mausoleum.[109] The Papal Chancery offered dispensations for monastic transfers both to individuals who genuinely desired to change their clerical status, and those who simply sought a place to retire and receive care, regardless of whether supplicants were actually suited to the religious lifestyle. Such authorizations ran counter to the edicts of canon law promulgated directly by the Curia. Conradus' case is particularly dramatic in this regard, as he was granted entrance to a *female* community, which, in theory at least, was absolutely prohibited to men. It is clear, however, that the papal institution was highly selective about to whom it offered such licence. Above all, the Church supported the powerful, whether they hailed from the clergy or laity. For these privileged few, resignation and 'retirement' to the monastery provided a strategic and practical route to ensure they received high-quality care in a safe environment until their dying day.

Conclusion

The Papal Chancery showed a genuine interest in providing care to those in need, including impaired clerics, as parts of its overarching remit of managing medieval society. To achieve its lofty goals, however, the Church first had to stigmatize impairment following certain criteria. For this purpose, the institution relied on provisions in canon law outlining the moral and ecclesiastical consequences of impairment, alongside medical knowledge which purportedly demonstrated the ways in which impairment concretely impacted clerics' suitability for office. The right to endorse and/or contravene laws relating to impairment was exclusively held by the Pope. This further legitimized the pontiff's authority over the clergy, as clerics were obliged to appeal to his judgment if they wished to modify the religious lifestyle in order to accommodate their impairment. In this context, hospitals played a relative significant role in the care of impaired

107 Gougaud, *Dévotions et pratiques ascétiques*, p. 129.
108 Volbert Sauerland (ed.), *Urkunden und Regesten*, n° 479.
109 See Miramon, "Embrasser l'état monastique".

and sick individuals. The ecclesiastical institution was instrumental to the foundation and upkeep of such therapeutic institutions from the eleventh to the fourteenth century. The petitions and papal letters emphasize the role of the papacy in the construction and endowment of such charitable institutions. Whilst this certainly serves to boost the Pope's reputation, it does not necessarily preclude the notion that the Chancery had an authentic interest in offering care to communities.

Whether the papal institution devoted its efforts to specialist institutions for impaired clerics, or into condition-specific hospitals like leprosaria, the Church's activities in this sphere reveal its flexibility in the application of monastic rules and canonical laws. What is more, institutional specialization – with leprosaria for lepers, or 'hostels of God' for the blind – suggests that assistance could be adapted according to an individual's unique circumstances. For the most privileged clerics, resignation could offer practical solutions to physical and/or mental impairment, and a means to secure ongoing financial support and care for the remainder of their lives, if they were awarded pensions or other material assistance. Supplicants from both the secular and regular clergy benefited from annuities and other special provisions transmitted by episcopal or pontifical favour that enabled them to live out their days with dignity. In their old age, they found safe refuge, for example, in monasteries which functioned something like retirement homes. The corpus demonstrates that the ecclesiastical institution also supported lower-ranked clerics with impairments, albeit to a lesser degree than their more illustrious colleagues, by transferring them to care facilities, either on a short-term or more permanent basis

Bibliography

Primary Sources

Benedictine monks (eds.), *Regestum Clementis papae V*, Bibliothèque des écoles françaises d'Athènes et de Rome, 1885.

Jerome Bertram (ed.), *The Chrodegang Rules: The Rules for the Common Life of the Secular Clergy from the Eighth and Ninth Centuries*, Ashgate, 2005.

Charles Bourel de La Roncière, Joseph de Loye, Pierre de Canival and Auguste Coulon (eds.), *Les registres d'Alexandre IV (1254–1261): recueil des bulles de ce pape*, Boccard, 1902.

Robert Digard, Antoine Fawtier, Maurice Faucon and Antoine Thomas (eds.), *Les registres de Boniface VIII: recueil des bulles de ce Pape publiées ou analysées d'après les manuscrits originaux des Archives du Vatican*, Bibliothèque des Écoles françaises d'Athènes et de Rome, 1884.

FRIEDBERG (ed.), *Corpus iuris canonici*, Akademische Druck- u. Verlagsanstalt, 1959.

Anne-Marie HAYEZ, Janine MATHIEU and Marie-France YVAN, *Urbain V: suppliques de 1362 à 1365 (années I à IV)*, [electronic version: *Ut per litteras apostolicas*], Brepols, 1978.

Leena LÖFSTEDT (ed.), *Gratiani decretum 1, Distinctiones*, Soc. Scient. Fennica, 1992.

Jean MARILIER (ed.), *Chartes et documents concernant l'Abbaye de Cîteaux, 1098–1182*, Éditions Cistercienses, 1961.

Jacques Paul MIGNE (ed.), *Patrologiae Cursus Completus, Series Latina*, Migne, 1844–1855.

Claude RIGUAUD (ed.), *Acta conciliorum et epistolae decretales, ac constitutiones summorum pontificum*, Imprimerie royale, 1714.

Philibert SCHMITZ and André BORIAS (eds.), *Règle de saint Benoît*, Brepols, 2009.

THOMAS AQUINAS, *Summa Theologiae II–II*, ed. By The Aquinas Institute and transl. by Fr. Laurence SHAPCOTE, URL consulted on 31 July 2021: https://aquinas.cc/.

Heinrich VOLBERT SAUERLAND (ed.), *Urkunden und Regesten zur Geschichte der Rheinlande aus dem Vatikanischen Archiv*, Vol. III, P. Hanstein, 1905.

Secondary Sources

Jole AGRIMI and Chiara CRISCIANI, "Charité et assistance dans la civilisation chrétienne médiévale", *in* Maria Laura BARDINET BROSO, Bernardino FANTINI and Mirko Drazen GRMEK (eds.), *Histoire de la pensée médicale en occident. 1, Antiquité et Moyen Âge*, Édition du Seuil, 1995, pp. 151–174.

Philippe ALBOU, *L'image des personnes âgées à travers l'histoire*, Glyphe & Biotem, 1999.

François BÉRIAC, *Histoire des lépreux au Moyen Âge: une société d'exclus*, Imago, 1988.

Nicole BÉRIOU and François-Olivier TOUATI, *Voluntate dei leprosus: les lépreux entre conversion et exclusion aux XIIe et XIIIe siècles*, Centro Italiano di studi Sull'altro Medioevo, 1991.

Elma BRENNER, *Leprosy and Charity in Medieval Rouen*, The Boydell Press, 2015.

Elma BRENNER and François-Olivier TOUATI (eds.), *Leprosy and Identity in the Middle Ages: From England to the Mediterranean*, Manchester University Press, 2021.

James BRODMAN, *Charity and Welfare: Hospitals and the Poor in Medieval Catalonia*, University of Pennsylvania Press, 2003.

Eliza BUHRER, "'But What is to Be Said of a Fool' Intellectual Disability in Medieval Tought and Culture", *in* Albrecht CLASSEN (ed.), *Mental Health, Spirituality, and Religion in the Middle Ages and Early Modern Age*, De Gruyter, 2014, pp. 314–343.

Isabelle COCHELIN, "*In senectute bona*: pour une typologie de la vieillesse dans l'hagiographie monastique des XIIe et XIIIe siècles", *in* Henri DUBOIS and Michel ZINK (eds.), *Les âges de la vie au Moyen Âge*, Presses de l'Université de Paris-Sorbonne, 1992, pp. 119–138.

Andrew T. CRISLIP, *From Monastery to Hospital: Christian Monasticism and the Transformation of Health Care in Late Antiquity*, University of Michigan Press, 2008.

Josephine M. CUMMINS, "Attitudes to Old Age and Ageing in Medieval Society", Philosophy thesis, University of Glasgow, Department of History, (Medieval) Faculty of Arts, 2000, pp. 220–221.

Ninon DUBOURG, "*Deo iudicio percusset* – l'idée de contamination d'après les suppliques et les lettres pontificales", *in* Sylvia CARARO (ed.), *Alter-habilitas. Perception of Disability Among People, Towards the Creation of an International Network of studies*, Alteritas, 2018, pp. 89–114.

Ninon DUBOURG, "Being a Leprous Cleric – In/ability to Hold a Benefice (XIIIth and XIVth centuries)", in Erin CONNELLY and Stefanie KÜNZEL (eds), *New Approaches to Disease, Disability and Medicine in Medieval Europe*, coll. *Studies in Early Medicine*, Archaeopress, 2018, pp. 62–77.

Pierre-Toussaint DURAND DE MAILLANE, *Dictionnaire de droit canonique et de pratique bénéficiale*, B. Duplain, 1770.

Arnaud FOSSIER, "La contagion des péchés (XIe–XIIIe siècle). Aux origines canoniques du biopouvoir", *Tracés. Revue de Sciences humaines*, 21 (2011), pp. 23–39.

Roberta GILCHRIST, *Medieval Life: Archaeology and the Life Course*, Boydell Press, 2018.

Elizabeth GONZALES, "L'heure de la retraite a sonné: les serviteurs de l'Hôtel du duc d'Orléans en fin de carrière (fin XIVe–fin XVe siècle)", *in Les serviteurs de l'État au Moyen Âge*, Éditions de la Sorbonne, 1998, pp. 257–268.

Louis GOUGAUD, *Dévotions et pratiques ascétiques du Moyen Âge*, Desclée De Brower & Cie, 1925.

Mirko Drazen GRMEK, "Le concept d'infection dans l'antiquité et au Moyen Âge, les anciennes mesures sociales contre les maladies contagieuses et la fondation de la première quarantaine à Dubrovnik", *in Rad Jugoslavenske akademije znanosti i umjetnosti, Razred za prirodne znanosti Prirodne znanosti*, Jugoslavenska akademija znanosti i umjetnosti, 1975, pp. 9–55.

Jean-Pierre GUTTON, *Naissance du vieillard, essai sur l'histoire des rapports entre les vieillards et la société en France*, Aubier, 1988.

Barbara F. HARVEY, *Living and Dying in England, 1100–1540: The Monastic Experience*, Clarendon Press, 2002.

Catherine HERMANN, "Lépreux et maladières dans l'ancien diocèse de Genève du XIIIe siècle au début du XVIe siècle", thesis presented to the Société savoisienne d'histoire et d'archéologie, Chambéry, 2009.

Jacques HOURLIER and Gabriel LE BRAS, *Histoire du droit et des institutions de l'Église en Occident. Les religieux, tome X, L'âge classique, 1140–1378*, Éditions Cujas, 1971.

Franz IRSIGLER and Arnold LASSOTTA, *Bettler und Gaukler, Dirnen und Henker: Außenseiter in einer mittelalterlichen Stadt; Köln 1300–1600*, Dt. Taschenbuch-Verl., 2010.

Clara JÁUREGUI, "Inside the Leprosarium: Illness in the Daily Life of 14th-Century Barcelona", *in* Erin CONNELLY and Stefanie KÜNZEL (eds.), *New Approaches to Disease, Disability, and Medicine in Medieval Europe*, Archaeopress, 2018, pp. 78–93.

Frédérique LACHAUD and Michael A. PENMAN, *Établir et abolir les normes: la succession dans l'Europe médiévale*, Brepols, 2008.

Sylviane LAZARD, "L'Ospedale di Santo Spirito à Rome: vers une spécialisation des lieux d'accueil?", *in* Alain MONTANDON (ed.), *Lieux d'hospitalité: hospices, hôpital, hostellerie*, Presses Universitaires Blaise Pascal, 2001, pp. 183–207.

Daniel LE BLÉVEC, "Les lépreux peuvent-ils vivre en société? Réflexions sur l'exclusion sociale dans les villes du Midi à la fin du Moyen Âge", *in* Claude CAROZZI, Daniel LE BLÉVEC and Huguette TAVIANI-CAROZZI (eds.), *Vivre en société au Moyen Âge: Occident chrétien, VIe–XVe siècle*, Publications de l'Université de Provence, 2008, pp. 281–292.

Chris G. LEWIN, *Pensions and Insurance Before 1800: a Social History*, Tuckwell Press, 2003.

Olivier MATTÉONI, *Servir le prince: les officiers des ducs de Bourbon à la fin du Moyen Age (1356–1523)*, Publications de la Sorbonne, 1999.

Irina METZLER, "Liminality and Disability: Spatial and Conceptual Aspects of Physical Impairment in Medieval Europe", *in* Patricia Anne BAKER, Han NIJDAM and Karine van't LAND (eds.), *Medicine and Space: Body, Surroundings and Borders in Antiquity and the Middle Ages*, Brill, 2012, pp. 273–308.

Irina METZLER, *A Social History of Disability in the Middle Ages: Cultural Considerations of Physical Impairment*, Routledge, 2013.

Georges MINOIS, *Histoire de la vieillesse en Occident: de l'Antiquité à la Renaissance*, A. Fayard, 1987.

Charles de MIRAMON, "Embrasser l'état monastique à l'âge adulte (1050–1200). Étude sur la conversion tardive", *Annales. Histoire, Sciences Sociales*, 54.4 (1999), pp. 825–849.

Élisabeth MORNET, "Âge et pouvoir dans la noblesse danoise (vers 1360–vers 1570)", *Journal des Savants*, 1 (1988), pp. 119–154.

Nicholas ORME, "Sufferings of the Clergy: Illness and Old Age in Exeter Diocese, 1300–1540", *in* Margaret PELLING and Richard M. SMITH (eds.), *Life, Death, and the Elderly: Historical Perspectives*, Routledge, 1991, pp. 62–73.

Carole RAWCLIFFE, *The Hospitals of Medieval Norwich*, Centre of East Anglian studies, 1995.

Joel T. ROSENTHAL, "Retirement and the Life Cycle in Fifteenth-Century England", *in* Michael M. SHEEHAN (ed.), *Aging and the Aged in Medieval Europe*, Pontifical Institute for Medieval Studies, 1990, pp. 173–188.

Michel ROUCHE, "La matricule des pauvres. Évolution d'une institution de charité du Bas Empire jusqu'à la fin du Haut Moyen Âge", *in* Michel MOLLAT (ed.), *Études sur l'histoire de la pauvreté*, Sorbonne, 1974, pp. 83–110.

Miri RUBIN, *Charity and Community in Medieval Cambridge*, Cambridge University Press, 2002.

Kirsi SALONEN, "What Happened to Aged Priests in the Late Middle Ages?", *in* Christian KRÖTZL and Katariina MUSTAKALLIO, *On Old Age, Approaching Death in Antiquity and the Middle Ages*, Brepols, 2011, pp. 183–196.

Antje M. SCHELBERG, "Leprosen in der mittelalterlichen Gesellschaft physische Idoneität und sozialer Status von Kranken im Spannungsfeld säkularer und christlicher Wirklichkeitsdeutungen", Thesis in medicine, University of Göttingen, 2003.

Shulamith SHAHAR, *Growing Old in the Middle Ages "winter clothes us in shadow and pain"*, Routledge, 1997.

Monique SOMMÉ, *Isabelle de Portugal, duchesse de Bourgogne: une femme au pouvoir au XVe siècle*, Presses universitaires du Septentrion, 1998.

Sheila SWEETINBURGH, *The Role of the Hospital in Medieval England: Gift-Giving and the Spiritual Economy*, Four Courts Press, 2004.

Bruno TABUTEAU, *Lépreux et sociabilité du Moyen Âge aux temps modernes*, Publications de l'Université de Rouen, 2000.

Bruno TABUTEAU, "Historical Research Developments on Leprosy in France and Western Europe", *in* Barbara S. BOWERS (ed.), *The Medieval Hospital and Medical Practice*, Ashgate, 2007, pp. 41–58.

Bruno TABUTEAU, "Vingt mille léproseries au Moyen Âge? Tradition française d'un poncif historiographique", *Memini. Travaux et documents*, 15 (2012), pp. 115–124.

Donna TREMBINSKI, "An Infirm Man: Reading Francis of Assisi's Retirement in the Context of Canon law", *in* Wendy J. TURNER and Sara M. BUTLER (eds.), *Medicine and the Law in the Middle Ages*, Brill, 2014, pp. 269–287.

Donna TREMBINSKI, *Illness and Authority. Disability in the Life and Lives of Francis of Assisi*, University of Toronto Press, 2020.

Conclusion

Abstract
As argued through this book, studying petitions and letters enriches our understanding of institutional and religious history: it sheds light on the Church's place in society and on the contemporary understanding of disability. Indeed, the process of supplication could erase the negative institutional effects of disability by actively including the disabled cleric within the ecclesial and Christian body. With this process, the Apostolic See thus created a metaphorical place conducive to negotiation, where disabled clerics could disclose their physical and/or mental difficulties to advocate for themselves, requesting accommodations from the institutional Church.

Keywords: Inclusion; Apostolic Penitentiary; Modern Canon Law; Modern Legislation

The petitions received and the letters issued by the Papal Chancery between the twelfth and fourteenth centuries attest to the recognition of disability by the pontifical institution. They record the existence of supplicants' physical or mental impairment and, on a case-by-case basis, authorize petitioners to adapt their duties, both as clerics and as Christians, according to their abilities. These documents are situated on the borderline between institutional edicts and lived experiences, between administrative theory and real-world practice. A petitioner's initial request set into motion an intense and complex epistolary exchange, highlighting the dynamism of all the actors involved, disabled supplicants and curial personnel alike. With the dispensation of grace, a privilege allowed only to the Pope, the Chancery established a system that allowed the Church hierarchy to govern the souls and bodies of all Christians, the clergy included. Indeed, grants of papal grace permitted the institution a greater degree of control over the clergy than ever before. Similarly, the petition process functioned as a formidable instrument by which the papacy exerted its authority throughout

Dubourg, N., *Disabled Clerics in the Late Middle Ages. Un/suitable for Divine Service?*
Taylor & Francis Group, 2023
DOI: 10.5117/9789463721561_CONC

Christendom, increasing the Church's already considerable sway over late medieval Christian society. Every step in the construction of the dialogue served papal authority: each protagonist, from the supplicant to the scribes, contributed to strengthening the Church's power. The perception of physical or mental conditions, including old age and chronic or terminal illnesses, allowed for the recognition of disability as a condition. The Church developed extensive administrative protocols out of necessity, as a means of effectively supervising the clerics in its employ, many of whom were scattered across the Christian world. This system was a bureaucratic extension, and reflection, of the control that the pontifical institution had established over Christian souls and bodies, demonstrated in particular by the Church's central role in determining questions of clerics' physical or mental incapacity.

The petition process was a way for supplicants to receive formal recognition of their disability. The effects of such recognition could be dramatic. It enacted a shift in supplicants' own sense of identity, and fundamentally transformed their relationship with the ecclesiastical institution. Such changes occurred initially at the individual level; identity remains above all a personal matter. Drafting a petition necessitated the supplicant present his life and circumstances, or a version thereof, to the discerning eye of his curial superiors. Such documents, then, operate to *constitute* the supplicant's identity as much as they reflect his identity more generally. The way in which a supplicant presented himself in a petition 'is not without effect on the construction of his self – if not moral, at least social'.[1] In this process, the individual submitted his newly fashioned identity for the judgment of the Chancery. If the petition were deemed worthy, the Chancery would essentially ratify the supplicant's disabled identity by issuing authoritative documents, the letters of response.[2] Notwithstanding the supplicant's agency in initiating the process and offering a specific version of his identity, the Apostolic See retained its superior authority, exerting substantial influence over the impaired bodies that submitted to its judgment. Grants of papal grace appear to have offered the optimal solution both for impaired petitioners and the Apostolic See. Indeed, the latter upheld the right of disabled petitioners to remain in the *ecclesia* (the Church), and recognized their specific differences, alongside the accommodations such differences necessitated. The papal institution established the prerequisites of bodily and mental normativity in its case-by-case administration of 'public assistance' and in its functional diagnosis, or minimal recognition

1 Fassin, "La supplique", p. 956 (my translation).
2 Tock, "Recours à l'écrit", p. 379.

of, 'medical' conditions as 'valid' impairments.[3] In this way, the Church 'manufactured' the disabled condition itself.[4] Papal letters possessed juridical value, transmitting the voice – and the authority – of the pontifical institution in hyper-local contexts. In the hands of successful petitioners, these documents ultimately functioned as a potent legal tool with which to circumvent established norms.[5]

The construction of identity was not simply an internal, individualistic endeavour, over which a petitioner had supreme control. Rather, the petitioner's disabled identity emerged in dialogue with the papacy, ever reliant on the gaze of the institutional other. Above all, the petition process determined the supplicant's disability based on his relative ability to fulfil his social role: in other words, his ability to retain the position in society he had enjoyed before the onset of his impairment, or before it demonstrably worsened. The supplicant's individual identity thus becomes a social artefact, a product of the way in which he now fits, or fails to fit, within the group to which he previously belonged. In the sources, the criteria used to constitute disabled identity are to a considerable degree collective. The petition process demonstrates the fluidity of the disability identity – and, arguably, of identities more generally – as each supplicant constructs a virtual identity which is temporary and fragile, emerging only in relation to the institution and for certain purposes. On another occasion, the same supplicant could, for instance, present himself in a very different light, put forward very different arguments in his case, and as a result be judged to be more or less disabled. The integration of impaired clerics into the Church, despite their mental or bodily 'defects', was not automatic. However, the flexibility of grace allowed impaired clerics to individualize themselves in petitions, and to thereby secure individualized accommodations afforded by the institutional recognition of their specific status.[6]

Petitions permitted disabled clerics to transgress the collective social identity accorded to them. With grants of grace, impaired clerics could remain active in the clergy, even if their physical or mental incapacity prevented them from participating in the community or undertaking clerical duties in the same way as an able-bodied person. Consequently, papal responses to the petitions testify to the Curia's desire to offer a variety of flexible adjustments

3 Abberley, "Disabled People", p. 55.

4 The use of the term 'make' is borrowed from a whole literature on public policy, presented in particular by Frigoli, "De la circulaire au guichet".

5 On the legal value of letters, see Oudin, "La pratique épistolaire médiévale"; Somerville and Brasington, *Prefaces to Canon Law Books*, p. 8.

6 On the individuation process through disability, see Oliver, *Understanding Disability*.

formulated to the specificities of each petitioner, in order to manage the clerics under its care in the most humane and administratively sensible manner. These documents are highly practical. They are a means, for example, to allocate clerics benefices that they are able to assume despite their disability, and to organize professional and/or social assistance to ensure petitioners' continued quality of life and the satisfactory management of Church affairs. As the preceding chapters highlight, the Pontifical Chancery adjusted its regulations for impaired clerics if they possessed desirable attributes that 'made up for' their physical limitations, such as a good education, or keen intellectual abilities. Similarly, the appointment of assistants demonstrates the legislative flexibility introduced by the grace system. The pontifical institution routinely appointed such professional helpmates to support disabled petitioners, thereby enabling the latter to stay in post and fulfil all associated requirements to a satisfactory degree, despite their physical or mental incapacities. Such protocols prevented the social exclusion of the most vulnerable disabled clerics, whether through spatial segregation or penury. The Church forestalled deleterious outcomes by ensuring disabled clerics had safe housing and adequate financial support. As a result, disabled clerics were able to live and work as members of the community, occupying public space in a well-defined and respectable ecclesiastical role. In this way, disabled clerics continued to be included in the ecclesiastical sphere, and thus in medieval society. Above all, petitioners in receipt of papal grace were recognized by the pontifical institution as entirely suitable for clerical office. Although their impairment meant that they could no longer fulfil their previous mission, disabled supplicants retained part of their clerical identity by incorporating their disability into it. As a result, their disabled bodies were normalized. The papal institution's treatment of impaired clerics went beyond a politics of simple inclusion. In fact, with dispensations of grace, the Pope actively enabled impaired clerics. Such grants, and the accommodations derived therefrom, functionally removed clerics' disability from the equation, rendering their bodies capable once more.

In addition, analysis of the dialectic between petitioners and the Chancery sheds light on the construction of theological authority in the Middle Ages. The Church was pulled between tradition – notably, respect for canon law – and innovation, in light of exigent circumstances faced by clerics in the here and now, as testified in the letters. The vocabulary used in the papal letters demonstrates the Chancery's significant expertise in the therapeutic field, thanks to a consistent culture, both theoretical and practical. The medical terminology deployed in these documents reveals that a scholarly understanding of impairment prevailed within the Church, and therefore illustrates the evolution of the concepts of impairment and disability in the period. In this way, the Church integrated nascent medical science into its culture, appropriating and reorienting it for the purpose of granting pontifical grace. The Church appointed doctors as experts and reproduced their discourse, thereby valorizing medical knowledge in all spheres of society. The pontifical institution represents the medium through which the social and political world imposed its view on the impaired body in the late Middle Ages. The Church's dominant position allowed it a real measure of flexibility, of which the letters in the corpus allow us only a partial glimpse. Nevertheless, it is evident that the Apostolic See played an essential role in defining disability in this period thanks to the authority conveyed in its correspondence with impaired petitioners, with its judgments circulated across Christendom. By extension, this institutional competence situated the Pope as the leading expert in defining physical and mental disability in the Middle Ages, occupying a role held by doctors in the modern world.[7]

A quick survey of the supplications sent to the Apostolic Penitentiary during the fifteenth century corroborates a number of the conclusions drawn from the present corpus.[8] First created by Innocent III (1198–1216) around 1200, the Penitentiary would come to take over some of the core responsibilities of the Papal Chancery. The latter was becoming overwhelmed, falling victim to the runaway success of the policy regarding dispensations of papal grace. During the reign of Benedict XII (1334–1342), the Penitentiary was staffed by specialized administrators. The increasing number of supplicants in daily correspondence with the Chancery necessitated the foundation of a special office reserved for issues relating to pontifical grace and justice. Something of a little sister to the Chancery, the Penitentiary also was responsible for granting pontifical pardons, in the form of absolutions, (minor) indulgences, dispensations, and licences.[9] The office thus dealt with important matters, and penitentiaries' power was not insubstantial, as they were endowed with pontifical authority to settle the matters at hand.

7 It is interesting to observe that in modern disability legislation pertaining to work regulations, all of these actions would be considered 'reasonable adjustments' that an employer would be expected to make for their staff. The church looked after its own personnel, much as in the modern public sector the civil servants can be in receipt of various benefits for incapacity. Even in what might be considered the medieval equivalent of the private sector it had become customary for retainers, artisans and even peasants to receive pensions by the latter Middle Ages.

8 This survey is based on the consultation of the volume *Matrimonialium et diversorum* 7, recorded during the pontificate of Pius II in 1459, but also on Stöhr, *Körpermakel – Arbeits(un) fähigkeit – Kirchenrecht*.

9 Consult Salonen, "The Decision of Pope Pius II".

Yet the Apostolic Penitentiary and its archives are little known, and have been neglected in scholarship, not the least because the penitential records were only relatively recently (re)discovered in the Vatican's collections.[10]

Petitions handled by the Penitentiary further enrich our knowledge of cases of clerical *defectus corporis* and *mentis*.[11] They allow us to observe the evolution of the Church's treatment of impaired petitioners and its recognition of their status. For example, the Penitential petitions testify to the institutionalization of the criteria of capacity and *claritas* (i.e., good reputation) as prerequisites for ordination. These criteria were established during the during the thirteenth and fourteenth centuries, as discussed in earlier chapters. The documentation received and produced by the Apostolic Penitentiary indicates, however, that they remained current in the fifteenth century and were consistent touchstones in papal adjudications of clerical impairment. They also explicitly classified the type of disability with which a supplicant lived, and identified its root causes. Petitions sent to the Penitentiary mention all manner of physical impairments – such as gibbosity, blindness, 'stains', limb loss, serious illness, and so on – that were understood to impact petitioners' capacity. Particular attention was paid to conditions that affected the supplicant's hands or eyes, unsurprisingly. These impairments appear again and again in both canon law and in the petitions of the Penitentiary, and are discussed with far more frequency than other conditions. This is due to the relative visibility of ocular and manual conditions, which would necessarily impact the supplicant's *claritas*, and the tendency for such impairments to detrimentally impact petitioners' capacity. Indeed, they are likely to be a problem in the context of promotion to higher orders, as they are the two parts of the body most 'in demand' and visible in religious ceremonies. The same criteria (sometimes even illustrated) can be found in the archives of the Congregation of the Roman Curia until the beginning of the eighteenth century.[12]

The petitions (with their verdict) preserved in the registers of the Penitentiary prove that determinations regarding individuals' exclusion from or inclusion in the *ecclesia* continued in the same way as they did in the Papal Chancery. Indeed, they still rest upon the extent to which the individuals' physical or mental impediments limited their active participation in worship and other Christian duties, such as pilgrimage, Lent, and so on. In fact,

10 They were mentioned by Göller, "Das alte Archiv" in 1913 and only became accessible to researchers in 1983.

11 Unfortunately, the letters written in response are not preserved before 1569.

12 Röder, *Der Körper des Priesters*.

analysis of the Penitential sources confirms several trends identified as early as the twelfth century. In the second half of the fifteenth century, the information contained in the petitions was still very much subject to the administrative tone and respect of the pontifical institution's writing rules. Sources from the Apostolic Penitentiary witness the continuation of tensions first observed in the Chancery's records in terms of the discursive exchange at play. The institutional office, whether the Chancery or the Penitentiary, expected a certain formalized discourse from petitioners, with the latter obliged to (re)formulate their own testimony appropriately. Petitioners from the twelfth to the fifteenth centuries had a similarly limited degree of discursive freedom in narrating their disability and formulating their requests.[13] In this context, the rhetoric used still leads to the categorization of the disabled and involves the recognition of the supplicants' conditions.

The documents under consideration afford privileged insight into the ways in which disability, as a category and a condition, came to be defined in the Middle Ages. This provides a premodern starting point for a conceptual trajectory which ultimately culminates in the emergence of the modern notion of disability in the twentieth century. Defining disability is a political action, an act of government. Criteria restricting the receipt of grace to only a select few were taken directly from canon law, a legislative corpus on which both the Papal Chancery and the Apostolic Penitentiary relied when determining grants of grace, licences, and absolutions. However, canonical legislation evolves with the times – in the medieval era, and so too in our modern times.[14] Regulations continued to prohibit the participation of priests with mental or bodily 'defects' in worship until the twentieth century. Indeed, this measure was reiterated in the 1917 Code of Canon Law promulgated by Benedict XV (1914–1922). This Code is, then, very close to the legislation contained in the Decree or the Decretals, as shown by the canon 984:

> Can. 984 2.° Those impaired in body who cannot safely because of the deformity, or decently because of the deformity, conduct ministry of the altar. To prevent the exercise of an order already legitimately received, however, it is required that the defect be more grave, nor can acts that can be rightly placed be prohibited because of this defect; 3.° Those who are

13 Eubel (ed.), "Der Registerband"; Lea (ed.), *A Formulary*; Schwalm, (ed.), *Das Formelbuch des Heinrich Bucglant*. See also Fossier, *Le bureau des âmes*.

14 The following remarks are based on a reflection with Henri-Jacques Stiker on recent developments in canon law.

> or were epileptics, insane, or possessed by the devil; but if after reception of orders they fall into these and it is certainly proved that they are free, the Ordinary can permit his subjects to exercise once again the orders already received.[15]

However, the 1917 provision was partially abolished by John Paul II in the 1983 Code of Canon Law, a relatively major update to ecclesiastical regulations which functions to this day as the Church's definitive legislative corpus. The updated Code authorizes the ordination of individuals with physical 'infirmities', while maintaining the exclusion of individuals with intellectual disabilities, as canons 1041 and 1741 testify:

> Can. 1041 The following are irregular for receiving orders: 1/ a person who labors under some form of amentia or other psychic illness due to which, after experts have been consulted, he is judged unqualified to fulfill the ministry properly; [...] 5/ a person who has mutilated himself or another gravely and maliciously or who has attempted suicide[.]
> Can. 1741 The causes for which a pastor can be removed legitimately from his parish are especially the following: [...] 2/ ineptitude or a permanent infirmity of mind or body which renders the pastor unable to fulfill his functions usefully.[16]

The text breaks with the tradition, handed down by Church Fathers, of excluding people with bodily 'defects' from the clergy, on the basis of their impairments and the *scandalum* their participation in worship could feasibly cause. Indeed, while canon 1741 illustrates that the criterion of capacity remains operative, the image of the disabled priest as irretrievably scandalous has faded from view. Canon 930 notes, for example:

> § 1. If an infirm or elderly priest is unable to stand, he can celebrate the eucharistic sacrifice while seated, but not before the people except with the permission of the local ordinary; the liturgical laws are to be observed.
> § 2. A blind or otherwise infirm priest licitly celebrates the eucharistic sacrifice by using any approved text of the Mass with the assistance,

15 Translation by Peters (ed.), *The 1917 or Pio-Benedictine Code of Canon Law*, p. 403.

16 Canon Law Society of America (eds.), *The code of canon law*, canon 1 040.1; canon 1 040.5 (repeated with a few words in canon 1044 2.2 to prohibit irregulars from exercising the orders received) and canon 1 741.2.

> if needed, of another priest, deacon, or even a properly instructed lay person.[17]

Crucially, clerics with recognized impairments no longer require papal grace to permit them to perform divine services. Rather, the focus is on supporting clerics in overcoming the challenges imposed by their impairment by making appropriate accommodations, including the appointment of an assistant. Such interventions do not necessitate an appeal to external ecclesiastical authorities. And if permissions are required, as with the 'infirm or elderly priest' in canon 930, they can be secured at the local level, from the cleric's own ordinand. Thus, the very notion of bodily or mental 'defect' disappears from the 1983 Code of Canon Law and is replaced by terminology for specific conditions (e.g., blindness, old age) or neutral expressions and descriptors (expansive 'infirmities', permanent disability, and so on). However, canon 1041 emphasizes that people with self-inflicted 'mutilations' are still not eligible, testifying that there is still an importance attached to the moral valency of certain impairments.

In theory, this new legislation allows the full integration of physically disabled clerics in the Church, without any obligation to secure pontifical grace. In truth, however, the picture is less rosy: impaired people continue to face substantive barriers to admission to the seminary and to holy orders.[18]

The difference between the 1917 Code and the 1983 Code reflects the 'end of a world', a palliative solution to the shortage of priests caused by the drastic decrease in priestly vocations.[19] The French clergy, as with their European counterparts more generally, have suffered from the decline in the practice of Catholicism since the mid-1960s.[20] On the one hand, the measures taken during the Second Vatican Council (1962–1965) radically transformed worshippers' relationship with the divine. On the other hand, though, the reforms did not offer the progress expected by some Catholics.[21] At the same time, the clerical profession has been transformed over the course of the late twentieth century. The earlier system, in which religious were also carers, teachers, and social workers, is becoming little more than a memory. Whilst remaining 'vocational' professions, these activities

17 Canon Law Society of America (eds.), *The code of canon law*, canon 930.

18 Kette, "Changer les mentalités".

19 The expression 'end of a world' is borrowed from Hervieu-Léger, *Catholicisme*, notably pp. 19–20.

20 Cuchet, *Comment notre monde*, p. 135.

21 For a review of Guillaume Cuchet's book, see Poutrin, "1965".

have been removed from the Church's broad remit, and are now typically run and managed by the state with a secular workforce.[22] The meaning of 'vocation' is evolving, no longer limited to religious vows. The 'exculturation' of Catholicism, that is, the stark decline in the religion's political and cultural influence, has diminished the role of clerics, and all religious, in both public and private spheres.[23] These are but a few of the reasons that the modern Church faces a crisis in recruiting new servants. This 'staff shortage' has undoubtedly contributed to the institution's decision to soften its clerical entrance requirements, and offer a warmer welcome to impaired entrants.[24]

The end of canonical regulations prohibiting the inclusion of impaired people in worship is also explained by changing attitudes towards impairment and disability among the faithful, and in society more generally. It reflects, for example, the semantic shift evident in most national and supra-national legislation in Europe and the Global North, with terms such as 'infirm' and 'infirmity' steadily displaced by 'disabled' and 'disability'. The legislation put in place by supra-national and national public policy from the 1980s onwards illustrates developments in the recognition and conceptualization of disability. Such statutes demonstrate that the definition of disability varies according to numerous factors: an individual's specific context, legislative objectives at play (e.g., if a law is targeted to improve health, intervene in workplaces, and so on), and the level of financial support committed by governments to a given endeavour.[25] For example, only a small proportion of disabled people qualify for governmental social assistance. In such cases, governments narrowly define disability in order to limit expenditure. By contrast, when cost is not an issue, such as in anti-discrimination law, a much more inclusive definition of disability predominates.[26] The first International Classification of Impairments (ICIDH) was published by the World Health Organization (WHO) in 1980 to consider the consequences and social dimensions of disability. It recognizes that disability has three effects: impairment (of function), incapacity (in the performance of activities),

22 Dubet, *Le déclin de l'institution*, 2002, especially p. 14 on priests and p. 35 on the changing direction of vocations.

23 The exit from political religion is linked to the democratic model, according to Gauchet, *Le désenchantement du monde*. Cultural exit is theorised by Hervieu-Léger, *Catholicisme*. The authors insist, however, on the persistence of beliefs, which go beyond the codes prescribed by religious institutions.

24 Denis, "Les religions en France", pp. 423–438.

25 Bolderson and Mabbett, *Definitions of Disability in Europe*, p. 24.

26 See Degener, "The Definition of Disability"

and disadvantage (in the conditions of social integration).[27] This landmark publication represents an important step forward in the global recognition of disability: it introduced the dimension of social disadvantage, which had never before been included in an official definition of disability.[28] In so doing, the policy document calls for, and facilitates, increasingly individualized care for disabled people, according to their unique circumstances and capacities. Indeed, legal categories in operation today differentiate disabled people according to their intrinsic individual characteristics, thanks in particular to the notion of vulnerability.[29]

Notwithstanding the substantive progress that has been achieved, activist researchers underscore that there is much left to do. For a start, the current understanding of disability lacks a global approach.[30] In 2001, the International Classification of Functioning, Disability and Health (ICF or ICIDH-2) was adopted, updating the 1980 ICIDH, in order to propose a common frame of reference (resolution WHA54.21). The new framework advocates accommodation and rehabilitation, focusing less on the diagnosis of disability and more on the lived experiences of disabled people. Authority to define disability is wrested from the hands of medical institutions, and returned to disabled people themselves, with the aim of supporting the greater integration of the disabled community in society.[31] Likewise, the United Nations emphasized the need to ensure disabled people are included fully in society in its most recent consideration of disability, dating to 2006.[32] The most recent communication from the WHO dates from 2011. In its World Report on Disability, the ICF is presented as a bio-psycho-social model, a compromise synthesizing individualistic and social models of disability, whilst also taking into account the role of environment:

> Disability is the umbrella term for impairments, activity limitations and participation restrictions, referring to the negative aspects of the interaction between an individual (with a health condition) and that individual's contextual factors (environmental and personal factors).[33]

27 World Health Organization, *International Classification*, p. 10.
28 Barral, "De l'influence des processus de normalisation", p. 23.
29 See Gittard, "Protection de la personne".
30 Roussel, "CIH-1/CIH-2".
31 Smart, "The Promise of the International Classification", p. 583.
32 Sherlaw and Hudebine, "The United Nations", p. 12.
33 World Health Organization, *World Report on Disability 2011*, p. 4.

International definitions of disability continue to proliferate, and the process of harmonization is ongoing. Nevertheless, there are connotative parallels between the papal system of categorizing disability in the Middle Ages, developed in order to grant graces, and the current system of assessing disability, an integral step in the allocation of governmental assistance to applicants deemed disabled 'enough', or disabled in the 'right way'. As studying the corpus of petitions and letters demonstrates, the cultural definition of disability developed by the medieval Church has more in common with our contemporary understanding of disability than we might first expect.

Bibliography

Primary Sources

CANON LAW SOCIETY OF AMERICA (eds.), *The code of canon law in English translation*, Collins, 1983.

Konrad EUBEL (ed.), "Der Registerband des Cardinalgrosspönitentiars Bentevenga: eine auf das kirchliche Bußwesen bezügliche Sammlung von Urkunden aus der Zeit von 1279–1289", *Archiv für Katholisches Kirchenrecht*, 64, 1890.

Henry Charles LEA (ed.), *A Formulary of the Papal Penitentiary in the Thirteenth Century*, Lea, 1892.

Edward N. PETERS (ed.), *The 1917 or Pio-Benedictine Code of Canon Law: In English Translation with Extensive Scholarly Apparatus*, P.J. Kennedy & Sons, 1918.

Jakob SCHWALM, (ed.), *Das Formelbuch des Heinrich Bucglant: an die päpstliche Kurie in Avignon gerichtete Suppliken aus der ersten Hälfte des 14. Jahrhunderts*, Gräfe, 1910.

WORLD HEALTH ORGANIZATION, *International Classification of Impairments, Disabilities, and Handicaps. A manual of classification relating to the consequences of disease*, WHO, 1980.

WORLD HEALTH ORGANIZATION, *World Report on Disability 2011*, WHO, 2011.

Secondary Sources

Paul ABBERLEY, "Disabled People, Normality and Social Work", *in* Len BARTON (ed.), *Disability and Dependency*, Falmer Press, 1989, pp. 53–66.

Catherine BARRAL, "De l'influence des processus de normalisation internationaux sur les représentations du handicap", *Handicap – revue des sciences humaines et sociales*, Les enjeux de la classification internationale des handicaps 81, 1999, pp. 20–34.

Helen BOLDERSON and Deborah MABBETT, *Definitions of Disability in Europe: A Comparative Analysis*, Londres, Brunel university, 2002.

Guillaume CUCHET, *Comment notre monde a cessé d'être chrétien. Anatomie d'un effondrement,* Seuil, 2018.

Theresia DEGENER, "The Definition of Disability in (German and) International Discrimination Law", *Disability Studies Quarterly*, 26.2 (2006) URL consulted on 31 July 2021: https://dsq-sds.org/article/view/696/873.

Pelletier DENIS, "Les religions en France depuis la fin de la Seconde Guerre mondiale. Crise ou recomposition?", *in* Alain TALLON (ed.), *Histoire du christianisme en France*, Armand Colin, 2014, pp. 423–438.

François DUBET, *Le déclin de l'institution*, Seuil, 2002.

Didier FASSIN, "La supplique. Stratégies rhétoriques et constructions identitaires dans les demandes d'aide d'urgence", *Annales. Histoire, Sciences Sociales*, 55.5 (2000), pp. 955–981.

Arnaud FOSSIER, *Le bureau des âmes. Écritures et pratiques administratives de la Pénitencerie apostolique* (*XIII*e–*XIV*e *siècle*), École française de Rome, 2018.

Gilles FRIGOLI, "De la circulaire au guichet. Une enquête sur la fabrique des populations vulnérables par les politiques publiques", *Déviance et Société*, 33.2 (2009), pp. 125–148.

Marcel GAUCHET, *Le désenchantement du monde, Une histoire politique de la religion*, Gallimard, 1985.

Vanessa GITTARD, "Protection de la personne et catégories juridiques: Vers un nouveau concept de vulnérabilité", thesis in Law, University Paris 2, 2005.

Emil GÖLLER, "Das alte Archiv der päpstlichen Pönitentiarie", *Römische Quartalschrift*, Supplementband 20, Festschrift A. de Waal (1913), pp. 1–19.

Danièle HERVIEU-LÉGER, *Catholicisme, la fin d'un monde*, Bayard, 2003.

Justin-Sylvestre KETTE, "Changer les mentalités en matière d'admission des personnes handicapées physiques au sacrement de l'ordre", *Revue de droit canonique*, 61/2 (2011), pp. 113–138.

Michael OLIVER, *Understanding Disability: from Theory to Practice*, Palgrave Macmillan, 2009.

Fanny OUDIN, "La pratique épistolaire médiévale, entre norme et liberté", *Camenulae*, 2 (2008), pp. 1–31.

Isabelle POUTRIN, "1965, l'année où les églises françaises se vidèrent", *Conversion/ Pouvoir et religion*, hypotheses.org, 6th june 2018 (URL consulted on 31 July 2021: https://pocram.hypotheses.org/2063#_ftnref7).

Brendan RÖDER, *Der Körper des Priesters: Gebrechen im Katholizismus der Frühen Neuzeit*, Campus, 2021.

Pascale ROUSSEL, "CIH-1/CIH-2: rénovation complète ou ravalement de façade", *Handicap – revue des sciences humaines*, Les enjeux de la classification internationale des handicaps, 1999, pp. 7–19.

Kirsi SALONEN, "The Decision of Pope Pius II in the Penitentiary Registers", in Andreas MEYER, Constanze RENDTEL and Maria Elisabeth WITTMER-BUTSCH (eds.), *Päpste, Pilger, Pönitentiarie. Festschrift für Ludwig Schmugge*, M. Niemeyer, 2004, pp. 515–530.

William SHERLAW and Hervé HUDEBINE, "The United Nations Convention on the Rights of Persons with Disabilities: Opportunities and Tensions Within the Social Inclusion and Participation of Persons With Disabilities", *ALTER – European Journal of Disability Research*, 9.1 (2015), pp. 9–21.

Julie SMART, "The Promise of the International Classification of Functioning, Disability, and Health (ICF)", *in* Arthur E. DELL ORTO and Paul W. POWER (eds.), *The Psychological & Social Impact of Illness and Disability*, Springer Pub. Co., 2007, pp. 582–596.

Robert SOMERVILLE and Bruce C. BRASINGTON, *Prefaces to Canon Law Books in Latin Christianity: Selected Translations, 500–1245*, Yale University Press, 1998.

Friederike STÖHR, *Körpermakel – Arbeits(un)fähigkeit – Kirchenrecht: Körperlich versehrte, kranke und alte Geistliche im spätmittelalterlichen Deutschen Reich und in Skandinavien*, Didymos-Verlag, 2020.

Benoît-Michel TOCK, "Recours à l'écrit, autorité du document, constitution d'archives en Occident", *in L'autorité de l'écrit au Moyen Âge* (*Orient-Occident*), Publication de la Sorbonne, 2009, pp. 379–384.

Index

For Product Safety Concerns and Information please contact our
EU representative GPSR@taylorandfrancis.com Taylor & Francis
Verlag GmbH, Kaufingerstraße 24, 80331 München, Germany